Psychological Perspectives in HIV Care

The care paradigm for people with HIV has shifted from managing progressive illness with a poor prognosis to managing a chronic condition. Despite this improvement, people living with HIV continue to experience considerable stresses, so promoting their holistic wellbeing is a key aspect of long-term care.

This book provides an accessible introduction for healthcare professionals who work with people living with HIV. It is designed to help readers understand how care in practice can be more person-centred and psychologically focused, whilst promoting compassion, health and wellbeing. Topics covered include self-awareness, attachment theories and communication as well as key aspects of providing care for people living with HIV, such as stigma in young adults, neurocognitive issues, the sexualized use of drugs, managing neuropathic pain, and the needs of older adults living with HIV.

Invaluable reading for health professionals working within multidisciplinary teams that provide care for people living with HIV, this book is also a core text for those studying in the area.

Michelle Croston is Senior Lecturer at Manchester Metropolitan University, UK, and has over 20 years of experience working within HIV care as a Specialist Nurse. She was previously the Chair of the UK's National HIV Nurses Association (NHIVNA).

Sarah Rutter is a Clinical Psychologist whose experience falls primarily within the field of physical health. She is Psychology Lead in the HIV Service at North Manchester General Hospital and the current chair of the British Psychological Society's Faculty of HIV and Sexual Health.

Psychological Perspectives in HIV Care

An Inter-Professional Approach

Edited by Michelle Croston and Sarah Rutter

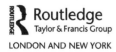
Routledge
Taylor & Francis Group

LONDON AND NEW YORK

First published 2020
by Routledge
2 Park Square, Milton Park, Abingdon, Oxon OX14 4RN

and by Routledge
52 Vanderbilt Avenue, New York, NY 10017

Routledge is an imprint of the Taylor & Francis Group, an informa business

British Library Cataloguing-in-Publication Data
A catalogue record for this book is available from the British Library

Library of Congress Cataloging-in-Publication Data
Names: Rutter, Sarah (Clinical psychologist), editor. | Croston, Michelle, editor.
Title: Psychological perspectives in HIV care : an inter-professional approach / [edited by] Michelle Croston and Sarah Rutter.
Description: Abingdon, Oxon ; New York, NY : Routledge, 2020. | Includes bibliographical references and index. | Summary: "This book provides an accessible introduction for healthcare professionals who work with people living with HIV"– Provided by publisher.
Identifiers: LCCN 2020011571 (print) | LCCN 2020011572 (ebook) |
ISBN 9780415792769 (hardback) | ISBN 9780415792783 (paperback) |
ISBN 9781315211404 (ebook) Subjects: LCSH: HIV-positive persons–Care. |
HIV-positive persons–Psychology. | HIV-positive persons–Medical care. |
HIV infections–Psychological aspects. | AIDS (Disease)–Psychological aspects. |
Medical personnel and patient.
Classification: LCC RC606.6 .P86 2020 (print) | LCC RC606.6 (ebook) |
DDC 362.19697/92–dc23
LC record available at https://lccn.loc.gov/2020011571
LC ebook record available at https://lccn.loc.gov/2020011572

ISBN: 978-0-415-79276-9 (hbk)
ISBN: 978-0-415-79278-3 (pbk)
ISBN: 978-1-315-21140-4 (ebk)

Typeset in Times New Roman
by Swales & Willis, Exeter, Devon, UK

Contents

vi *Contents*

Tables

Figures

Contributors

India Amos is a lecturer in Counselling and Psychotherapy at the University of Salford and a Chartered and HCPC-registered Counselling Psychologist working within HIV services. Her research has included investigating post-traumatic growth experiences among people living with HIV.

Sarah Blackshaw is a clinical psychologist with a special interest in chronic physical health conditions. She has previously worked in the field of HIV and sexual health and is currently working within a specialist service providing biopsychosocial interventions to patients experiencing chronic pain. Sarah is currently a member of the British Pain Society and is interested in exploring lived experiences of pain.

Kathryn Bourne is a Clinical Psychologist with experience of research and clinical work within physical health settings. Her current role is at Greater Manchester Mental Health NHS Foundation Trust, where she has a split post working into the Pennine Acute Hospitals NHS Trust HIV service at North Manchester General Hospital, and also the Manchester University NHS Foundation Trust Sleep Service at Wythenshawe Hospital.

Tomás Campbell is a Chartered Clinical Psychologist with the HCPC, an Associate Fellow of the British Psychological Society (BPS), and a Chartered Scientist and a Fellow of the Royal Society of Medicine. Tomas spent two years working in an HIV programme in Zambia and has since developed links with the only dedicated adolescent HIV clinic in Africa. He is especially interested in the neuropsychological aspects of HIV disease, addressing the effects of HIV stigma and working with adolescents.

Roland Chesters became a campaigner for disability rights after being diagnosed with HIV in 2006. Roland is a trained peer mentor for Positively UK, a trainer for gay men's health project GMFA and one of Terrence Higgins Trust's positive voices.

Michelle Croston has over 20 years of experience working within HIV care as a Specialist Nurse, including previously holding the position of Chair of the National HIV Nurses Association (NHIVNA). Her research interests focus around person-centred care for people living with HIV.

Michelle currently works as a Senior Lecturer at Manchester Metropolitan University and has recently joined Gilead Sciences' Outcomes Service and Support Team, which explores strategies to improve patient outcomes.

Stuart Gibson is a clinical psychologist from Canada, who has been teaching, conducting research and providing clinical services in HIV and sexual health for more than 20 years.

Stuart served as the Chair of the Faculty for HIV & Sexual Health with the British Psychological Society for many years. His current NHS appointment is at Barts Health in East London, where he is the Head of Psychology in Infection & Immunity – one of the country's largest psychology services for sexual health and HIV.

Catherine Heaton is a Senior Physiotherapist with a special interest in pain. She has worked widely across the NHS in a variety of different pain services. Catherine is an active member of the Pain Relief Foundation, which is dedicated to improving the quality of life for people living with chronic pain.

Rusi Jaspal is Pro Vice-Chancellor for Research, and Professor of Psychology and Sexual Health at De Montfort University, Leicester, UK. He is also an Adjunct Professor of Minority Research at Åbo Akademi University, Turku, Finland. Rusi is a Chartered Psychologist and Fellow of the British Psychological Society. He has written over 100 articles and book chapters focusing mainly on the social psychological aspects of sexual identity, sexual health, and behaviour among gay men.

Emma Jones is a senior lecturer at the University of Central Lancashire. She is the course leader of an MSc and other programmes exploring the term 'personality disorder'. Emma has previously worked as a nurse in a secure hospital. Emma has an MSc in personality disorder research, PGCert in health and social care education, and is currently studying a Professional Doctorate in Health.

Alexander Margetts is a Clinical Psychologist and BABCP accredited CBT therapist with experience in working with individuals presenting with common mental health difficulties, especially in the context of physical health and neurocognitive issues. He has worked in HIV & Sexual Health at Chelsea & Westminster Hospital for the past decade.

Angelina Namiba has been living with HIV for more than two decades, she has been an instrumental advocate in the HIV sector for over 17 years, and has worked on different initiatives ranging from one-to-one support and treatment advocacy to managing service delivery. Angelina is currently the patron of the National HIV Nurses Association, and a community representative for the British HIV Association, National AIDS Trust and Safe Kenya

James Meeks is a Senior Lecturer in Sexual and Reproductive Health and a registered nurse at the University of Central Lancashire in Preston. His specialist interests are HIV and gay men's health. He is the course leader for the MSc Sexual Health Studies and teaches across the undergraduate and postgraduate provision. He's an editor of the *HIV Nursing Journal* and is currently completing his PhD exploring the role of others in men who have sex with men following a diagnosis of HIV.

Gemma Paszek has worked within Paediatric Care at Alder Hey Hospital, Neurological, Acute Medicine and Diabetes Services, as well as Primary Care Psychology Services and Complex Cases in Greater Manchester. In addition to her current clinical roles in HIV, respiratory and sleep services, Gemma holds a teaching role and contributes to the physical health modules on the Manchester Clinical Psychology Doctorate course.

Merial Rattue is a psychology graduate from Oxford Brookes, with extensive experience working in mental health. Merial is a trained counsellor and mindfulness teacher. She promotes self-awareness as a key to unlock internal stigma and tackle intersectionality. Merial was diagnosed HIV positive in 2001 and shares her experiences as part of the 4M mentor mother's network. Merial is also a representative for UKCAB on the BHIVA Guidelines Committee, Psychological Standards Writing Group and Kings Fund.

Caroline Ridley is a registered adult nurse, health visitor and sexual health nurse, and has recently worked as a nurse educator at Manchester Metropolitan University, where her research and teaching interests included community nursing, public health and sexual health. Caroline was awarded one of the first 50 Fellowships of the Institute of Health Visiting and is currently working as a Children's Safeguarding Nurse Specialist at East Cheshire NHS Trust.

Sarah Rutter is a Clinical Psychologist with a particular interest in the complex psychological issues within HIV. As well as her present role as Psychology Lead in the HIV Service at North Manchester General Hospital, Sarah is also the current Chair of the British Psychological Society's HIV Care and is an honorary teacher at the University of Liverpool.

Hoo Kee Tsang leads the Pain Medicine Department at the Royal Liverpool and Broadgreen University Hospitals NHS Trust. Dr Tsang is a member of the local clinical ethics committee. He is a keen advocate for a psychologically informed approach to pain management.

Sam Warner is a Chartered and Consultant Clinical Psychologist with a specialist interest in sexual violence. Sam holds an honorary lectureship in the School of Society and Health, Salford University, and has been engaged by the Department of Health and British Government as an expert in mental health on both national and international sexual violence projects.

Shaun Watson has worked in HIV care since qualifying in 1989. During his career Shaun has facilitated many self-management programmes for people living with HIV. Shaun was the chair of NHIVNA between 2017 and 2020 and is passionate about HIV nurse education, speaking to a variety of different audiences to improve outcomes for people living with HIV, both in the UK and overseas.

Acknowledgements

We would like to thank the authors who have contributed to the chapters within the book. Thank you for your tireless hard work and dedication to improving the quality of life for people living with HIV, without which this book would not have been brought to publication. We are very grateful to Routledge for publishing our work, without which our thoughts and ideas would have remained dreams.

Sarah would like to thank all family and friends who have supported her to reach this point. Particular gratitude goes to her partner Michael, for feeding her during stressful times, and her mother, Pat, who has been there each step of the way.

Michelle would like to thank her daughter Harriet, mum Pauline, and dad Mike, for their endless support and words of encouragement.

Michelle and Sarah would also like to acknowledge each other, in terms of the mutual support required and offered throughout this process, which formed the basis of a productive, meaningful and resilient partnership.

Finally, we would like to thank all the people living with HIV, whose stories, reflections and experiences have driven the focus of this book. You continue to encourage us to provide the best care possible.

Introduction

The considerable advancements in HIV treatment (antiretroviral therapy: ART) mean that people diagnosed with the condition are now living much longer, healthier lives. If the diagnosis of HIV is made fairly soon after acquisition and treatment is commenced with immediate effect, a normal lifespan can now be expected. The care paradigm for people living with HIV has changed therefore from managing a condition with a poor prognosis and high risk of transmission, to one of managing a long-term chronic health issue. According to Public Health England, in the UK, the UNAIDS worldwide target of 90–90–90 (90% of people living with HIV to be diagnosed; 90% of those diagnosed to be on treatment; 90% of those on treatment to have an undetectable viral load) has been achieved. This means that a significant proportion of people living with HIV are not able to transmit the condition to others, given that an undetectable viral load means the virus is untransmittable (U=U).

Whilst these developments are, of course, highly welcome, new challenges have arisen in response to these changes, many of which are psychosocial in nature. These can include factors that impact on patients' health-related quality of life, such as the burden of lifelong adherence to antiretroviral therapy, telling people about their HIV status and aging. Such issues, which are often inter-related, can have a significant influence on psychological and emotional wellbeing, and monitoring patients' holistic wellbeing is an important, although often a complex, aspect of long-term care. On the back of this, calls have been made to extend the framework to include a fourth 90, which focuses on people living well with HIV. It is within this arena that the importance of providing holistic care is underlined.

Healthcare professionals are under increasing pressure to demonstrate that the care they deliver is supported by best evidence, and that it is delivered in a compassionate and person-centred way. For those working in HIV services, this can be challenging, as people who are living with HIV can have needs that are complex and diverse. There is growing evidence that physical health is strongly linked to psychological and emotional wellbeing, and therefore attention to these factors is essential for optimum health outcomes. It follows then that healthcare professionals who are providing care for people living with HIV can provide more effective support if they have an enhanced understanding of the psychological issues that can be experienced when living with this condition.

Just as patient needs are diverse and individual, the healthcare professionals providing care draw from their own personal experiences and have a unique style of care delivery. For those whose experiences are deeply rooted in the medical model, working in an area such as HIV, which has a strong presence of psychosocial needs, may be unfamiliar. Changing the way we think about providing care can be challenging and cause a sense of uncertainty. It is hoped that this book will help provide readers with increased knowledge of salient psychological issues for the HIV population and suggest helpful frameworks to support a shift in thinking or reinforce the style of care already developed. However daunting looking at care differently may feel, in the experience of the authors, we can reassure you that the rewards are worth the efforts.

The book aims to provide an accessible overview of key concepts that can help a range of healthcare professionals to understand how HIV care within clinical practice can be more person-centred and psychologically focused, while promoting medical care that is compassionate and supports an individual's quality of life. As HIV care evolves and people living with HIV access their treatment in a variety of different healthcare settings, it is hoped that this book will appeal to readers from different disease areas with an interest in holistic care approaches.

When compiling the chapters, the authors have taken into consideration the main themes arising within the HIV population. This has been influenced by 'experts by experience' who have shared their stories, the HIV literature, and anecdotal evidence from clinical practice. The book opens with an exploration of a variety of healthcare experiences provided by people who are living with HIV. This sets the scene for the following chapters, which focus in on specific issues. Given that the book advocates interdisciplinary approaches to meet what can often be a complex interplay of needs, a range of professionals from different disciplines have been invited to offer their perspective. Alongside the 'experts by experience', the professions include nursing, clinical, counselling and academic psychology, physiotherapy and medicine.

Features of the book

Each chapter is structured to enable the reader to reflect on the theories and concepts discussed within the chapter and consider how this may relate to clinical practice. There is an initial overview of the salient points that will be covered in the chapter, and the main body of the text is punctuated with a mixture of reflection points, activity boxes, case studies and resource boxes to aid your learning. This book is not intended to be used as a workbook, so we would recommend that any written reflections or activities be recorded in a separate notebook for future reference.

The book can be used in a variety of different ways. The reader may choose to focus on chapters that relate to their own clinical practice and interests, or they may choose to read the book in its entirety. Wherever possible, we have tried to guide you to the chapters that are linked, by using cross-referencing to support the overlapping issues, concepts and theories being explored. However the reader chooses to approach the book, we hope that it can add value to everyday clinical practice.

An overview of the chapters

This book is made up of 11 chapters and a brief outline of each follows. This is to give the reader the opportunity to acquire a taste of the perspectives on offer, before deciding how they might engage with the text.

Chapter 1: The good, the bad and the ugly: how do people living with HIV experience care in the health system? Throughout the first chapter, India and Roland explore the changes in HIV care through the eyes of people living with HIV. The participants candidly share their experiences of receiving care in a variety of different health and social care settings. India and Roland explore the commonly expressed psychological challenges of living with HIV in order to share with the reader ways to improve outcomes for people living with HIV when accessing a variety of different services. The reflection boxes throughout the chapter ask the reader to consider any experiences they have had of providing care for people living with HIV and how the care they deliver could be improved as a result of hearing the participants' stories.

Chapter 2: Self-awareness in HIV care explores the concept of self-awareness and how this relates to the care of people living with HIV is discussed. Throughout the chapter Caroline provides useful insight into the concept of self-awareness, what self-awareness means for healthcare professionals, and how this can be effectively used when developing therapeutic relationships with people living with HIV. The activities within the chapter help the reader to explore how the core value of respect is demonstrated within relationships and the impact that this core value can have when communicating with others. The reader is encouraged to explore their own sense of self and how they may consider developing their own self-awareness to improve outcomes for people living with HIV.

Chapter 3: Seeing the whole person: a biopsychosocial perspective in HIV provides guidance for healthcare professionals who do not have an in-depth understanding of mental health to enable them to adopt a holistic approach to providing care for people living with HIV. Gemma and Kathryn discuss the use of different models in healthcare and ask the reader to reflect on how healthcare is generally delivered using a biomedical model and how this traditional approach may be enhanced by considering a biopsychosocial approach to understanding patient needs. The case studies within the chapter encourage the reader to draw on the theory that has been discussed to explore how care could be delivered differently to improve patient outcomes. The reflection points throughout the chapter help the reader to consolidate their learning and begin to consider how they can link the theory that has been highlighted with the chapter to their clinical practice.

Chapter 4: HIV diagnosis: the impact on mental health and wellbeing encourages the reader to explore how living with HIV can affect someone psychologically and emotionally and offers helpful strategies relating to informing someone of their HIV diagnosis. Throughout the chapter the reader is encouraged, through the use of reflective exercises and case studies, to consider the effects an HIV diagnosis has on a person's mental health and wellbeing. James and Emma introduce the reader to communication models that might be helpful to consider when delivering complex and difficult news to a person, such as giving a positive HIV test result.

Chapter 5: Navigating stormy waters: difficult conversations in HIV care acknowledges the personal and professional challenges associated with communicating complex and sensitive information. The chapter highlights the significance of good communication linked to patient outcomes and provides frameworks to promote therapeutic communication. The activities within the chapter encourage the reader to consider the relevance of authentic and genuine responses when developing therapeutic relationships. Empathy is explored as a fundamental requirement when creating an effective clinical encounter. Throughout the chapter, Michelle and Stuart help the reader, through the use of reflection, to consider how their communication styles and behaviours are conducive to, or perhaps block, effective communication.

Chapter 6: Traumatic beginnings, complicated lives: attachment styles, relationships and HIV care addresses how adverse early experiences can have a negative impact on HIV health and wellbeing outcomes. It uses attachment and trauma theory to consider why people with difficult histories can struggle to manage their self-care and might experience distress in some healthcare relationships. The chapter acknowledges the importance of staff being aware of their own attachment styles as well as the influence of the context of healthcare delivery. Sarah and Sam utilise case studies and reflective tasks throughout to help the reader make sense of the material presented. Recommendations are made regarding person-centred clinical interventions that are rooted in the understanding of attachment-related needs. The concept of interdisciplinary working is then considered as a potential 'safe base' from which people with complex needs can begin to feel cared for, and eventually learn to care for themselves.

Chapter 7: Chemsex among men who have sex with men: a social psychological approach explores the sexualised use of psychoactive drugs commonly referred to as 'chemsex'. The practice of chemsex is understood to most often occur within the men who have sex with men (MSM) population. Throughout this chapter, Rusi explores multiple factors that make chemsex a distinct phenomenon amongst the MSM population. He utilises social psychological theory to help understand the issues that underpin the practice of chemsex and proposes a model on which to base clinical interventions. The reflective exercises and case studies enable the reader to consolidate the theoretical knowledge gained within the chapter and then apply this knowledge to their own clinical practice.

Chapter 8: The seemingly intractable problem of HIV-related stigma: developing a framework to guide stigma interventions with young people living with HIV thinks about stigma and HIV generally, before focusing in on how it impacts the younger generations. Within this chapter, Tomas explores the development and maintenance of HIV-related stigma. The impact that stigma has on young people living with HIV is highlighted in particular, followed by suggestions for clinical interventions. The reader will be introduced to frameworks that can help address stigma-related issues within the workplace to empower young people to manage their relationships and wider wellbeing. Tomas provides a thought-provoking chapter that is an essential read for healthcare professionals working with people living with HIV.

Chapter 9: Multidisciplinary management of neuropathic pain in HIV care provides practical advice on how to assess someone presenting to the clinical consultation with neuropathic pain. The chapter provides a comprehensive overview of the common presenting features associated with neuropathic pain, providing useful tips for healthcare professionals when making a diagnosis. Sarah, Hoo Kee and Catherine provide an interdisciplinary overview of how to provide holistic care for people living with HIV who are experiencing neuropathic pain. Throughout the chapter the reader is encouraged to consider the quality of life issues that living in chronic pain brings. The reflection points and case studies augment the theories that are being discussed within the chapter and help the reader to explore how they can improve quality of life for people living with HIV who are experiencing neuropathic pain.

Chapter 10: The psychological impact of ageing with HIV explores the increasing phenomenon of the complexities that people living with HIV are facing as they begin to age. The chapter explores different definitions of ageing alongside what this might mean for individuals' care needs. Shaun and Alexander advocate for increased interdisciplinary working to promote safe care and successful ageing for people living with HIV. The reflection points throughout the chapter are designed to help healthcare professionals consider what the evolving needs of an ageing cohort could potentially be as we voyage into unknown health and social care territory with the first group of people living with

HIV to age. The case studies at the end of the chapter draw the chapter's learning points together, helping the reader to consider the issues explored within the chapter in a real-world setting.

Chapter 11: Neurocognitive issues for adults in HIV care. Within this final chapter Tomas and Alexander explore the effects HIV can have on the brain and brain function. Adults living with HIV can experience neurocognitive issues and, within this chapter, the complex issues around neuropsychological assessments are discussed and practical suggestions are offered to the reader when considering the type of screening to use in clinical practice. The reflective exercises within the chapter explore what challenges people may face when living with cognitive difficulties and the case studies help the reader to consolidate their learning.

Overall aims of the book

As stated above, the book aims to cover a range of areas relevant to HIV care and is designed to be widely accessible. However, it does not claim to be exhaustive and readers may wish to deepen their knowledge by following up on relevant references and resources. Many of the chapters are co-written, sometimes by professionals from different clinical disciplines, and therefore a variety of perspectives are shared. There is both overlap and divergence between the chapters, and the editors have provided cross-referencing to assist the reader in further exploration of issues, if they choose not to read the book in full. The overall intent is to provide a broad description of approaches to HIV care, and it is likely that some chapters will appeal more to some readers than others. This will perhaps be influenced by the reader's own clinical background and experiences, and it is hoped that there will be something of interest for any healthcare professional interested in the area of HIV. Additionally, although chapters are focused on HIV, some of the concepts and approaches can be extended to other areas of care provision. Whether the reader works specifically in an HIV speciality or would just like to learn about HIV-related issues so they can effectively support someone living with the condition, the book provides a helpful framework for compassionate and effective practice.

1 The good, the bad and the ugly

How do people living with HIV experience care in the health system?

India Amos, Roland Chesters, Angelina Namiba and Merial Rattue

---

Chapter description

What it is like to live with HIV in the global north has changed dramatically over the last two decades. There have been significant developments in the treatment and prevention of HIV, and the healthcare landscape continues to evolve. This chapter intends to highlight some of the impact of such changes on people living with HIV, who are accessing healthcare in the United Kingdom (UK). Initiating conversations with the contributors to this chapter commenced by asking them to recount part of their story using healthcare services that was particularly poignant, memorable or important to them – what stands out to you? was the question. The good, the bad and the ugly encounters with health and social care came forth in response. Through sharing and discussing some of their helpful and hindering experiences of health services, HIV or otherwise, what could be seen as some of the common psychological challenges associated with living with HIV were also illuminated. This chapter aims to bring attention to the lived experience of people living with HIV and the care they receive; to consider what works – and what does not. The contributors to this chapter have all helped to achieve this aim. Other first-hand accounts of healthcare experiences, published elsewhere, have also been drawn upon.

Reflection boxes have been included throughout the chapter and are an invitation to explore and consider any experiences you may have of providing care for people living with HIV. Perhaps you work in an HIV service. If you do not work in HIV services specifically, it is possible that you might be in a position of working with someone living with the diagnosis. How does the content of this chapter apply to you in the context that you work?

Firstly

Jesse reminds us that 'everyone living with HIV has a completely different story and a very different approach in how they see and think of their HIV status'. The collection of perspectives here offers an insight into some of the experiences, but not all. That is to say that the issues raised are not exhaustive or necessarily representative of everyone's perspective. Similarly, as the readers of this chapter, you too will bring a range of unique experiences personal to you.

Reflection box 1: capturing initial thoughts and feelings

Before you continue reading, consider the following:
What comes to mind for you upon reading the title and introduction to this chapter?
What might you be expecting to read about as you move through the content?
Make a note of what you consider could be the good, the bad and the ugly of experiences of healthcare for people living with HIV.

At the time of diagnosis

Consistent across the conversations with the contributors to this chapter was the support required at the time of diagnosis. Irrespective of time since diagnosis, age, sexuality and gender, the overwhelming response to diagnosis has been reported in the literature (Walker, 2019), and speaking to Bella there was an acute sense of the shock and distress that was felt upon being diagnosed:

> When I got diagnosed with HIV in March 2008, I was totally devastated and felt that my whole world had been blown apart.
>
> (Bella)

An HIV diagnosis can be sudden and unexpected. In Bella's case the sensation of her world, as she knew it, having been 'blown apart' evokes an image of destruction.

For Jack, a participant in a study by Flowers, Davis, Larkin, Church, and Marriott (2011) feelings of worthlessness and loss were apparent:

> Close friends, family, anybody, even new people that I'd meet; I just felt that I couldn't, I suppose I felt quite, quite worthless because I didn't have the, [sighs] I felt like I'd lost something, I just found everything so tiring, I didn't have anything to give, I didn't feel that I had anything worthwhile to kind of contribute, I don't know, I was just kind of like shell shocked I suppose.
>
> (p. 1382)

Jack's sigh is almost audible as you read his account. When an HIV diagnosis is sudden and unexpected, it can be experienced as traumatic. Shock, numbness and distress are commonly cited as initial responses. A 20-year-old participant in a qualitative research study investigating experiences of motherhood recalled the time they were diagnosed with HIV very clearly:

> It was a big shock, and things got kinda blurry. I just remember going into my mother's bedroom and going to bed. I stayed there for like 2 to 3 days. I was diagnosed in my formative years; you're not really the same person after diagnosis.
>
> (in Sanders, 2008, p. 4)

Similarly, Judith comments on the defining moment she was diagnosed:

> I got my positive result and life has never been the same since.

Reflection box 2: response to being diagnosed

The excerpts above provide an insight into the major impact an HIV diagnosis had on them.

Why might the people quoted here have responded in the way they did about being diagnosed with HIV?

A dramatic change was felt by Bella, Judith and the participant from the study by Walker (2019). Making sense of diagnosis seems, for some, to be via the separation of their lives into the temporal categories of before and after the event. There is a sense of *who I was*, then *what happened* and *who I am now*. A key theme developed in the analysis of the experience of receiving a diagnosis of HIV was 'unwelcome and problematic changes in identity' (Flowers, Davis, Larkin, Church, & Marriott, 2011, p. 138). This was experienced as an identity crisis for some, in which parts of the self were considered to have died and a mourning process for the lost aspects of identity commenced. The everyday experience of living with HIV can encompass a series of unfolding stresses for the individual, including starting treatment, managing side effects, sharing HIV status with others and anticipating and/or experiencing HIV-related stigma. Together these can call into question the coherence of one's life and personhood, and can cumulatively constitute a traumatic stressor (Hefferon, Grealy, & Mutrie, 2009). James Meeks and Emma Jones in Chapter 4 explore the impact that HIV has on mental health.

Whilst the current HIV treatment context consists of very *effective treatments* that enable people, predominantly those diagnosed early in the course of the infection, to live a long and healthy life, diagnosis and starting treatment can nonetheless be experienced as a life-transforming event. This is not to be underestimated. People living with HIV have reported that the way in which HIV results were given to them made the testing process more difficult, upsetting, or disturbing (Hult, Maurer, & Moskowitz, 2009). For one participant in a qualitative research study, the diagnosis was experienced as being made in a 'scripted and impersonal' fashion:

> I was surprised there wasn't much conversation ... the person who did it just handed me a couple of brochures about places where I could go.
>
> (Hult, Maurer, & Moskowitz, 2009, p. 186)

It could be said that individuals may struggle to comprehend the meaning of a positive test result when they are first diagnosed. In the same study, one participant said:

> from that point on, I couldn't hear anything. I mean, they try to talk to you, they try to counsel you, they try to tell you everything's okay. I don't know what they said. I don't remember. I just remember sitting there going, 'Uhh ... uh, uh, yeah ...' just my mind was just shut down.
>
> (Hult, Maurer, & Moskowitz, 2009, p. 187)

Sarah Rutter and Sam Warner explore the psychological effects of trauma further in Chapter 6.

Noelly's account of her experience shines a different light on what it is like to be diagnosed with HIV. A found poem has been constructed from Noelly's interview transcript. Please see Gabriel, Lee, and Taylor (2018) and Amos (2019) for discussion on the process of creating found poetry.

Reflection box 3: a found poem by Noelly

'What really stands out'
What really stands out is going for my HIV test
not in a bad way
just that I remember
I was really scared
took me a long time before I went
I remember walking in
I was on my own
lining up and getting into the room where the nurse had to take my blood
clearly it said on the sheet HIV
I could see the nurse looking at me
I don't know whether it was
I would say pity
I could see she felt for me
I was there
you know, really worried
and everything you know
I remember that memory very well
just going all the way up to the hospital
the journey was very long and sitting there all by myself
that kind of stands out for me
Reflective questions:
What is your response to this poem?
Do any of the words, phrases, sections stand out to you?
Note down any immediate thoughts, feelings or bodily sensations.

It is worth noting here the words that Noelly uses: *'not in a bad way'*, she says, when recalling the time of her diagnosis. She remembers it but she seems keen to state that her recollection is not because it was felt exclusively as damaging. Perhaps there is an assumption that the person receiving the diagnosis will respond negatively. Could this be why the nurse working with Noelly looked at her with *'pity'*? The power of diagnosis in transforming self and relationships highlights it to be, as Jutel (2009) deems, 'a powerful social tool' (p. 289). There is no doubt that some people experience significant distress in response to being diagnosed. However, it seems it could be harmful if healthcare professionals assume that this will be the case.

Giving an HIV positive test result requires time and skill to provide the emotional support that the experiences shared here suggest are needed. Rayment, Asboe, and

Table 1.1 The language of HIV

Rule 1: positive words	Rule 2: person-first language	Rule 3: avoid the language of war
Focus on using positive words such as 'promoting health' (two positive words) rather than 'ending disease' (two negative words).	It is important to use language that puts people first. Using language that puts people first acknowledges people living with HIV as fellow human beings.	Describing HIV in militaristic ways such as immune cells as soldiers fighting HIV, or ending HIV as elimination, killing or the scourge of AIDS or using these words may lead people to think those living with HIV have to be 'fought' or 'eliminated'.

Adapted from 'The language of HIV: a guide for nurses' by Watson, Namiba and Lynn, *HIV Nursing* (Watson, Namiba, & Lynn, 2019); 19(2).

Sullivan (2014) report that in an ideal circumstance a confirmed positive test result would be delivered face to face by the team or clinician who conducted the test, and that this would take place in a confidential environment with clear language being used. Watson, Namiba, and Lynn (2019) draw attention to the power of language and provide a useful overview of the preferred language of HIV. Table 1.1 summarises three rules that the authors encourage practitioners to observe.

Historically, disclosure has been the termed used to describe the process of telling someone about their HIV status. If you look at the definition of disclosure, it is often referred to as the action of making new or secret information known (Watson, Namiba, & Lynn, 2019). In many definitions of disclosure, the word secret often appears, which brings with it implications of confession, revelation and biblical connotations.

The term disclosure is loaded with legal and negative terminology and reinforces self-stigma and the underlying belief that the person living with HIV is doing something wrong. Therefore we encourage people to use words like 'telling' or 'sharing' to reduce stigma and to reduce the implications that something is being hidden.

When referring to a person, avoid using the word 'infectious' as this can be associated with words like 'dirty' or 'tainted' and can imply that someone is contaminated. Using more neutral words such as 'acquire' or 'transmit' say the same thing but carry different feelings for people (Watson, Namiba, & Lynn, 2019).

The use of stigmatising language unfortunately still exists both in the media and in published academic articles. Challenging others on their use of inaccurate terminology can possibly evoke feelings of anxiety. Not challenging the use of inaccurate language can perpetuate stigma and discrimination (Leahy, 2018).

Chapter 5 delves further into the navigation of difficult conversations that can occur within HIV care.

It may seem reasonable to think that following diagnosis, therapeutic intervention such as counselling or psychological therapy would be an appropriate next step. For some people this may well be what they want and need. However, the psychological processing of an HIV diagnosis can take time and not everyone perceives the benefit of talking therapy at such an early stage. For example, Neil did not:

> I was diagnosed and was still coming to terms with my diagnosis of HIV. I felt unready really to go deep with any talking and turned down further sessions at that point.
>
> (Neil)

How someone responds to their HIV diagnosis will depend on many contributing factors, including access to support, knowledge, previous experience of trauma and other psychosocial factors (Pence et al., 2012). The range of mental, emotional, physical and behavioural reactions associated with a trauma response (see Chapter 6) are considered part of a normal reaction and, for a lot of people, these thoughts, feelings and behaviours reduce naturally as they psychologically adjust to living with HIV. To offer psychological intervention at this point has the potential to pathologise that process. Ensuring that the medical implications of the diagnosis are understood might be the primary focus for a healthcare professional involved in HIV testing and diagnosis. Regardless, for the overwhelming majority of people, this process of adjustment is most successful when they feel listened to and heard by those supporting them.

Reflection box 4: checking-in

Engaging with the lived experiences of being diagnosed is one way in which to improve the process in which an HIV positive test result is given (Schrooten et al., 2001).
In what way might your engagement with the experiences shared so far in the chapter support you in your professional role?
How might you understand your response and apply it in your practice context?
What skills might be considered useful in supporting someone at the time of diagnosis?

Feeling heard

Hardavella, Aamli-Gaagnat, and Frille (2017) acknowledge that:

> Bad news may be broken in a nonempathetic way, messages may be given to the nurses over the patient's head while interrupting the consultation, difficult words may be used that the patient does not understand, and the patient may feel excluded from conversations with almost no concern showed for their feelings and emotions. Often, what is everyday routine clinical data to the healthcare practitioner may be completely unfamiliar to the patient, giving the impression that the clinician is cold and unsympathetic to the individual's emotions as they try to come to terms with the diagnosis and its implications.
>
> (p. 131)

Neil recalls his engagement with psychological services in which he felt dismissed:

> I did feel at the time that the psychologist had seen it all before and was more concerned to tell me that I wasn't going mad and get me off his books, although that might have been my impression at the time. It made me feel that other people were more important than me as they were in greater difficulty.

Medical doctors in practice report a lack of training in clinical empathy (Buckman, Tulsky, & Rodin, 2011). However, there is a substantial literature to support the claim that doctor–patient relationships strengthen as a result of the detection of emotional cues and expression of empathy by doctors to the patients they work with (Flickinger et al., 2016) (see Chapters 5 and 6 for the importance of relationships and communication). What results is a feeling of being heard, supported and accepted. In turn this can have a major impact on subsequent retention in care. Hardavella, Aamli-Gaagnat, and Frille (2017) go on to provide some top tips for dealing with challenging situations within the patient–doctor dyad that may be found useful. Chapter 5 explores these tips further.

It has already been highlighted that the way people are given an HIV diagnosis can greatly impact the individual's experience, as well as their decision-making in relation to treatment down the line. These are findings well documented in the literature (Evans et al., 2015), and is why Martin Buber's work provides a valuable framework in which to consider how to communicate with the people you work with. The discomfort felt by some healthcare providers in disclosing positive test results, or in some cases even offering a patient an HIV test, have been brought to light (Conners et al., 2012; Mitchell, Bushby, & Chauhan, 2011). It is worth saying here that the effect of delayed diagnosis can result in avoidable loss of life (May et al., 2011) and late diagnosis of HIV remains an important clinical and public health issue in the UK (Chadwick & Freedman, 2019). A national audit of late diagnosis highlighted that a third of individuals diagnosed with advanced HIV had earlier missed opportunities for diagnosis documented (Byrne et al., 2018). It was identified that most of these missed opportunities were due to clinicians not offering an HIV test, as opposed to patients declining to have one.

The emotional requirements for professionals involved in provider-initiated HIV testing and diagnosis can be experienced as stressful. Feeling inexperienced in giving an HIV diagnosis, not knowing how patients will respond and managing the ethical dilemmas related to disclosure were all cited as factors contributing to the emotional work required, in addition to organisational contexts in which nurses and midwives felt overworked and under-supported (Evans et al., 2015). What is going on for someone internally has an impact on the way in which they relate to others (please see Chapters 2, 5 and 6).

People waiting to receive their HIV test results have noticed when healthcare professionals were upset, nervous or crying when communicating the diagnosis. One person said:

> When he came back, he was crying. He told me that, 'I'm sorry, you tested positive.' … And, he's crying, I'm like, 'Okay, I need to calm myself down, 'cause I gotta take care of him!'
>
> (Hult, Maurer, & Moskowitz, 2009, p. 186)

This points to the importance of supervision for professionals involved in managing complex issues such as testing and diagnosing (Horwood, Voce, Vermaak, Rollins, & Qazi, 2010).

In response to the poem created from Noelly's narrative, perhaps you have considered what constitutes a helpful encounter with a healthcare professional for someone living with HIV. Particular attitudinal qualities may come to mind. When asked about experiences of a particularly good interaction with services, and what made it so, these were some of the responses from contributors:

She [sexual health advisor] talks to me like a human being and has even cried with me.

(Bella)

This other doctor in the same clinic was just so nice, so friendly, so patient and understanding … they [doctor] took the time and listened … it was the first time since my diagnosis that I felt I had some control of my own care … that I was able to choose what I was able to do. I almost cried as it felt that someone was actually listening to me. There is something about being listened to and understood and having some autonomy in your own care … being treated like a human being who's quality of life matters.

(Jesse)

What made it helpful was she [psychiatrist] understood how I was feeling and she did not talk much but she listened to me.

(Kya)

Being able to talk freely without it turning into a tick box exercise … someone who would just listen and not necessarily give you answers as sometimes you just need to talk.

(Mason)

Reflection box 5: what helps?

What do you notice Jesse, Kya and Mason are talking about in relation to helpful experiences they have had in healthcare?
What does the word autonomy mean to you?

Empathy, authenticity and honesty

People have different ways of interacting with others, so the expectation that there is a set of prescribed responses to be adhered to is certainly not what is advocated. However, not feeling heard can leave an individual feeling misunderstood, unaccepted and unsupported by others, and as a result might be less likely to foster self-acceptance. Empathy is distinctive from sympathy, with the latter perhaps defined as 'feeling sorry for someone'. Empathy is the attempt to 'understand how it feels for another person, imagining what it would be like to stand in their shoes, feel how they feel and see the world through their eyes'.

Reflection box 6: what is empathy?

Carl Rogers (1975), in his development of the person-centred therapeutic approach, reflected on empathy as both 'an unappreciated way of being' and 'possibly the most potent and certainly one of the most potent factors in bringing about change and learning' (p. 3). Empathy could be said to refer to the process of seeking to understand the world of another person – as they experience it, or what could be described as the internal frame of reference of another.

Can you recall a time when you experienced empathy from someone else?

What happened?

How did you know it was empathy?

Note down your responses to these questions

Empathy requires authenticity – another quality that was prized by the contributors to this chapter. For example, An said:

> I think clarity is really important … it's about having a grown-up conversation, be honest with people and do not make assumptions that people will not understand, you need to be honest with them.

An expresses the need for clarity. This could refer to the provision of clear and accurate information that is imparted to people living with HIV that could support them in their treatment decisions. It could also refer to a 'way of being' with people that is characterised by honesty, authenticity and genuineness. A human connection is what is important – a way of relating that is characterised by reciprocity and mutuality; communicating person to person. This is what philosopher Martin Buber (1988) described as the difference between I–It and I–Thou methods of relating in his work to understand the nature of dialogue. In the I–It relationship, the person relates to the person in a functional manner, like the way one might relate to an object. In contrast, the I–Thou relationship is typified as a two-way relationship, between persons all of whom are actively engaged with each other in a shared effort to enter into an authentic relationship. In establishing and maintaining a human connection to the person you are working with, you are someone 'with' the person as opposed to someone doing something 'to' them. Given the descriptions provided by Bella, Jesse, Kya and Mason, what transpires to be the most helpful experience at the time of diagnosis is someone who can tune in to the emotion/s being felt by the individual who has been diagnosed. Noelly put it succinctly when she explained that it is not what the healthcare professional feels like that matters, but what the person living with HIV feels like: *'What is more important for people living with HIV is how they deal with living with the virus.'* HIV care is for life, and so the importance of good care to maintain quality ongoing relationships is paramount. Good care requires time and the ability to apply a patient-centred approach, in which communicating empathy both verbally and non-verbally is central. HIV-related stigma is an important aspect to consider when thinking about the nature and quality of the working relationships, as it is well known that this is a persistent issue for the HIV population (see Chapter 8).

HIV-related stigma

Stigma in society

The most stressful problems reported by people living with HIV/AIDS are related to navigating challenging social situations, including discrimination, stigma, confidentiality, and sharing HIV status (Pakenham & Rinaldis, 2002). It affects the quality of life and mental health of people living with HIV and is also related to disengagement from HIV care and treatment (Donovan & Durey, 2018; Varni, Miller, McCuin, & Solomon, 2012).

So, what is stigma, and why is the impact of HIV-related stigma so significant? Perhaps the words 'stereotypes', 'prejudice' and 'discrimination' come to mind. Respectively, these could be said to be the cognitive, affective and behavioural manifestations of stigma. Erving Goffman defined stigma, in his seminal work, as 'an attribute that is deeply discrediting' (1963, p. 3). Associated with a deviation from a constructed ideal or expectation, stigmatising attitudes can evoke feelings of fear and revulsion towards stigmatised groups, and in the context of HIV, can sometimes result in the 'unfair and unjust treatment of an individual based on his or her real or perceived HIV status' (UNAIDS, 2003), known as discrimination. Stigma could be said to challenge one's humanity and contribute to an exercise of power (Dovidio, Major, & Crocker, 2000).

Reflection box 7: reflecting on your personal experience

You are invited to think about a time in your life when you felt isolated or rejected for being seen to be different from others, or when you saw other people treated this way.
What happened? How did it feel? What impact did it have on you?

Since Goffman's work, stigma has continued to be studied within social psychology. Research has sought to understand the mechanism in which categories are constructed and linked to stereotyped beliefs (Link & Phelan, 2001), as well as the extent to which stigma generates and perpetuates health inequities (Hatzenbuehler, Phelan, & Link, 2013). Stigma continues to be significantly problematic for people living with HIV today. The following reaction to HIV diagnosis from a male pinpoints some of what the stereotyped, group-based beliefs can be about people living with HIV:

> This only happens to promiscuous sluts having BB [bareback] chem sex every weekend … I felt dirty, infected, unclean and scared of the future and what people, friends and family would think of me.
>
> (in Walker, 2019, p. 102)

The evidence suggests that stigma is created and sustained by social structures as well as interpersonal processes (Hatzenbuehler & Link, 2014). The consistent message across the corpus of data is the negative impact stigma has on the lives of those people identified as possessing an attribute (real or perceived) that is linked to a negative social identity (Crocker, Major, & Steele, 1998). The majority of respondents who participated in a study on contemporary experiences of HIV diagnosis in the UK (Walker, 2019) articulated how, in their view, the social dimensions of HIV are what separates it from other long-term health conditions. Participants suggested that other long-term health conditions generated more sympathy as they were not associated with shame or stigma in the same way as HIV is possibly, as it is related to sex, drugs and a legacy of when death was almost certain. A participant diagnosed within six months of taking part in the study reported:

> I knew little about HIV when I was diagnosed. I thought someone had just told me I had 5 years to live. Now I know it is a manageable long-term condition, you can have babies and you suppress the virus to UD [undetectable] levels. The only

problem is the stigma attached to it. Had I been diagnosed with some other illness I would have told my mom and close family members. I would have told my now ex-boyfriend.

(in Walker, 2019, p. 106)

This extract from Walker (2019) illustrates the power of stigma in silencing people, and unfortunately the act of concealment and 'keeping secrets' can exacerbate feelings of shame, which in turn leads to people feeling ashamed and then increases stigma.

Reflection box 8: HIV-related stigma

There are considered to be different ways in which HIV-related stigma can manifest. Earnshaw and Chaudoir (2009) highlight the following in their framework:

Enacted stigma: actual experience of stigma and discrimination based on HIV status.

Anticipated stigma: also known as felt or perceived stigma, relating to the expectation of being stigmatised by others because of HIV status.

Internalised stigma: self-directed stigma in which negative assumptions about what it means to be living with HIV are accepted by the person living with HIV.

Some of the ways that HIV-related stigma might negatively affect the wellbeing and/or healthcare of persons living with HIV have already been raised.

Can you think of any other effects of HIV-related stigma on people living with HIV?

Telling others about their HIV status may seem a frightening experience for someone living with HIV who anticipates they may be judged negatively or treated unfairly as a result. It is not uncommon for people living with HIV to feel reluctant to share their status with the medical professionals they have support from:

I know a lot of women and men who are still not able to tell their HIV status to their GP because they have fear.

(Noelly)

A fear of stigma and confidentiality breaches can silence individuals. Perhaps this is not surprising. After all, HIV-related stigma is a reality. If someone expects to be stigmatised, and potentially discriminated against, in their interactions with others, avoiding circumstances in which this may occur seems an understandable response. This notion becomes increasingly concerning when it is considered that HIV-related stigma extends to healthcare settings too.

Stigma in healthcare

In accordance with the Equality Act 2010, people living with HIV are entitled to fair access and equitable care. However, experiences of HIV-related stigma exist beyond personal relationships, and are also experienced in interactions with medical and mental health service providers (Elford, Ibrahim, Bukutu, & Anderson, 2008).

Reflection box 9: HIV-related stigma in healthcare

Earlier in the chapter, an empathetic way of being with others was raised as a central ingredient to helpful encounters with professionals. Stigma could be said to be the expression of bias and can therefore block/impede/get in the way of empathising with someone.

Consider the following:

What assumptions might a healthcare professional make about someone who has been diagnosed with HIV?

In what ways might a healthcare professional discriminate against someone living with HIV?

Here are some examples of how HIV-related stigma can manifest in a healthcare setting:

When Jordan first went for an HIV test, he was asked by the doctor why he was requesting it and what profession he was in. When Jordan responded, he was told by the doctor: 'You can't be a police officer if you are a homosexual, and it will have to be reported to the police that you have been for an HIV test.'

Judith was delayed dental treatment for a year after visiting the practice to enquire about a problem with her gums. Judith attended for several appointments; however, she was refused treatment, being directed to back to her GP time and time again.

Can you put yourself in their position and imagine how this must have felt?

A number of studies have reported on the acts of discrimination experienced in healthcare environments towards people living with HIV. These have been enacted in numerous ways, including breaches of confidentiality, humiliating practices by health care professionals (for example 'double gloving'), and refusal of treatment as demonstrated in Judith's story. In fact, the Positive Voices Survey (2017) found that one in nine (11%) people living with HIV in the UK have been denied healthcare or delayed a treatment due to their HIV status. Displays of negative attitudes or prejudice occur, as shown in Jordan's case, drawing attention to how HIV-related stigma is often experienced intersectionally alongside other attributes that may also generate marginalisation, including a person's gender, ethnicity and social class (Boucher et al., 2019).

Jordan went on to share how his fear of stigma and discrimination impacted on his decision to engage with care. When he moved to a different area, he highlighted his preference to remain registered with his current GP practice – as it was more 'personable'. He reflected on the 'fear of having to tell people at another practice about his diagnosis' and the thought that crossed his mind: *'If I am ill, I'd rather just be ill than go there.'* A further finding from the Positive Voices Survey (2017) highlighted that 18% of people living with HIV had avoided healthcare when they needed it because of fear of being treated differently from other patients.

Jesse recalled experiences of having his confidentiality breached in a healthcare setting. His experience visiting his GP is shared here first of all:

I went in for a random thing … I can't remember what and my folder was on the front desk … and it had HIV on the front of it in red marker pen … it was on the front desk where everyone checks in for everyone to see … you could see my name on it … it made me feel so violated … so … I was to you know be treated differently … that made me feel awful.

The use of a red marker pen stands out here. For some, the colour red has long been associated with danger. It attracts attention and can signify threat. Jesse's use of the word 'violation' suggests a traumatic experience in which a boundary was crossed.

A question emanating from discussions with people living with HIV was, 'what is it with dentists?' Recall Judith's experience of seeking dental treatment and being denied, described earlier in this section. Jesse also described his experience of registering with his local dental practice once they became aware of his HIV status:

When we handed her back the forms, her tone very much changed … we are quite a busy dental surgery … funny, appointments are quite difficult for us … you would have to call on the day to see if we could fit you in at the beginning or at the end … which we knew what that was code for.

Reflection box 10: making sense of Jesse's experience

Jesse describes how it felt for him to see his folder on the front desk marked in red pen with the letters HIV.
How might you feel if you saw sensitive information about you on display?
Jesse described the communication he received from the dental receptionist as 'code'.
What do you think Jesse is describing here?
What is the message being implied?

In Jesse's interaction with the dental receptionist, it is suggested, though not directly expressed, that his appointment will need to be scheduled either side of routine appointments. There is no scientific reason why Jesse's appointment should be scheduled in this way. Implicit messages such as this are harmful and such practices are unlawful and clinically unnecessary. Advancements in HIV treatment mean that HIV will not be transmitted by people who are virally suppressed Undetectable=Untransmittable (U=U), therefore appointments throughout the day should be made available to all. Thankfully, a fruitful dialogue appears to be taking place within the discipline of dentistry, in which stigmatising experiences of people living with HIV in this context are being illuminated, including the challenges faced with registering with dental practices and being refused treatment (Levett, Slide, & Mallick, 2009). Methods to tackle this issue are also at the forefront, particularly in the context of staff training (Okala et al., 2018). For example, the *BDJ Team*, which is a peer-reviewed online magazine supported by the British Dental Association, recently published an article outlining the key facts that primary care dental teams need to know about blood-borne viruses (Lala, Harwood, Simon, Lee, & Jones, 2018). There is a need to raise culturally sensitive awareness and develop educational tools to address stigma. Okala et al. (2018) emphasise that training should focus on the ways to support patients after sharing of their HIV status. The authors suggest it should include training on:

ensuring confidentiality, using non-discriminatory language, booking appointments at any time of day, having up-to-date knowledge of current antiretroviral therapy, treatment outcomes for people living with HIV and comorbidities likely to affect patients who have been living with HIV for a number of years and who have been on long-term antiretroviral therapy.

(p. 150)

It could be safe to say that the recommendations made by Okala et al. (2018) are relevant to the training of healthcare teams working in HIV services or otherwise.

The psychological impact of shame, stigma and HIV are discussed in more depth in Chapter 8.

Healing suffering

As has already been indicated earlier in the chapter, receiving a diagnosis of HIV, or any other chronic disease, is often characterised by negative psychological outcomes such as helplessness, guilt, anxiety and depression (Richardson et al., 2001). In addition, trauma responses have been increasingly recognised as an important factor associated with HIV diagnosis (LeGrand et al., 2015). Kevin and Jane's stories are presented here to provide an insight into the impact of such a response.

Kevin's story

Kevin was 18 when he received his HIV diagnosis. He contracted HIV from his first sexual partner, who was older than him and was unaware of her own HIV status until Kevin was diagnosed.

Kevin was a self-confessed bad boy, who liked taking risk and had experimented with drugs, which led him to being involved in a local gang. For years Kevin struggled with being in the gang and was very fearful that the other members of the gang would find out his HIV status. Due to this fear of people finding out about his status, Kevin refused to take medication.

As Kevin's immune system began to decline, he started to lose weight and was eventually admitted onto the ward very unwell with pneumonia.

A subjective sense of loss of control is commonly associated with a trauma response. In Kevin's story so far, there is a sense of the build of fear he experienced – his anxiety about those around him becoming aware of his HIV status and what that might mean for him. The shame that Kevin experienced led him to conceal his status to such an extent that he felt too fearful of taking the necessary medication to support his immune system. Perhaps by not taking up antiretroviral treatment, Kevin was attempting to regain a sense of control over what he felt he had lost since being diagnosed. Inevitably, his refusal to take medication had significant consequences for his physical health. It could be argued that this constituted a further loss of control – over his body as he became increasingly unwell.

Jane's story

Jane was diagnosed HIV positive after a long period of unexplained illness. She had been admitted to a variety of different hospitals and been exposed to numerous tests, biopsies and procedures. This had led to mistrust between Jane and the medical team, as Jane felt that the team were not looking after her properly as she continued to deteriorate. Eventually Jane was offered an HIV test. She recalled that the team at the time felt that this was an unlikely diagnosis as she was young (23) and white British. Looking back on this, Jane felt that the doctors' attempts to reassure her were not medical in origin and were more moralistic. At the time of her HIV diagnosis her immune system was low and she had multiple HIV-related opportunistic infections.

Once Jane received her diagnosis, she was transferred to a specialist unit for inpatient care. During her admission Jane became very withdrawn and felt very anxious about her diagnosis. She reported feeling a sense of loss of the future that she had hoped for. The nursing team and psychologist engaged with Jane to explore the distress that she was feeling.

Janoff-Bulman (1992) conceptualises the psychological impact of trauma as emanating from the shattering of fundamental assumptions a person has about the world and about the self. The assumption that the world is kind and that the self is good and capable can shift. As a result of trauma, the world can suddenly be perceived as unsafe and scary, and the self may be unable to cope or perhaps even to blame. As Jane reflects, the loss she felt for her imagined future led her to withdraw from support.

Awareness of trauma responses to HIV diagnosis is becoming increasingly more important when providing psychological support for people living with HIV. Feelings of fear, guilt, shame, anxiety and low mood can exist in the everyday life of living with HIV. Kya states that *'a good service in my experience is where a consultant or a healthcare specialist recognises the need for a patient to be referred onto psychological or psychiatric services'*. Increasing understanding of the relationship between physical and mental health can ensure that individual need is recognised and appropriate referrals made (Naylor et al., 2016). In Chapter 6, Sarah Rutter and Sam Warner explore the relationship between trauma and physical and mental health.

Let's see how Kevin and Jane's stories develop.

Kevin's story continued …

During his admission to hospital, he discussed his concerns with the specialist nurse. As the therapeutic relationship developed, it gave Kevin the opportunity to explore his diagnosis and his hopes for the future. During this time Kevin began to rethink his diagnosis and stated that he felt that his HIV diagnosis had given him the opportunity to re-evaluate what was important to him. This resulted in Kevin agreeing to take antiretroviral therapy.

Kevin reported that he had never felt happier contributing to society in such a positive way. During his clinic visit Kevin was very candid and stated that he felt that his diagnosis had changed his life in a positive way, and had he not had the opportunity to rethink his life as a result of his diagnosis, he would have ended up in prison or dead.

Despite being happy in his work life, Kevin expressed a desire to have a committed relationship and to one day become a father. Kevin felt that due to his HIV diagnosis that neither were possible. To help Kevin explore these issues further, he was referred for clinical psychology.

Two years after his hospital admission and support from the specialist nurse and clinical psychologist, Kevin was delighted to announce that he and his partner were expecting their first child.

Jane's story continued …

Jane mentioned that she had always wanted to become a nurse and was at the start of her nurse training when she became unwell. Jane felt devastated and worried that because of her diagnosis she would not be able to complete her nursing course.

As Jane became physically better, she decided that she was going to use her desire to become a nurse to help with her recovery and decided to set this as a goal. Jane wanted to restart her nurse training within one year of diagnosis.

Jane responded well to treatment and her immune system recovered well. Jane was still very anxious about her HIV diagnosis and the stigma that she had received prior to being transferred to the specialist unit. Jane engaged in a series of sessions with the HIV clinical psychologist and specialist nurse with regards to the issues that she was experiencing. This was mainly around her desire to become pregnant and end the current relationship that she was in. Jane felt a sense of conflict and was concerned that she would never have the future she had hoped for.

One year after diagnosis, Jane recommenced her studies at the university. At first, she found this challenging. She managed to complete her course and graduated with a first-class honours degree. After Jane had qualified as a nurse, she felt a strong passion and motivation to 'give something back'. For Jane, this meant that she was going to use her training and qualifications to work with people living with HIV to improve standards of care. Over a period of time, Jane became a very passionate HIV activist and would attend clinic appointments with stories about her work – always protecting confidentiality when she did so.

Four years after her initial diagnosis, Jane attended clinic and she informed the team that she was pregnant. She had finally managed to leave her old partner and fell in love with a man whom she had met via a friend.

Reflection box 11: healing suffering

What is different about these sections of Kevin's and Jane's stories?
What has shifted for Kevin and Jane, and how might you make sense of this?

Whilst the negative psychological impact related to HIV positive status is well documented, there is growing empirical evidence to substantiate the profound and positive change that people living with HIV can experience following their diagnosis. This has come to be known as post-traumatic growth, or experiences of benefit-finding (Tennen & Affleck, 1998), or thriving (O'Leary & Ickovics, 1994). Such experiences appear to occur amongst people who share the common factor of a struggle with adversity following a traumatic experience. Subsequently, the individual is propelled 'to a higher level of functioning than which existed prior to the event' (Linley & Joseph, 2004, p. 11). A systematic review of qualitative research (Amos, 2015) explored the experiences of post-traumatic growth among 203 people living with HIV across eight research studies. It supported what has been identified as being the central domains in which positive transformations in beliefs and behaviour are manifested when experiencing post-traumatic growth, including: (i) improved relations with others; (ii) identification of new possibilities for one's life; (iii) increased perception of personal strength; (iv) spiritual growth; and (v) enhanced appreciation of life (Tedeschi & Calhoun, 1996).

Kevin's and Jane's stories highlight the complexities involved in receiving an HIV diagnosis and the positive outcomes that can occur. A re-evaluation of life goals and a motivation to live in accordance with what was deemed most meaningful to Kevin propelled him towards living a value-guided life. Jane's story illuminated how she managed to stay focused on her goals as a way of adjusting to her HIV diagnosis. She appeared to recognise her potential for acquiring knowledge and caring for others, and this was realised in her decision to train to be a nurse.

Reflection box 12: promoting growth

Think about a time you have had a challenging experience.
Were there any positives that came from what was a difficult situation?
Within your professional role, how could you support Kevin and Jane?
What are the implications for practice considering Kevin's and Jane's stories?

With the recognition of both traumatic stress and traumatic growth responses to HIV diagnosis, the attempt to untangle the relationship between these two concepts has become a focus (Bluvstein, Moravchick, Sheps, Schreiber, & Bloch, 2013; Schuettler & Boals, 2011). Practitioners working in HIV services may benefit from increased awareness of the potential for post-traumatic growth to occur among the individuals they work with. Furthermore, the facilitation of growth may be considered as a clinical intervention different from interventions designed to alleviate distress. Healthcare professionals may wish to consider how they can support people living with HIV to 'find their own vehicles of change' (Woodward & Joseph, 2003, p. 281). A strengths-based approach that recognises and emphasises people's personal strengths and capabilities, rather than their limitations, is advocated. In addition, acknowledging an individual's resilience, where appropriate, and drawing attention to how that person has survived and surpassed difficulties in their life can help to instil hope. The participants in Woodward and Joseph's study reported 'experiences of an awakening, validating, nurturing, liberating and mastery nature' (p. 275) were important in bringing about positive change. Healthcare professionals may like to reflect on how such experiences may be facilitated. In the final section, the framework of care, in which all that has been discussed so far occurs, is explored.

An inter-professional approach: working together towards meaningful change

Early access to treatment reduces susceptibility to opportunistic infection associated with AIDS and increases life expectancy. In order to maintain this, a consistent and continuous delivery mode of health, treatment and social care that is in line with clinical treatment guidelines (British HIV Association, 2018) is required. Working in isolation does not work, whilst inter-professional working enables preventative care (BHIVA, 2018). Crowley (2013) discusses how the restructuring of the National Health Service in the UK has led to a significant decrease in third sector services available to people living with HIV, such as voluntary and community organisations and charities. In addition, the funding cuts imposed on local authorities has resulted in the removal of HIV provision in some places altogether (Dalton, 2018). This, as Dalton (2018) labels it, culminates in a 'postcode lottery' when it comes to the provision of HIV support services. Research completed by the National AIDS Trust (2016) reported that service users want to be supported by HIV specialist provision and that being part of a community was vital for psychological and physical wellbeing. The contributors to this chapter were generally of the view that continuity of care was of the utmost value to them.

Roland has experienced both the one-stop-shop service offered by his clinic when he was diagnosed in 2006 and the current fragmented offer. He comments:

> It's like moving from being chauffeur driven in a Bentley to being put behind the steering wheel of a juggernaut, never having driven one before. I feel like I am now the one having to do all the steering work, chasing up appointments and referrals, being the messenger between clinic, GP and other specialists, sometimes transmitting messages that I have no understanding of. Before I felt safe and secure in the knowledge that someone was actually in control of my care. Now, it seems that I have to be in control. But I am not qualified or competent enough to assume that control and indeed it is not the position I want to be in. Of course, I want to be fully participant in the management of my condition, but I don't want to be the one leading on it.

This seems to emphasise the importance of supported empowerment via the joining-up of healthcare services working together to create a secure framework. This makes sense given how physical and mental health are interchangeable and entwined (refer to Chapter 3). Bella reflects on how interdisciplinary working significantly benefits service users, using her local support centre as an example: *'We have an amazing working relationship with our clinic and I think that this combination works. They have the medical side and we have the holistic side and the two combined work.'* Unfortunately, this model of healthcare management has come to be an exception.

Kya's experience in primary care brought to her attention that *'the practitioner had little or no knowledge about some of the issues facing a person living long term with HIV'*. Fragmentation in HIV care can result in people feeling batted back and forth between their GP and their HIV consultant. What can result is people feeling like they have been missed – a part of a bigger system of care, however not treated as an individual with individual needs. This experience can act as a trigger for people with complex histories that include abuse and neglect (please refer to Chapter 6). For example, Neil and Jesse shared how experiences of being ignored and dismissed had significant repercussions for their mental health:

> I have recently had to go back to my old HIV medication as a result of an interaction with my antidepressants. I think that this could have been picked up before as it sent my mental health and depression into a tail-spin …
>
> (Neil)

> I was put on to Atripla, which has efavirenz in it, which is a medication that caused me a great number of horrible side effects. I had insomnia, migraines, visual and auditory hallucinations. I had anxiety attacks which went on for the best part of nine months. I had spoken to my doctor about it a couple of times but he kept saying, 'But you are doing fine; your viral load and CD4 count are doing well. Just keep at it.'
>
> (Jesse)

Jesse's extract highlights that the HCP was only focusing on the physical aspects of his care and did not consider the wider impact that these side effects were having on Jesse's life.

At its most severe, people can be left feeling entirely on their own. When Billy was asked what issues he faced with the healthcare support he received, he said:

> I don't have health care support, it doesn't exist, I just have my GP. I am my own doctor and it's ridiculous because sometimes what I have to go through, we want our own doctor, for prevention. More designed for our sort of things because the problems are still there, it's not like oh everybody take prep, HIV is gone, what about the ones who are left over, there is a lot. I got friends who lost benefit, people living in poverty and they don't understand, I didn't find help because things start to shut down, now many people have lost everything.

This quotation outlines how the lack of interdisciplinary working and specialist services can result in feeling like there is no support at all. Respectfully supporting the autonomy of people living with HIV in navigating their care decisions does not imply that they take on the role of care coordinator. As Neil reports: *'a service should be joined up more and practitioners should talk to each other, GP, mental health team etc.'*

In a population in which one in three people accessing HIV are over the age of 50 (Public Health England, 2016), cross-disciplinary collaboration provides an effective healthcare management model that can support all people living with HIV. Ageing with HIV is explored further in Chapter 10. Services working in isolation can be particularly detrimental for those people living with one or more additional conditions co-occurring with HIV (for example HIV and diabetes). Earlier in this chapter, the experience of feeling heard was highlighted as being one of the most important factors in what is considered to be good care. The consequences of not listening are starkly illuminated in Mason's account:

> I was concerned that the HIV treatments were affecting my diabetes. In 2000 I had an incident where my diabetes nearly killed me and I still didn't feel heard …

A national audit completed by Croston (2016) reported a lack of mental health support in many UK services providing HIV care. It was reported that 'There was no mental health professional member (psychologist, mental health nurse, liaison psychiatrist or social worker) in 21 (40%) teams' who participated in the study. In light of the current care context described here, it is perhaps not surprising that people living with HIV cite HIV support in the community as *'raising awareness and providing the psychological services that the hospital service can no longer provide' (Bella)*. Despite the reduction in third-sector HIV services, participation with community HIV services for people living with HIV is considered by many as very helpful to their needs.

M recalls the positive experience he had accessing community support services:

> I felt better with the group of people living with HIV because I could open up, I had more to share.

As has been reiterated throughout the chapter so far, 'one size does not fit all'. For example, whilst some may find peer support very effective, others may be less keen to engage in this mode of support provision. Once again, the importance of remaining patient-centred is restated.

Summary

Returning to the title of this chapter, how might the good, the bad and the ugly of experiences with HIV care be summarised?

Reflection box 13: what does HIV care look like today?

Having engaged with this chapter, consider the following questions:
What is it that stands out to you?
How do you think about HIV care?
If you do not work within HIV care specifically, what would you be mindful of if
you were to work with someone living with HIV?

The good (what works)

• Accessible services without restrictions
• Ways of relating – listening, seeking to understand from the perspective of the
  person living with HIV, communication of empathy
• Timely referrals that reflect the individual's needs
• Clear and thoughtful communication of diagnosis
• Supporting autonomy in treatment decision-making
• Training for healthcare staff that includes awareness of stigma, transmission routes
  and U=U
• Peer-support

The bad (what does not work)

• Working in 'silos' – resulting in poor assessment and treatment of co-morbidities
• People living with HIV finding themselves in the role of coordinating care

The ugly (what is unacceptable)

• Stigmatising and discriminatory practice – use of stigmatising language, non-
  adherence to best practice guidelines
• Withdrawal from treatment

The lasting impact of a good interaction with health services is clear from Noelly's
reflections on her experiences in maternity care, Jesse's experience in his HIV clinic and
Kya's experience in an appointment with a psychiatrist:

> The midwife was just … I still remember her to this day … she was just incred-
> ible … she was … she was reassuring. I think for me she made my pregnancy jour-
> ney much more bearable and much more pleasant than it could have been otherwise
> if I had not had her as a midwife.
>
> (Noelly)

> Once I was stable and on the medication and happy, they were happy for me to be
> seen by the nurses twice a year. It's more relaxed, more chatty, more friendly and it
> has just made the whole experience a lot quicker and friendly and less like I was

dealing with a serious condition, more that it was a regular friendly health check and I think that has made the whole thing a lot less onerous; a lot more easy to manage.

(Jesse)

The staff member I saw was like a light at the end of a tunnel that I never thought I would exit. After so many years of struggling, she was the first to confirm I was not imagining things and actually confirmed that the way I was feeling. She was very caring and put things into place before letting me go home. She liaised with my HIV consultant and my GP and suggested a treatment regime. What made it helpful was she understood how I was feeling and she did not talk much but she listened to me.

(Kya)

The quality of the relationship with professionals is what stands out as being particularly important to people living with HIV accessing healthcare. At present, when someone is diagnosed with HIV, this means they will be involved with HIV care services for life. This means in your role as someone (potentially) supporting someone living with HIV, in whatever capacity, you contribute vitally to that experience. In the following chapters, some of the issues raised here will be explored in more depth. You are invited to take the voices of the people presented in this chapter with you as you venture further into this book and consider in more detail how your practice can promote the health and wellbeing of people living with HIV.

Helpful resources

- British HIV Association (2018). Standards of care for people living with HIV in London, Retrieved from www.bhiva.org/file/KrfaFqLZRlBhg/BHIVA-Standards-of-Care-2018.pdf
- British HIV Association and Medfash (2011). Standards for psychological support for adults living with HIV, Retrieved from www.bhiva.org/file/BbShtfyMFNKCz/Standards_for_psychological_support_for_adults_living_with_HIV.pdf
- Changing Perceptions: Talking about HIV and attitudes. National AIDS trust accessed at www.nat.org.uk/publication/changing-perceptions-talking-about-hiv-and-attitudes march 2020.
- Kall (2018). *Met and unmet health, welfare and social needs of people accessing HIV services: Findings from the Positive Voices 2017 Survey.* Public Health England. Retrieved from http://regist2.virology-education.com/presentations/2018/3healthyliving/06_kall.pdf
- Poindexter, C. C. (2002). Research as poetry: A couple experiences HIV. *Qualitative Inquiry, 8*(6), 707–714.
- Terrence Higgins Trust (2017a). *Uncharted Territory: A Report Into the First Generation Growing Older with HIV.* tinyurl.com/jajnv4d
- Shaw, L. et al. (2015). *Living Confidently with HIV: A self-help book for people living with HIV.* Oxford: Oxford Development Centre.
- Chesters, R. (2018). *Ripples from the Edge of Life.* London: Silverwood Books.

References

Amos, I. (2019). "That's what they talk about when they talk about epiphanies": An invitation to engage with the process of developing found poetry to illuminate exceptional human experience. *Counselling and Psychotherapy Research*, *19*(1), 16–24.

Amos, I. A. (2015). What is known about the post-traumatic growth experiences among people diagnosed with HIV/AIDS? A systematic review and thematic synthesis of the qualitative literature. *Counselling Psychology Review*, *30*(3), 47–56.

Bluvstein, I., Moravchick, L., Sheps, D., Schreiber, S., & Bloch, M. (2013). Posttraumatic growth, posttraumatic stress symptoms and mental health among coronary heart disease survivors. *Journal of Clinical Psychology in Medical Settings*, *20*(2), 164–172.

Boucher, L. M., O'Brien, K. K., Baxter, L. N., Fitzgerald, M. L., Liddy, C. E., & Kendall, C. E. (2019). Healthy aging with HIV: The role of self-management support. *Patient Education and Counseling*, *102*(8), 1565–1569.

British HIV Association. (2018). Standards of care for people living with HIV in London. Retrieved from www.bhiva.org/standards-of-care-2013.aspx/.

Buber, M. (1988). *The knowledge of man*. New Jersey: Humanities Press International.

Buckman, R., Tulsky, J. A., & Rodin, G. (2011). Empathic responses in clinical practice: Intuition or tuition? *Canadian Medical Association Journal*, *183*(5), 569–571.

Byrne, R., Curtis, H., Sullivan, A., Freedman, A., Chadwick, D., & Burns, F. (2018) *A national audit of late diagnosis of HIV: Action taken to review previous healthcare among individuals with advanced HIV*. On behalf of the BHIVA Audit and Standards Sub-committee.

Chadwick, D. R., & Freedman, A. (2019). Treating late HIV diagnosis as a patient safety issue in the UK. *The Lancet HIV*, *6*(6), 346–348.

Conners, E. E., Hagedorn, H. J., Butler, J. N., Felmet, K., Hoang, T., Wilson, P., Klima, G., Sudzina, E., & Anaya, H. D. (2012). Evaluating the implementation of nurse-initiated HIV rapid testing in three Veterans Health Administration substance use disorder clinics. *The International Journal of STD & AIDS*, *23*(11), 799–805.

Crocker, J., Major, B., & Steele, C. M. (1998). Social stigma. In D. Gilbert, S. Fiske, & G. Lindzey (Eds.), *The handbook of social psychology* (Vol. 2, pp. 504–553). Boston: McGraw Hill.

Croston, M. (2016). A national nurse-led audit of the standards for psychological support for adults living with HIV. *HIV Medicine*, *17*, 3–5.

Crowley, N. (2013). Lost in austerity: Rethinking the community sector. *Community Development Journal*, *48*(1), 151–157.

Dalton, D. (2018). Cutting the ribbon? Austerity measures and the problems faced by the HIV third sector. In P. Rushton & C. Donovan (Eds.), *Austerity policies* (pp. 7–10). Cham: Palgrave Macmillan.

Donovan, C., & Durey, M. (2018). "Well that would be nice, but we can't do that in the current climate": Prioritising services under austerity. In P. Rushton & C. Donovan (Eds.), *Austerity policies* (pp. 197–220). Cham: Palgrave Macmillan.

Dovidio, J. F., Major, B., & Crocker, J. (2000). Stigma: Introduction and overview. In T. F. Heatherton, R. E. Kleck, M. R. Hebl, et al. (Eds.), *The social psychology of stigma* (pp. 1–30). New York: Guilford Press.

Earnshaw, V. A., & Chaudoir, S. R. (2009). From conceptualizing to measuring HIV stigma: A review of HIV stigma mechanism measures. *AIDS and Behavior*, *13*(6), 1160.

Elford, J., Ibrahim, F., Bukutu, C., & Anderson, J. (2008). HIV-related discrimination reported by people living with HIV in London, UK. *AIDS Behaviour*, *12*(2), 255–264.

Equality Act 2010. (2010). Retrieved from www.legislation.gov.uk/ukpga/2010/15/contents (accessed 15 August 2019).

Evans, C., Nalubega, S., McLuskey, J., Darlington, N., Croston, M., & Bath-Hextall, F. (2015). The views and experiences of nurses and midwives in the provision and management of provider-initiated HIV testing and counseling: A systematic review of qualitative evidence. *JBI Database of Systematic Reviews and Implementation Reports*, *13*(12), 130–286.

Flickinger, T. E., Saha, S., Roter, D., Korthuis, P. T., Sharp, V., Cohn, J., … Beach, M. C. (2016). Clinician empathy is associated with differences in patient–clinician communication behaviors and higher medication self-efficacy in HIV care. *Patient Education and Counseling*, *99*(2), 220–226.

Flowers, P., Davis, M. M., Larkin, M., Church, S., & Marriott, C. (2011). Understanding the impact of HIV diagnosis amongst gay men in Scotland: An interpretative phenomenological analysis. *Psychology & Health*, *26*(10), 1378–1391.

Gabriel, P., Lee, J., & Taylor, R. (2018). Evidence-based poetry: Using poetic representation of phenomenological research to create an educational tool for enhancing empathy in medical trainees in the management of depression. *Journal of Poetry Therapy*, *31*(2), 75–86.

Goffman, E. (1963). *Stigma: Notes on the management of spoiled identity.* Englewood Cliffs, NJ: Prentice-Hall.

Hardavella, G., Aamli-Gaagnat, A., Frille, A., Saad, N., Niculescu, A., & Powell, P. (2017). Top tips to deal with challenging situations: Doctor–patient interactions. *Breathe*, *13*(2), 129–135.

Hatzenbuehler, M. L., & Link, B. G. (2014). Introduction to the special issue on structural stigma and health. *Social Science & Medicine*, *103*, 1–6.

Hatzenbuehler, M. L., Phelan, J. C., & Link, B. G. (2013). Stigma as a fundamental cause of population health inequalities. *American Journal of Public Health*, *103*(5), 813–821.

Hefferon, K., Grealy, M., & Mutrie, N. (2009). Posttraumatic growth and life threatening physical illness: A systematic review of the qualitative literature. *British Journal of Health Psychology*, *14*(2), 343–378.

HIV Positive voices survey. (2017). Department of Health accessed via https://assets.publishing.ser vice.gov.uk/government/uploads/system/uploads/attachment_data/file/857922/PHE_positive_voi ces_report_2019.pdf march 2020.

Horwood, C., Voce, A., Vermaak, K., Rollins, N., & Qazi, S. (2010). Routine checks for HIV in children attending primary health care facilities in South Africa: Attitudes of nurses and child caregivers. *Social Science & Medicine*, *70*(2), 313–320.

Hult, J. R., Maurer, S. A., & Moskowitz, J. T. (2009). "I'm sorry, you're positive": A qualitative study of individual experiences of testing positive for HIV. *AIDS Care*, *21*(2), 185–188.

Janoff-Bulman, R. (1992). *Shattered assumptions: Towards a new psychology of trauma.* New York: Free Press.

Jutel, A. (2009). Sociology of diagnosis: A preliminary review. *Sociology of Health and Illness*, *31*, 278–299.

Lala, R., Harwood, C., Simon, S. E., Lee, A., & Jones, K. (2018). Blood borne viruses-key facts for primary care dental teams. *BDJ Team*, *5*(5), 18075.

Leahy, B. (2018). Language used to convey HIV infection risk is important. *Lancet HIV*, *5*, 272.

LeGrand, S., Reif, S., Sullivan, K., Murray, K., Barlow, M. L., & Whetton, K. (2015). A review of recent literature on trauma among individuals living with HIV. *Current HIV/AIDS Reports*, *12*, 397–405. doi:10.1007/s11904-015-0288-2

Levett, T., Slide, C., Mallick, F., & Lau, R. (2009). Access to dental care for HIV patients: Does it matter and does discrimination exist? *The International Journal of STD & AIDS*, *20*(11), 782–784. doi:10.1258/ijsa.2009.009182

Link, B. G., & Phelan, J. C. (2001). Conceptualizing stigma. *Annual Review of Sociology*, *27*, 363–385.

Linley, P. A., & Joseph, S. (2004). Positive change following trauma and adversity: A review. *Journal of Traumatic Stress*, *17*(1), 11–21.

May, M., Gompels, M., Delpech, V., Porter, K., Post, F., Johnson, M., … Hill, T. (2011). Impact of late diagnosis and treatment on life expectancy in people with HIV-1: UK Collaborative HIV Cohort (UK CHIC) Study. *The BMJ*, *343*, d6016.

Mitchell, L., Bushby, S. A., & Chauhan, M. (2011). An audit highlighting a lack of awareness of the UK national guidelines for HIV testing, 2008. *The International Journal of STD & AIDS*, *22*, 753–754.

NAT. (2016) *The importance of HIV support services: Report from the survey of HIV support service providers*. Unpublished. National AIDS Trust.

Naylor, C., Das, P., Ross, S., Honeyman, M., Thompson, J., & Gilburt, H. (2016). *Bringing together physical and mental health: A new frontier for integrated care*. London: The Kings Fund.

Okala, S., Doughty, J., Watt, R. G., Santella, A. J., Conway, D. I., Crenna-Jennings, W., ... Benton, L. (2018). The people living with HIV STIGMA survey UK 2015: Stigmatising experiences and dental care. *British Dental Journal, 225*, 143–150.

O'Leary, V. E., & Ickovics, J. R. (1994). Resilience and thriving in response to challenge: An opportunity for a paradigm shift in women's health. *Women's Health: Research on Gender, Behavior, and Policy, 1*, 121–142.

Pakenham, K., & Rinaldis, M. (2002). Development of the HIV/AIDS stress scale. *Psychology and Health, 17*(2), 203–219.

Pantelic, M., Steinert, J. I., Park, J., Mellors, S., & Murau, F. (2019). 'Management of a spoiled identity': Systematic review of interventions to address self-stigma among people living with and affected by HIV. *BMJ Global Health, 4*(2).

Pence, B. W., Mugavero, M. J., Carter, T. J., Leserman, J., Thielman, N. M., Raper, J. L., & Whetten, K. (2012). Childhood trauma and health outcomes in HIV-infected patients: An exploration of causal pathways. *Journal of Acquired Immunodeficiency Syndromes, 59*, 409–416.

Public Health England (PHE). (2016) Retrieved from www.gov.uk/government/uploads/system/uploads/attachment_data/file/602942/HIV_in_the_UK_report.pdf (accessed 16 August 2019).

Rayment, M., Asboe, D., & Sullivan, A. K. (2014). HIV testing and management of newly diagnosed HIV. *The BMJ, 349*, 27–32.

Richardson, J., Barkan, S., Cohen, M., Back, S., FitzGerald, G., Feldman, J., & Palacio, H. (2001). Experience and covariates of depressive symptoms among a cohort of HIV infected women. *Social Work in Health Care, 32*(4), 93–111.

Rogers, C. R. (1975). Empathic—An unappreciated way of being. *The Counseling Psychologist, 5*, 2–10.

Sanders, L. B. (2008). Women's voices: The lived experience of pregnancy and motherhood after diagnosis with HIV. *Journal of the Association of Nurses in AIDS Care, 19*(1), 47–57.

Schrooten, W., Dreezen, C., Fleerackers, Y., Andraghetti, R., Finazzi, R., Caldeira, L., & Eurosupport Group. (2001). Receiving a positive HIV test result: The experience of patients in Europe. *HIV Medicine, 2*(4), 250–254.

Schuettler, D., & Boals, A. (2011). The path to posttraumatic growth versus posttraumatic stress disorder: Contributions of event centrality and coping. *Journal of Loss and Trauma, 16*(2), 180–194.

Tedeschi, R. G., & Calhoun, L. G. (1996). The posttraumatic growth inventory: Measuring the positive legacy of trauma. *Journal of Traumatic Stress, 9*(3), 455–471.

Tennen, H., & Affleck, G. (1998). Personality and transformation in the face of adversity. In R. G. Tedeschi, C. L. Park, & L. G. Calhoun (Eds.), *Posttraumatic growth: Positive changes in the aftermath of crisis* (pp. 155–165). Hillside, NJ: Lawrence Erlbaum.

UNAIDS. (2003). UNAIDS fact sheet on stigma and discrimination. Retrieved from http://data.unaids.org/publications/Fact-Sheets03/fs_stigma_discrimination_en.pdf.

Varni, S. E., Miller, C. T., McCuin, T., & Solomon, S. E. (2012). Disengagement and engagement coping with HIV/AIDS stigma and psychological wellbeing of people with HIV/AIDS. *Journal of Social and Clinical Psychology, 31*(2), 123–150.

Walker, L. (2019). 'There's no pill to help you deal with the guilt and shame': Contemporary experiences of HIV in the United Kingdom. *Health, 23*(1), 97–113.

Watson, S., Namiba, A., & Lynn, V. (2019). NHIVNA best practice: The language of HIV: A guide for nurses. *HIV Nursing, 19*(2), BP1–BP4.

Woodward, C., & Joseph, S. (2003). Positive change processes and post-traumatic growth in people who have experienced childhood abuse: Understanding vehicles of change. *Psychology and Psychotherapy: Theory, Research and Practice, 76*(3), 267–283.

2 Self-awareness in HIV care

Caroline Ridley

Chapter description

This chapter will raise awareness of the concept of practitioner self-awareness and its importance when caring for people living with HIV. Having read the chapter, the reader will be able to: discuss the concept of self-awareness and its links to therapeutic communication, analyse the importance of self-awareness when developing relationships with people living with HIV, and discuss ways to develop self-awareness.

Introduction

Relationships are central to the delivery of safe and effective care and may be described as 'the way in which two or more people are connected and regard each other' (Oxford English Dictionaries 2017). Within healthcare, the nature of the relationships professionals have with patients is constantly evolving. The paternalistic approach, in which the professional dominates the agenda, sets goals and makes decisions and in which the patient's voice remains quiet, is arguably out of step with the demands and expectations of a modern society. The white paper *Equity and Excellence: Liberating the NHS* (DH 2011) sets out the government's vision of an NHS where patients and the public come first and where 'no decision about me without me' is the norm. Advances in healthcare also mean more choice about how and where care is delivered and have triggered the emergence of the consumerist model in which individuals are empowered to be active participants in decision-making. Just as the paternalistic model can be criticised for excluding the patient's perspective, the consumerist model can limit the care professional's participation in decision-making without appreciating the benefits of their expertise – and this too may be unproductive. The optimal model appears to be one of mutuality or collaboration that is grounded in mutual respect and trust between healthcare professionals and patients. Each party brings vital expertise to the relationship; the healthcare professional is the 'medical' expert and the patient is the 'personal' expert and each can support the other to develop a shared body of knowledge that becomes the foundation for a mutually agreeable plan of care and treatment (Greenfield 2001). This relationship might be regarded as what Spichiger et al. (2005) call 'relational care' – one that involves connection, interdependence and collaboration (Dupuis et al. 2016). In these relationships sit those buzzwords of partnership, empowerment, engagement, responsiveness, participation and respect.

Whilst respect as a concept can be hard to distinguish from other concepts, including liking or accepting someone, in healthcare literature it seems to relate to acknowledging the patient as a unique individual with valid concerns, ideas and rights. Respect within therapeutic relationships brings mutual benefits; care professionals demonstrate more positive communication behaviours and patients in return are more likely to share psychosocial information that can assist in care planning (Flickinger et al. 2016). In relation to HIV, Beach et al. (2006) found associations between antiretroviral therapy (ART) adherence and feeling known as a person by their clinician. Where there is mutual respect, other studies have also shown more positive outcomes and greater overall satisfaction with care and health-related quality of life (Beach et al. 2005; Arbuthnott and Sharpe 2009; Oetzel et al. 2015).

Activity

Identify someone you feel shows you respect. What do they say or do that makes you feel respected? How does their respect for you influence your behaviour towards them?

A mutually respectful relationship envisages professionals and patients will support and value each other and work together to understand what is important to the individual in relation to decision-making about care and treatment. This approach to care demands a level of self-awareness on the part of the professional because 'only by understanding how we are seen can we make sure we're sending the right signals' (Gosling 2009, p. 1). Developing or enhancing our self-awareness serves to raise self-esteem, promote efficiency in our practice and promote our personal health and wellbeing (Freshwater 2002), and is the best possible start to understanding others (Rungapadiachy 1999).

Self-awareness

Self-awareness has been defined as a conscious process in which we consider our 'understanding of ourselves' (Rawlinson 1990). Knowing ourselves as professionals in a mutual relationship with people in our care helps ensure those particular facets of our person and personality enhance rather than detract from a therapeutic relationship (Luft 1969). Rungapadiachy (2008) refers to self-awareness as a state of 'general self-knowledge' and Williams (2003) suggests that self-awareness can also be a momentary state of self-consciousness. A few individuals might be described as naturally self-aware (Fletcher and Baldry 2000), and Church (1997) argues that self-awareness can be conceptualised both as a personality trait and an acquired skill, leading us to believe we can all improve our ability in this regard if we want to. Rasheed (2015, p. 12) reminds us, however, that 'knowing about oneself is not an easy task; it is a painful and time-consuming process requiring continuous effort'. Becoming self-aware has no 'saturation point' (Rungapadiachy 1999). It means understanding our own position on life, our beliefs, values, conscious and unconscious biases, prejudices, needs and wants. As care professionals we should be constantly striving to be more cognisant of those aspects of ourselves that impact on our therapeutic relationships with others and identifying personal factors and emotions, and separating them from the patient's presenting problem enables care professionals to meet those needs more effectively (Forrest 2012).

Rungapadiachy (1999) proposes three layers of self-awareness:

1. Superficial – for example, our age and gender.
2. Selective – those things we feel we need to be aware of such as how we dress, our expressed attitudes, our accent and style of language we choose to use.
3. Deeper awareness – those issues known only to ourselves. Our 'private self' – those aspects of ourselves we choose to hide from others.

So why is it important to understand ourselves in this way? What are the benefits and are there any drawbacks associated with self-awareness? Regarding the latter, Duval and Wicklund (1972) suggest that dwelling on ourselves as objects can lead to feelings of negativity as we realise how far short we fall from our ideals, and Williams (2003) highlights how in a therapeutic relationship, self-awareness can lead to more of a focus on oneself and less on the patient. Neither does being self-aware guarantee improvements in care, but the general position seems to be that it is only when we know ourselves that we can begin to know others. The Roman philosopher Seneca said that whilst 'other men's sins are before our eyes, our own are behind our backs'. The process of self-awareness enables nurses to examine their own value positions so these biases and prejudices are not projected onto others who do not share similar values. For example, a nurse may be angry at what they believe to be immoral behaviour, and these beliefs may reveal themselves in hostile language or disinterested behaviour with a service user. This can lead to the service user feeling anxious and questioning their own behaviour. They may stop talking, which in turn can lead to their most important healthcare needs not being met.

Self

Knowing ourselves begins with a self-concept – a belief about ourselves based on a set of unique characteristics (Baumeister 1999). Rogers (1959) presents self-concept as having three different components:

- **Self-image** – the view we have of ourselves. Self-image is developed over time and can be shaped by external forces such as the media, peers and family influences. Gosling (2009) reminds us of our personal bias towards thinking we are decent and competent, and therefore self-image may not always reflect reality.
- **Self-esteem** – a subjective and mobile phenomenon; how much value we have of ourselves; the extent to which we like, accept or approve of ourselves. Our evaluation of self may be positive or negative (or perhaps a mix of both?).
- **Ideal self** – what we wish we were really like and a likely motivator for individuals to change, improve and achieve. A mismatch between our self-image and our ideal self can influence self-esteem and feelings of self-worth, yet Adler (1963) reminds us that we are both the artist and the picture and can recreate ourselves over time.

Activity

Take a few moments to reflect on your own concept of self. What aspects of your ideal self mirror those of your self-image? How can you 'close the gap'?

Self-awareness and caring for people with HIV

Caring for those affected by HIV demands an honest, sensitive and empathic approach, which has been explored in the previous chapter. Professionals are charged with responsibilities associated with battling stigma, discrimination and negative stereotyping, telling others about their HIV diagnosis and contact tracing, issues around sexuality, sexual risk-taking behaviour, harm reduction and the onward transmission of HIV. Meeting these responsibilities means knowing a patient intimately, and professionals may naturally worry about saying the 'right or wrong thing', saying too much or too little, or unleashing emotional responses they feel unprepared to handle. Jung (1963, p. 33) declared that the professional must 'keep watch over himself … over the way he is reacting to his patients', but it is not always easy to predict what patients will want to talk about. Working closely with people who are experiencing challenging circumstances in their lives will often evoke an emotional response (see Chapter 5). The term 'emotional labour' has been described as involving the generation or suppression of feelings that support others to feel cared for in a safe place (Hochschild 1983). Emotional labour can often encompass conflicting emotional responses. Ellis and Bochner (1999, p. 7) argue we should be willing to be 'uncomfortable and vulnerable', but is this too much to ask, especially of novice practitioners? Is exposing vulnerability necessarily a way of improving outcomes for patients? At its most skilled, emotional labour includes managing negative feelings in a way that results in a neutral or positive outcome (James 1993), yet the complexities of adopting a person-centred approach to caring for people with HIV means the emotional labour can be intense. Distancing oneself physically and emotionally from the patient is perhaps understandable. Emotional distancing, however, has been shown to have a negative effect on care provision, with an increased likelihood that social- and health-related problems might be neglected (Michaelsen 2012). If we do not know our own self, we are more likely to feel vulnerable when patients express themselves (Jourard 1971). So by developing skills of self-awareness, professionals may be able to respond in a more appropriate way, thus helping the patient at the same time as protecting themselves from feelings of discomfort or embarrassment.

Case study

A service user who has tested positive for HIV becomes very distressed and tells you his life is not worth living. He knows he will have to tell his wife of 15 years, but suspects he acquired HIV from a man he has sex with regularly outside of the marriage. His wife does not know about this relationship.

A clinician who is self-aware will understand how their personal attitudes and beliefs affect their behaviour. Potential feelings of shock, anger, blame, disgust or perhaps complacency and even approval may compromise the consultation. Being self-aware can enable the clinician to successfully discriminate between what feelings are theirs and what belong to the service user. Being self-aware can make the clinician feel capable of managing a therapeutic relationship. The clinician's raised consciousness means the service user will be supported to problem-solve and take action based on objective and personalised support. Advice given will be well considered rather than spontaneous and potentially unhelpful. It will be about the service user and not about the clinician.

Rungapadiachy (1999) suggests there are three dimensions to self-awareness that are active in Rogers' (1959) concept of self discussed earlier. These are: cognitive (the thinking aspect of the individual); affective (the feeling aspect of the individual); and behavioural (the actions of the individual, both verbal and non-verbal). Each dimension relates to the other, and is explored within the next chapter, but unless people make a conscious effort to recognise their inner thoughts and feelings, they may remain unknown to them.

If we are more aware of our thoughts and feelings, we can monitor them and use them to guide our actions in positive and affirming ways (Croston 2016).

Reflection box

How often do you consider your own thoughts, feelings and behaviours? Do you ever think that your thoughts or feelings control your actions in positive or negative ways?

Have there been times when you have said or done things that you regret? What feelings or thoughts were directing these actions at that time?

Imagine for example an individual caring for a gay male who has acquired HIV through unprotected intercourse with his HIV-positive partner. One potential approach to this individual's situation is described in Figure 2.1.

Healthcare professionals who consider the medical, social, organisational and personal factors related to an individual with HIV can improve their understanding of the complexity of the patient's circumstances (see Chapter 3). Perhaps this individual did not know his partner was HIV positive. Perhaps this individual was a victim of coercive power and control within an intimate relationship. Perhaps this individual chooses to engage in risk-taking behaviours for reasons known only to himself (see Chapter 7). Perhaps this individual is

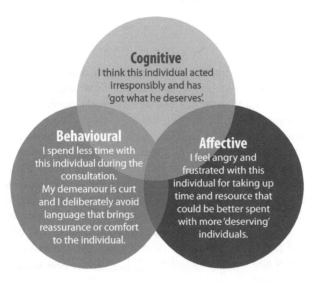

Figure 2.1 An example of a cognitive, affective behavioural cycle

ignorant of the risks associated with unprotected sex. If the clinician thinking, feeling and behaving in the ways outlined in Figure 2.1 failed to consider these potential influences and factors, how is care compromised and is this an appropriate way to manage this individual?

Activity

Reflect on a patient you have cared for who is living with HIV or any other long-term condition and consider the following:

- an occasion when your thoughts about something related to this individual influenced your feelings or behaviour
- an occasion when your behaviour towards this individual influenced your feelings or thoughts
- an occasion when your feelings towards this individual influenced your behaviour or thoughts.

What was the impact of these interrelated thoughts, feelings or behaviour on care for that individual? Can you think of any additional factors that might have impacted on that individual at the time you were caring for them? How do you feel now having completed this activity?

Developing self-awareness

'The curious paradox is that when I accept myself just as I am, then I can change.' Many care professionals would benefit from self-awareness development. One tool professionals can use is the Johari window, a model developed in the 1950s by American psychologists Joseph Luft and Harry Ingham (Luft and Ingham 1961). This model encourages individuals to explore aspects of themselves including feelings, experiences, attitudes, skills, motivating factors, intentions and thoughts in relation to others from four perspectives: **open** (what is known by the person about him/herself and is also known by others); **blind** (what is unknown by the person about him/herself but which others know); **hidden** (what the person knows about him/herself that others do not know); and **unknown** (what is unknown by the person about him/herself and is also unknown by others). Like a window pane, the four quadrants are initially represented as equal in size but can change as people develop self-awareness and learn more about themselves (see Table 2.1). Becoming more self-aware facilitates growth of the open and hidden areas and diminution of the blind and unknown areas.

Activity

Draw your own Johari window and make notes in each section in relation to self.

OPEN – this can include your likes or dislikes, feelings and behaviours you willingly share with others.

BLIND – This is hard to complete because this is what others know about you that you don't know yourself, but we can learn more about ourselves by seeking multiple perspectives. It requires you to ask people to share those feelings and thoughts with you. You might be able to imagine how others see you by reflecting on ways people behave towards you in certain situations. For example, do people take advantage of you because they see you as a 'soft touch' or 'passive'? Do you notice in a group of friends that you always get what you want, perhaps because you come across as bossy or intractable?

HIDDEN – This area exists because others know how you behave, but they don't always know your intentions or feelings. What do you know about yourself that you choose to keep private? Why? For example, are you afraid people will stop liking you if you tell them your personal beliefs? Is this an aspect of self you can develop or change to allow you to be more 'yourself' in some relationships with others? Would this make you feel happier or more relaxed?

UNKNOWN – This is the most challenging area to consider as it relates to those areas of self unknown to anyone, including you. Perhaps you can consider how satisfied you are with life and begin to consider why you feel as you do. Is there something you have always wanted to do but have not had the courage to try? Maybe you have hidden talents or skills as yet unearthed.

Table 2.1 Johari window (draws on Luft 1969)

	Known to self	*Not known to self*
Known to others	**OPEN AREA** What you show to others. Public knowledge. This area can grow as the other areas become smaller.	**BLIND AREA** What you don't know about yourself that others know; your 'blind spots'. Feedback from others can help reduce this area.
Not known to others	**HIDDEN AREA** Your sensitivities, fears, hidden agendas, manipulative intentions, secrets. The private zone. The information you can choose or not to share. Hidden information and feelings can be revealed and move into the open area through self-disclosure. Trust is important within relationships to facilitate this process.	**UNKNOWN AREA** Your unconscious area. May also include repressed feelings related to traumatic events or abilities, aptitudes or talents never unearthed or tested. Self- or mutual discovery can serve to decrease this area.

Once you have a better understanding of yourself in a personal context, you might like to repeat the exercise in a professional context thinking about you in relation to your patients. For example, how do patients seem to behave when in a consultation with you? Are they relaxed? Do they confide in you? Are they different with other staff? Reflecting in this way might help you see more clearly any 'blind spots' in relation to your professional self. It might equally affirm your positive sense of self and motivate you to continue in the ways you are working.

Interdisciplinary and team self-awareness

In practice we cannot meet the holistic needs of the individual with HIV alone. We work in multi-professional teams and recognise that attitudes towards patients will vary. Not all care professionals' attitudes are positive (Walusimbi and Okansky 2004; Pickles et al. 2011; Ozakgul et al. 2014), yet we are expected to work cooperatively, share our skills and knowledge and respect those of others. We need to recognise when to ask for advice or support, as working to the boundaries of our own roles keeps people safe. We need to be able to communicate effectively and efficiently. One dimension of a team is the degree to which members have shared knowledge, experiences, norms and values and are aware of their commonalities (Wilson and Pirrie 2000). The Johari window can be used as a tool for developing self-awareness within your team. The aim is to develop the 'open area' for every person because, when we work in this area with others, we are at our most effective and productive and the team is at its most productive too. The open space facilitates good communication and cooperation, as well as freedom from distractions, mistrust, confusion, conflict and misunderstanding (Chapman 2003). Established teams have the advantage; the open area may be large. People know each other well. A feeling of safety and 'comfortableness' facilitates disclosure, and feedback from colleagues may have helped reduce the size of the hidden and blind areas. Perhaps through mutual discovery of the team's talents the unknown area has also reduced. For new teams the window will look different. The open and blind panes will be smaller. It takes time to get to know people and the hidden area may be large. People need to build confidence and trust, and if the person lacks self-knowledge or self-belief, the unknown areas may be the largest. Team leaders and managers can endeavour to create an environment that encourages self-discovery and self-awareness. Jack and Miller's (2008) self-development awareness tool is another way practitioners can facilitate the development of self-awareness. Their model is presented in three stages: the 'now' stage; the 'transitional' stage; and 'the re-group' stage. It invites practitioners to ask reflexive questions during each stage.

Stage 1 – the now stage:

- Who am I? (Consider your thoughts, feelings and behaviours.)
- What do I know about myself and what do I show to others? (Consider your past experiences and the impact of contextual factors, such as culture, ethnicity, religion and relationships with others.)
- What is it I would like to be more aware of? (Perhaps you want to know more about how others see you. Ask other people what they 'see' and try to solicit their opinions directly. This takes courage but is important, because if you try to guess what others think of you, you may find it impossible to disregard all the things you know about yourself to which others don't have access (the hidden window in the Johari tool).)
- What has triggered this desire to change? (This might relate to personal or professional frustrations or feelings of discomfort, irritation or unease.)

Stage 2 – the transition stage:

- What strengths/limitations do I have already? (This will require a certain amount of honesty and may be informed through feedback from others.)
- What do I need to develop? (This is a proactive stage and you may choose to seek help from others to help you. Managers, colleagues and patients can all offer valuable insight into your areas for development.)
- What are the opportunities and threats to my development? (You may have to think about previous experiences that were helpful and not so helpful. Be willing to move on from past experiences that were unhelpful or are causing conflict with your areas for development. Use positive experiences as a platform on which to grow and develop.)

Stage 3 – the regroup stage:

- Where am I now? (What new knowledge have I gained about myself and the situation? Be mindful of where this new knowledge came from.)
- What has changed about me and the way I am in the situation? (Do I think, feel, behave differently now in these situations? These different ways of being and behaving are the new 'now stage'.)
- How do we grow? Where do we go from here? (Getting an outsider's perspective through stages 1 and 2 provides us with new information. How can we use this new information to move forwards into a new way of being?)

Jack and Miller (2008)

The model as a tool for interdisciplinary working

The Jack and Miller (2008) model can be used to support effective interdisciplinary team working. An example is how this model was successfully used during the HIV team's peer supervision session. It was highlighted that the team were struggling to meet the needs of a patient who was experiencing multiple health and social care challenges. The team utilised the stages within the model to explore the current strengths and limitations of the team. They also explored how they might need to develop as a team to effectively support the patient, taking into account what support they may need to make the changes required to provide the care for the patient. As a result of undertaking the stages in the Jack and Miller (2008) model, the team were able to learn from what they had discovered in order to work more collaboratively to provide the patient with the care that they needed.

Self-awareness as a tool for caring

It seems clear that as we become more mindful of our strengths and areas for development, we are better able to appreciate our own acts and omissions in relation to care for people with HIV and take positive steps towards redressing the balance. We must then begin to extrapolate what it feels to be someone else and how it must feel to be a user of healthcare services. Rungapadiachy (2008) argues that successful engagement with others requires us to use our 'self' as agents of three key therapeutic interventions: empathic understanding, social and emotional intelligence.

Empathic understanding

Empathic understanding or empathy (Nelson-Jones 2000) is the ability to see the world from another person's view. Unlike sympathy, which is relating to another as though they were us and we were experiencing the situation (Miller and Nambiar-Greenwood 2011), empathy is relating to the other person and understanding *their* experience. It is the ability to understand an individual's private world *as if* it were your own without necessarily experiencing the feelings. It is a human to human connection that relates to Rogers' (1959) definition of humanism as a 'mode of thought in which human interest, values and dignity are taken to be of primary importance'. Building empathy requires effort that deepens one person's engagement with the experiences and suffering of another (Aronson 2014). Professionals who use more empathic communication are rewarded for that effort as they elicit more relevant information from patients (Maguire et al. 1996) and help people with HIV overcome hurdles such as stigma and discrimination (Parker and Aggleton 2003) and barriers to trust (Saha et al. 2010).

To be truly empathetic we need to know people's medical and psycho-social history, and this means focusing our attention on that individual, acknowledging and actively listening to verbal and observing non-verbal cues. The feminist psychologist Blythe Clinch refers to 'connected knowing', a process that requires us to use our imagination to get behind the other person's eyes and look at it from that person's point of view. Being empathic requires us to suspend our personal beliefs and judgements but be willing to use self-disclosure where appropriate (Moss 2012). This is not the same as being more interested in ourselves than in others, rather it is a means of sharing experiential encounters that engender shared interpretations, interests and values (Cohen 2017). For example, 'I remember when I went for health screening myself; I know how it made me feel' might enlighten a patient's anxiety about HIV testing. However, sharing is a fine balance as it can pose problems; for example, if there is too much self-disclosure or it comes too soon in the relationship, there is a risk that the patient may feel invalidated or not fully understood. However, it can help to build trust, and once one person engages in self-disclosure, it is implied that the other person will do so too. This is known as the norm of reciprocity and can help both people understand each other more. Still, it is important to remain within professional boundaries (refer to Chapter 5 for more information on this aspect of care).

Tentative, open questioning develops people's stories and reflection helps to clarify what has been said to develop a clearer understanding. These ways of building an empathic rapport require practice with friends, family members and colleagues, and becoming more empathic requires us to be self-aware. Whilst empathic understanding may be seen as an individual ability, the end result is improved rapport. Professionals are tasked with managing those interactions and relationships we have with patients, and knowing what, when, how and where to say things that support positive outcomes (Rungapadiachy 2009).

Social and emotional intelligence

Social intelligence relates to what happens as we interact and connect with each other. Professionals need to have a feel for how to behave in a consultation with their patients; they need to have a feel for what to say and do and when to say and do it; in other words, they need to 'act wisely' (Thorndike 1920) in order for their interactions to be successful. Emotional intelligence relates to our individual human capacities that help us manage emotions and build those relationships with others. On occasion we may find ourselves overwhelmed by our own emotions and feeling as if we are swimming against the tide. Sometimes we need to acknowledge the need for help and support and may even need to take a break in order to remain effective in practice. Emotions can influence how we react and respond to and treat other people, and emotional intelligence helps us recognise that challenging dimension of our work and develop and maintain the skills necessary to handle the diversity of emotions in a professional manner. In practical terms, it means being aware that emotions can influence behaviour and impact people (positively and negatively) – and learning how to manage those emotions, especially when we are under pressure, supports better outcomes for everyone involved.

Activity

Emotion can be overt or hidden. Make a list of the number of different emotions you have felt today. Write down why you felt this way and what you did about it. Is there anything else you could have done to relieve any negative emotions?

Emotional intelligence as conceptualised by Mayer and Salovey (1997) is presented as a 16-step developmental model that can be summarised within four themes (see Figure 2.2).

Utilising self-awareness

It is useful to reflect on the model in Figure 2.2. In healthcare we should all be able to recognise emotions accurately; many professionals can use emotion to guide care planning.

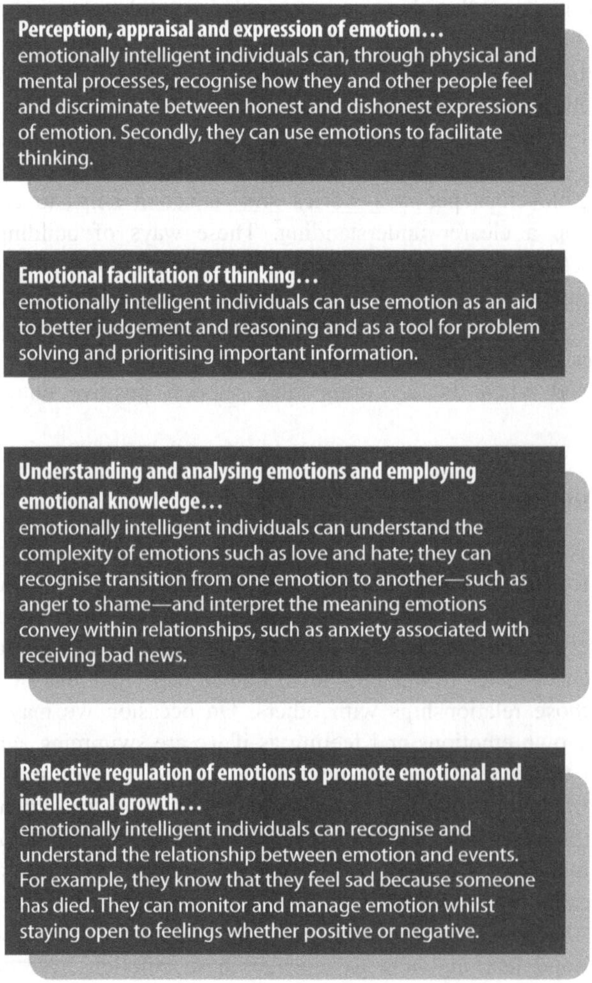

Perception, appraisal and expression of emotion…
emotionally intelligent individuals can, through physical and mental processes, recognise how they and other people feel and discriminate between honest and dishonest expressions of emotion. Secondly, they can use emotions to facilitate thinking.

Emotional facilitation of thinking…
emotionally intelligent individuals can use emotion as an aid to better judgement and reasoning and as a tool for problem solving and prioritising important information.

Understanding and analysing emotions and employing emotional knowledge…
emotionally intelligent individuals can understand the complexity of emotions such as love and hate; they can recognise transition from one emotion to another—such as anger to shame—and interpret the meaning emotions convey within relationships, such as anxiety associated with receiving bad news.

Reflective regulation of emotions to promote emotional and intellectual growth…
emotionally intelligent individuals can recognise and understand the relationship between emotion and events. For example, they know that they feel sad because someone has died. They can monitor and manage emotion whilst staying open to feelings whether positive or negative.

Figure 2.2 Emotional intelligence 16-step model categorised into four themes (adapted from Mayer and Salovey 1997)

Basic cues, such as words or phrases suggesting particular emotions, and non-verbal cues including expressions of emotion, such as sighing or frowning (Del Piccolo et al. 2006), can be picked up on. Taking the cue seriously will validate the patient's concerns and there-fore help build trust that enables the concern to be addressed. If we shrink away when emo-tions are at the fore, people are less likely to have respect for or confidence in us, whereas 'weathering the storm' builds respect and professional confidence (Thompson 2006, p. 133). In face-to-face interactions with patients, we are well placed to spot these important cues – Egan's (1998) SOLER technique is a useful tool to help (see Chapter 4).

In healthcare, the more people who are involved in a situation, the more emotionally charged things can become. There is a tendency to panic in these volatile or emotionally charged situations, but responding with fear or anger can serve to make things worse. The emotionally intelligent individual working at the highest level will be able to manage emotions properly, but for many of us still developing the skills associated with emotional intelligence, tools such as SAGE and THYME (see Table 2.2), a mnemonic that acts as an aide-memoire for a structured conversation with a person in distress or

Table 2.2 Sage and Thyme mnemonic – an aide-memoire for a structured conversation with a person in distress (adapted from the SAGE and THYME model (UHSM 2012))

S – Setting	The environment can aid or diminish dialogue. Create some privacy. Ensure people can sit down. Consider her feelings. She may be upset, shocked and angry. Is the room private and free from interruptions? Is seating conducive to therapeutic dialogue?
A – Ask	You need to let people get things off their chest. Ask them what they are concerned about. As Moss (2012) says, 'some people just need a good listening to'. Acknowledge her feelings and begin by inviting her to talk about these. Be mindful of your non-verbal messaging. Listen well.
G – Gather	Gather all of the concerns. Keep notes. Explain this helps you remember what they have said. It demonstrates you are taking this seriously. People may have many concerns, and the most important concern may be the last they tell you. As they tell you something, ask, 'Is there something else you are concerned/worried/angry/upset about?' Keep asking until all her concerns have been expressed. Keep notes and explain why; you don't want to forget anything and want to make sure everything of concern is recorded
E – Empathy	Recognise and acknowledge what they are feeling. Respond sensitively. Try to avoid losing your 'professional balance' (Moss 2012) by becoming part of their problem. Offer undivided attention. Don't trivialise her feelings. Respond to the words and the emotions behind the words. Allow quiet times and don't feel you have to have an immediate answer. Reflect back and ask clarifying questions.
and	
T – Talk	Find out about any existing support systems they have. As care staff we cannot do it all and patients will need to make use of other support mechanisms. 'Who do you have to talk to or support you?' Who can she talk to when she leaves the clinic?
H – Help	Find out how these support mechanisms/people have helped already. It is useful to know what has been effective and what you can recommend as part of an ongoing system of care and support. What has she found helpful in her past when she has been upset, angry or anxious? Signpost appropriately to services that will help her adjust to her diagnosis.
Y – You	People have knowledge about themselves, so invite them to tell you what they think would help them in that situation. Let her be a partner in care. Be empowering in your approach

(Continued)

Table 2.2 (Cont.)

M – Me	You might be able to help in ways previously unknown. Ask the person what they would like you to do. You may need to signpost to other services as the best sources of support whilst being honest about the limits of your role. You may devise a plan of action that leads to you concluding the conversation.
	Be honest about what is available and consider the skills of the wider interdisciplinary team. One person will not meet all her needs. Get practical by writing things down for her, giving other information such as contact details of services, leaflets, web addresses and so on.
E – End	Summarise and close. Ask, 'Can we leave it there?' Notice how emotions have changed.
	Acknowledge her feelings once more. Offer reassurances about services that can help. Arrange a follow-up as appropriate.

with concerns, can help (UHSM 2012). 'SAGE' gets the user into the conversation and 'THYME' helps them to create a good ending.

Case study example: SAGE and THYME

A young woman was told by her partner to get tested for HIV. She was faithful in her relationship. He was not. She has been tested and is HIV positive. She is talking to the healthcare worker at the sexual health clinic about treatment.

Resource box

Carl Rogers (1959) http://journalpsyche.org/revisiting-carl-rogers-theory-of-personality/; www.psychologytoday.com/blog/what-would-aristotle-do/201505/how-be-empathetic

---

Summary

This chapter has focused on the concept of self-awareness and the need for practitioners working in all healthcare disciplines to have a better understanding of themselves in order to better understand others. Self-awareness is the foundation for building successful relationships with people with HIV and their families. It is a skill we can develop on an individual and interdisciplinary team basis. With a better understanding of our own attitudes, beliefs and values, we can deliver person-centred effective care.

References

Adler, A. (1963) *Understanding human nature* (Translated by Walter Beran Wolfe). London: Allen and Unwin.

Arbuthnott, A., and Sharpe, D. (2009) The effect of physician patient collaboration on patient adherence in non-psychiatric medicine. *Patient Education and Counseling, 77(1)*, 60–67.

Aronson, L. (2014) Examining empathy. *The Lancet, 384(9937)*, 16–17.

Baumeister, R.F. (Ed.) (1999) *The self in social psychology.* Philadelphia, PA: Psychology Press (Taylor & Francis).

Beach, M.C., Kerly, J., and Moore, R.D. (2006) Is the quality of the patient-provider relationship associated with better adherence and health outcomes for patients with IV? *Journal of General Internal Medicine, 21 June (6)*, 661–665.

Beach, M.C., Sugarman, J., Johnson, R.L., Arbelaez, J.J., Duggan, P.S., and Cooper, L.A. (2005) Do patients treated with dignity report higher satisfaction adherence and receipt of preventive care? *The Annals of Family Medicine, 3(4)*, 331–338.

Chapman, A. (2003) Johari window: A model for self-awareness, personal development, group development and understanding relationship. Online: https://apps.cfli.wisc.edu/johari/support/Johar iExplainChapman2003.pdf. Accessed 14-01-2019.

Church, A.H. (1997) Do you see what I see? An exploration of congruence in ratings from multiple perspectives. *Journal Applied Social Psychology, 27*, 983–1020.

Cohen, E.D. (2017) How to be empathic. Online: www.psychologytoday.com/blog/what-would-aris totle-do/201505/how-be-empathetic Accessed 18-3-17.

Croston, M. (2016) Self awareness and HIV nursing HIV nursing 16 47-51 Online: https://e-space. mmu.ac.uk/617062/ Accessed March 2017.

Del Piccolo, L., Goss, C., and Bergvik, S. (2006) The fourth meeting of the verona network on sequence analysis; concensus finding on the appropriateness of provider responses to patient cues and concerns. *Patient Education and Counselling, 60*, 313–325.

Department of Health. (2011) *Equity and excellence: Liberating the NHS*. London: DH.

Dupuis, G., Jonas-Simpson, K., and Mitchell. (2016). *Relational caring. Handout prepared for toward relationalcare:* A hands-on workshop exploring relationality through theatre presented at walk with me: Changing the culture of aging in Canada, Edmonton, AB Online: https://uwaterloo. ca/partnerships-in-dementia-care/sites/ca.partnerships-in-dementia-care/files/uploads/files/relatio nal_caring-final.pdf Accessed 14-01-2019.

Duval, S., and Wicklund, R.A. (1972) *A theory of self awareness*. New York: Academic Press.

Egan, G. (1998) *The skilled helper. A problem management approach to helping* (6th ed.). Pacific Grove, CA: BrooksCole.

Ellis, C., and Bochner, A. (1999) Bringing emotion and personal narrative into medical social science health. *An Interdisciplinary Journal, 3(2)*, 229–237.

Fletcher, C., and Baldry, C. (2000) A study of individual differences and self awareness in the context of multi source feedback. *Journal of Occupational and Organizational Psychology, 73*, 303–319.

Flickinger, T., Saha, S., Roter, D., Korthuis, P.T., Sharp, V., Cohn, J., Eggly, S., Moore, R.D., and Beach, M.C.L. (2016) Respecting patients is associated with more patient-centred communication behaviors in clinical encounters. *Patient Education and Counseling, 99*, 250–255.

Forrest, C. (2012) Working with 'difficult' patients. *Primary Health Care, 22(8)*, 20–22.

Freshwater, D. (Ed.) (2002) *Therapeutic nursing. Improving patient care through self awareness and reflection*. London: Sage.

Gosling, S. (2009) *Mixed signals*. Online: www.psychologytoday.com/articles/200909/mixed-signals. Accessed 14-01-2019.

Greenfield, J.A. (2001) Medical decision making: Models of the doctor patient relationship. *Health-care Communication Review Online Edition, 1(1)*, 1–2.

Hochschild, A. (1983) *The managed heart*. Berkeley, CA: University of California Press.

Jack, K., and Miller, E. (2008) Exploring self-awareness in mental health practice. *Mental Health Practice, 12*, 31–35.

James, N. (1993) Divisions of emotional labour: Disclosure and cancer. In: Fineman, S. (Ed.) *Emotion in organisations* (pp. 260–270). London: Sage.

Jourard, S. (1971) *The transparent self*. New York: Litton.

Jung, C.G. (1963) *Memories, dreams, reflections*. New York: Pantheon.

Luft, J. (1969) *Of human interaction*. Palo Alto, CA: National Press.

Luft, J., and Ingham, H. (1961) The Johari Window; a graphic model of awareness in interpersonal relations. *Human Relations Training News, 9*, 6–7.

Maguire, P., Faulkner, A., Booth, K., Elliot, C., and Hillier, V. (1996) Helping cancer patients disclose their concerns. *European Journal of Cancer*, *32A*, 78–81.

Mayer, J.D., and Salovey, P. (1997) What is emotional intelligence? In: Salovey, P. and Sluyter, D.J. (Eds.) *Emotional development and emotional intelligence* (pp. 3–31). New York: Basic Books.

Michaelsen, J.J. (2012) Emotional distance to so-called difficult patients. *Scandinavian Journal of Caring Sciences*, *26(1)*, 90–97.

Miller, E., and Nambiar-Greenwood, G. (2011) The nurse-patient relationship. In: Web, L. (Ed.) *Nursing communication skills in practice* (pp. 20–32). Oxford: Oxford University Press.

Moss, B. (2012) *Communication skills in health and social care* (2nd ed.). London: Sage.

Nelson-Jones, R. (2000) *Six key approaches to counselling and therapy*. London and New York: Continuum.

Oetzel, J., Wilcox, B., Avila, M., Hill, R., Archiopoli, A., and Ginosser, T. (2015) Patient-provider interaction, patient satisfaction, and health outcomes: Testing explanatory models for people living with HIV/AIDS. *AIDS Care*, *4(March)*, 1–7.

Oxford English Dictionaries. (2017).

Ozakgul, A., Sendir, M., Sender Atav, A.S., and Kiziltan, B. (2014) Attitudes towards HIV/Aids patients and empathic tendencies: A study of Turkish undergraduate nursing students. *Nurse Education Today*, *34*, 929–933.

Parker, R., and Aggleton, P. (2003) HIV and AIDS related stigma and discrimination; a conceptual framework and implications for action. *Social Science and Medicine*, *57(July 1)*, 13–24.

Pickles, D., King, L., and deLacy, S. (2011) Culturally construed beliefs and perceptions of nursing students and the stigma impacting on people living with AIDS: A qualitative study. *Nurse Education Today*, *49*, 39–44.

Rasheed, S.P. (2015) Self-awareness as a therapeutic tool for nurse/client relationship. *International Journal of Caring Sciences*, *8*, 211–216.

Rawlinson, J.W. (1990) Self awareness: Conceptual influences, contribution to nursing, and approaches to attainment. *Nurse Education Today*, *10(2)*, 111–117.

Rogers, C. (1959) A theory of therapy, personality and interpersonal relationships as developed in the client-centered framework. In: Koch, S. (Ed.) *Psychology: A study of a science. Vol. 3: Formulations of the person and the social context* (pp. 106–120). New York: McGraw Hill.

Rungapadiachy, D.M. (1999) *Interpersonal communication and psychology for health care professionals*. Edinburgh: Elsevier.

Rungapadiachy, D.M. (2008) *Self-awareness in health care*. Basingstoke: Palgrave Macmillan.

Rungapadiachy, D.M. (2009) *Interpersonal communication and psychology for healthcare professionals: Theory and practice*. Oxford: Butterworth/Heinemann.

Saha, S., Jacobs, E.A., Moore, R.D., and Beach, M.C. (2010) Trust in physicians and racial disparities in HIV care. *AIDS Patient Care STDS*, *24(July 7)*, 415–420.

Spichiger, E., Walhagen, M.I., and Benner, P. (2005) Nursing as a caring practice. *Scandanavian Journal of Caring Science*, *19*, 303–309.

Thompson, N. (2006) *People problems*. Basingstoke: Palgrave Macmillan.

Thorndike, E.L. (1920) Intelligence and its uses. *Harper's Magazine*, *140*, 227–235.

UHSM. (2012) *Sage and Thyme*. Online: www.sageandthymetraining.org.uk/sage-thyme-model-and-benefits-1. Accessed 06-04-17.

Walusimbi, M., and Okansky, J.G. (2004) Knowledge and attitude of nurses caring for patients with HIV/AIDS in Uganda. *Applied Nursing Research*, *17*, 92–99.

Williams, E. (2003) The relationship between momentary states of therapist self-awareness and perceptions of the counselling process. *Journal of Contemporary Psychotherapy*, *33(3)*, 177–186.

Wilson, V., and Pirrie, A. 2000 *Multidisciplinary teamworking. Beyond the barriers? A review of the issues*. Online: www.researchgate.net/publication/265232384_Multidisciplinary_Teamworking_Beyond_the_Barriers_A_Review_of_the_Issues 14-01-2019.

3 Seeing the whole person

A biopsychosocial perspective in HIV care

Gemma Paszek and Kathryn Bourne

Chapter description

People are made up of interrelating, multifactorial complex sets of phenomena. This chapter acknowledges the uniqueness that an individual brings to the care setting and provides an overview of the biopsychosocial approach to care delivery. The chapter highlights that this approach to care delivery seeks to explore the 'whole person', instead of providing care for the people that only focus on separate elements (physical health, psychological wellbeing, sexual health, spiritual health). The biopsychosocial approach to care delivery focuses on the person holistically, taking into consideration the interrelating components that impact on a person's health. This chapter will provide guidance for healthcare professionals, without in-depth experience in mental health, to adopt a holistic approach to the care they provide for people living with HIV. It will highlight the importance of recognising and responding to the complex interactions between biological, psychological, and social factors, to improve a patient's experience and advance healthcare delivery.

Introduction

HIV is a complex chronic long-term condition and the needs of a person living with HIV are undeniably best met by a compassionate biopsychosocial approach to care. The biopsychosocial model encourages a perspective that seeks to view the 'whole person' within the systems that surround them. The person's lived experience of HIV is a multifaceted interplay of both physical and mental/emotional factors that are influenced by the sociocultural/political context. It is therefore imperative that they are both given adequate consideration by the care team. Historically, delineation between 'physical health' and 'mental health' has left patients feeling dismissed, and their care package could be seen as fragmented. The biopsychosocial model supports interdisciplinary working as it guides a clinician to take into account a patient's attitude towards their illness, personality style, emotional responses, behavioural changes, social milieu, relational transitions, as well as biological and physiological changes, in understanding the lived experience of the condition.

Why do we have models in healthcare?

A model, at its most basic, is a belief (or set of beliefs) about the way things are. Models in this sense permeate every aspect of daily life. Sometimes models are obvious and explicitly labelled as such. For example, we often hear about companies' 'business models' in which they explain how the company aims to make its money by making a product for 50p and then selling it for £1.50 to cover other costs such as labour and overheads and, of course, to make a profit. But there are also less obvious models we use every day that have become so internalised that we do not think about them. We have a 'model' of how pedestrian crossings work: as a pedestrian, if I want to cross a busy road safely, I walk to the nearest crossing, I push the button, I wait for the green man, the cars stop at a red light, and I safely reach my destination.

Models help us understand how things work (according to the degree to which we believe in the model, at least). They are therefore incredibly useful in helping us know how to behave in a given situation and what to expect from any given course of action. For example, if I walk across the busy road without using the crossing or looking for traffic, my risk of being hurt is high. If I use the crossing correctly and look for cars, my risk of being hurt is minimised.

Models in healthcare work in the exact same way. Although they are perhaps a little more detailed, in essence they help the healthcare professional know what the important questions to ask are, how to understand the information in terms of identifying illness, and how to respond in terms of treatment. Further extending this, the healthcare professional knows what treatment response to look for and how to adapt treatment as necessary (i.e. increase the dose, switch treatment, stop when symptoms clear).

The biomedical model

The dominant model of modern Western medicine is undoubtedly the biomedical – or medical – model. In doing research for this chapter, it was surprisingly difficult to find any universal much quoted definition of the biomedical model. The idea that it needs no explanation is perhaps telling of the status it achieved as a kind of 'universal truth'. Nonetheless, the following definition is offered: at its most reductionist, the biomedical model of health and medicine asserts that all types of disease and illness are caused by changes in biological variables. These changes can occur for a number of reasons. They can be innate: a person born with sickle cell disease produces irregular-shaped red blood cells that do not last as long, carry less oxygen, and can get 'stuck' in blood vessels, all of which can contribute to lack of oxygen, damaged organs, and pain. They can be caused by changes that occur over time: a mutated gene in a cancer patient. They can be acquired unexpectedly from an external cause: a cyclist who comes off her bike at speed, breaking her wrist. We get ill because something abnormal happens in our body, or to our body, and nothing else needs consideration.

The biomedical thus gives rise to a number of assumptions (Ogden, 2012; Wade & Halligan, 2004): (1) health is a dichotomy: you are well or you are ill. There is no in between. (2) Presumably an illness or disease should affect everybody in the same way, with little interpersonal differences, save from other biological variables. (3) The patient is a passive victim of illness; it is not their fault they became ill. (4) Responsibility of healing lies solely with the physician. (5) Nothing wider than biological factors of illness matter.

Reflection point 1

Think about the above assumptions of a purely biomedical model and think about people you have worked with who had the same diagnosis. Consider the following questions:

- Were there any differences in how their illness affected them physically?
- What about the emotional impact? Did everyone react the same way?
- Were there any differences in the wider implications for different people? For example, impact on work life or family life?
- Can you think of any examples where the same illness required different treatment in different people? If so, why?
- Can you think of any times a patient has dome some additional helpful things to aid recovery on top of what the medical team has prescribed?

The dominance of the medical model is in no small part due to its undoubted success in the advancements of treatments and healthcare. Vaccinations are a good example of this. Polio is a childhood disease that predominately affects children under 5. It is highly contagious and can lead to irreversible muscle paralysis and even death. The World Health Organization (WHO) website (2017) reports: 'Polio cases have decreased by over 99% since 1988, from an estimated 350 000 cases then, to 37 reported cases in 2016.' Moreover, the model gave the medicine a scientific, rigorous research method that provided a framework for this continual advancement, especially as technology advances, allowing us to hypothesise and test out ideas in more and more ways.

Criticisms and a move away from the biomedical model

Despite the obvious success medicine had as a result of the biomedical model, its narrow focus began to become a sticking point that led to some questioning its universal utility. A major turning point for this was growing unrest and uncertainty within the field of psychiatry, which inspired George Engels to challenge the model (1977, 1980), and suggest a different approach. Engels reported that psychiatry was in the middle of a crisis and there were concerns from within the field that it 'has become a hodgepodge of unscientific opinions, assorted philosophies ... mixed metaphors ... propaganda and politicking'. Thus the question being asked within psychiatry was: should it remain part of medicine and strictly adhere to a medical model of mental health; or should it break away into its own, completely separate discipline? This is not the place to recount his paper in detail (if you are interested, check out the reference list), but in brief, Engels proposed that the question was not, 'is the biomedical model appropriate for psychiatry?', but rather, 'is the biomedical model appropriate for medicine as a whole anymore?' Engels' main criticism, unsurprisingly, was that the model was too narrow in its focus on only the biological variables. Moreover, he argued that as well as the model's successes, there were other reasons that the model remained dominant and unchallenged. In fact, he went as far as to argue that the biomedical approach had gone beyond the status of a scientific model in that, in science, a model needs to be revised or abandoned if it cannot fully account for new data. He accused the biomedical model of becoming a dogma, in that it was being treated as un-arguable truth where, as evidenced by the psychiatry debate, things had to be forced to fit or were thrown out of the model.

Engels (1977) highlights the fact that modern Western science was developing in a time when Christianity and the church were a powerful part of the establishment. Doctors were given permission by the church to use bodies for dissection purposes to further their knowledge. However, there was a tacit understanding that whilst healing ailments of the body was the job of medical practitioners, healing the 'soul' – which in modern terms could be conceptualised as psychological, emotional, and social difficulties – was firmly the job of the church. This may in part explain why the model had to develop to be so focused on biology alone. As the field of medicine grew and developed with each discovery and success, the biomedical model became the norm for Western medicine. Thus it was understandably hard for professionals and patients alike to think about it in any other terms, as this was all that had been known.

Another reason to be mindful of focusing solely on the biological is that it creates a hierarchy in which the healthcare professional has all the knowledge about illness and treatment, and therefore the power, and the patient has none. Thus it could be argued that some groups, including medical professionals and big pharmaceutical companies, have a vested interest in keeping medicine exclusively biological.

Engels therefore advocated for a new approach for medicine that built on and included what worked well from the biomedical model, but also accounted for the wider processes and factors that undoubtedly influence illness and healthcare. The majority of medical professionals today welcome a more flexible approach that allows them to consider the complexities of modern healthcare that impact on the immediate biomechanical issues at hand.

The biopsychosocial model

Engels proposed a biopsychosocial model that, as its name suggests, widens the traditional approach to medicine to include the effects of psychological and social factors on health. Figure 3.1 shows what is meant by each of the terms. A model that tries to incorporate these additional factors is more compatible with agreed definitions of what it actually means to be healthy. The WHO (1948) defines health as 'a state of complete physical, mental, and social well-being and not merely the absence of disease or infirmity'. These days, people are more aware and accepting of the idea that there is a 'mind–body link' (as opposed to mind–body dualism of the biomedical model).

Prior to Engels' work, earlier attempts to incorporate the role of the mind into modern, Western medicine came in the early part of the 20th century, when psychoanalysts such as Dunbar (1947), Alexander (1950), and Freud (1953) started to use the term 'psychosomatic' within the medical context. The term psychosomatic in its most literal translation from its Greek origins relates to the link between mind *(psyche)* and body *(soma)*. In reality, however, over time the term became synonymous for cases where traditional medicine could not explain physical symptoms – and the assumption therefore was that it must be 'all in their head'. Freud in particular developed his theory of 'neuroses', which he defined as physical or psychological symptoms that were manifestations of repressed, unconscious anxiety. To put this into an oversimplified example, imagine a young man who presents as having totally lost his voice for no obvious medical reason. The psychoanalytic understanding of this, as described above, might propose that the symptom is an unconscious display of his anxiety at never being listened to by his parents when growing up, nor by his wife now.

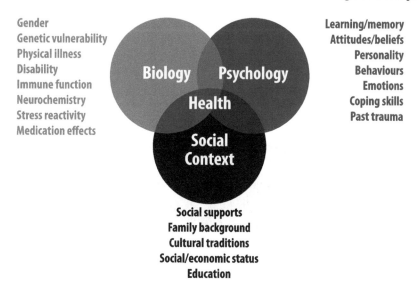

Gender
Genetic vulnerability
Physical illness
Disability
Immune function
Neurochemistry
Stress reactivity
Medication effects

Biology   Psychology

Health

Social
Context

Learning/memory
Attitudes/beliefs
Personality
Behaviours
Emotions
Coping skills
Past trauma

Social supports
Family background
Cultural traditions
Social/economic status
Education

Figure 3.1 The biopsychosocial model
(adapted from Bronfenbrenner, 1992)

Whilst this work very much developed in a positive way to progress our understanding of how the mind and mental health can impact on physical health, the idea of psychosomatic illnesses could often risk being misconstrued and misused by some in a pejorative way to dismiss, discredit, and disempower patients, who would be labelled things such as 'neurotic', 'hypochondriacs', and, at worst, 'malingerers'.

Why should medicine consider psychological and social factors?

Biopsychosocial

By looking at the biopsychosocial model from the perspective of each part, we can begin to understand how each factor relates to one another, and why it all needs to be considered as part of a holistic approach to healthcare. Let us first consider what is perhaps the most obvious, and least contentious, aspect of the model: the vast majority of healthcare providers and the general population will appreciate that living with a long-term health condition, or the after effects of a physical traumatic injury, can have an impact on a person's psychological wellbeing and social world. If we accept the above definition of health, healthcare services are not doing their jobs if they treat the biological aspects of illness in isolation. Consider hormone therapy as a treatment for prostate cancer as an example. Some patients may have to take hormones for up to three years post-radiotherapy to prevent the cancer returning, or others may have it as a single long-term palliative treatment to slow the progress of the disease where it is incurable, or they opt not to have radiotherapy or surgery. Focusing solely on the biological factors, an oncology team may consider the treatment very successful if they see no recurrence of disease, or its progression is significantly slowed: job done. A common side effect of hormone treatment, however, is loss of sex drive and sexual dysfunction. What if this leads the patient to feel

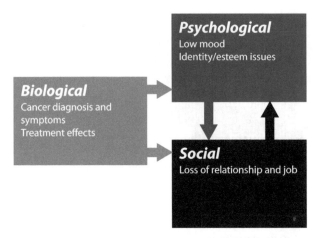

Figure 3.2 The impact of the biological on the psychological and social

embarrassed and that he is 'not like a man anymore'? What if he struggles to be close to his partner and pushes him or her away, leading to the breakdown of the relationship? What if he becomes low in mood and loses motivation to go to work? What if he loses his job and can no longer afford his mortgage payments? Is this still a job well done? The answer, of course, is clearly no. Cancer is a good example of healthcare where the wider impacts of the disease are well known and there is a lot of additional provision available, such as psychological support to help people adjust both to life with and life after cancer, and also financial advice to help people access benefits they are entitled to whilst they are in treatment, recovery, or palliation. This simple relation has been depicted in Figure 3.2.

Biopsychosocial

Second, we move round to the psychological aspect. The above section and example tell us why it is important to consider psychological factors, because biological issues can have a negative impact on wellbeing; but this is only one half of a bidirectional story. There is evidence that psychological factors can have a direct impact on physical health (see also Chapter 6). There is a considerable body of work that demonstrates that people who experience more positive emotions live longer (Diener & Chan, 2011) and are less likely to develop a range of health conditions later in life, including cardiovascular disease, mental health difficulties, and alcohol-related liver disease (Diener & Chan, 2011). The reverse of this is that low levels of well-being have been linked with depression (Keyes & Magyar-Moe, 2003), which in turn has been consistently linked with poorer outcomes in physical health (e.g. Musselman & Nemeroff, 2000). To put this into a working example, one of the most well-researched examples of this is heart disease. Evidence has shown that people with depression have the worst outcomes in this area in terms of increased symptomology and mortality rates. In part, this can be explained by the mediating role of some key social factors that may result from being depressed. For example, people who are depressed are likely to be less physically active and to engage in lifestyle factors such as smoking and increased alcohol intake, which in turn impact directly on the biology of the heart disease. The research shows, however, that a direct

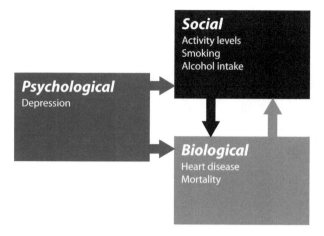

Figure 3.3 The impact of the psychological on the biological and social

relationship between depression and heart disease exists, even when these and all other relevant factors are controlled for. This has been illustrated in Figure 3.3.

There are other ways in which psychological factors can impact on healthcare. For example, it might be that the individual knows they need to be more active and smoke less, but she has crippling agoraphobia and social anxiety which prevents her from leaving the house and being active. She also finds smoking calms her down when she gets anxious. A narrow biological assessment would not uncover these factors and a narrow biological treatment would not address these factors, which would ultimately undermine medical efforts to help bring about any meaningful long-term change.

Lastly, we need to think about how health difficulties and treatments sit within the wider social context of an individual's life. Although an 'illness' may be identifiable by the biological symptoms the patient reports, and these biological symptoms may be directly treatable with traditional medical approaches, social factors may have played a more important part in the development and maintenance of the health condition, and left unaddressed can affect the success of medical treatment. A good example of this is type II diabetes, where lifestyle factors such as weight, diet, and stress can all contribute to the development of the disease and impact on disease trajectory. Focusing on a narrow biomedical view would mean asking about the patient's symptoms, hypothesising the symptoms are indicative of type II diabetes, running confirmatory tests, and then prescribing insulin use as required and giving vague advice to 'eat more healthily and lose weight'. A more in-depth biopsychosocial approach to assessment might help a clinician to understand more about the contributing psychological and social factors. For example, it may uncover social factors such as the individual living in a very low-income household, which makes it very hard to afford 'healthy' food. Moreover, they may have little knowledge about what a healthy, balanced diet looks like. Taking it a step further, if their finances are so desperate, they may be struggling to feed their

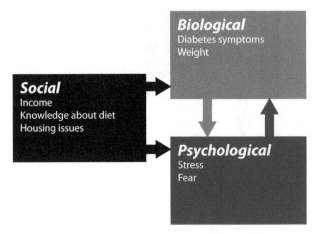

Figure 3.4 The impact of the social on the biological and psychological

children, pay the rent, heat their house, and so on. If an individual is living in constant fear of eviction, how easy is it for them to focus on remembering to take their insulin or learn new eating habits? This relationship is demonstrated in Figure 3.4.

Reflection point 2: case study

Read the case study of Esther below. See if you can answer the questions by thinking about what we have discussed in this chapter so far.

Esther is a 28-year-old woman originally from the Democratic Republic of Congo. She grew up in a supportive family and attended school, where she did well but was disowned by her family when she refused to enter into a marriage her family had arranged when she was 15 years old. Threatened with violence, she was forced to flee her home and unfortunately became a victim of trafficking and forced prostitution in another part of the country. Esther was raped by 'customers' on a daily basis and became pregnant after a short while. It was whilst she was accessing maternity care that she discovered she was HIV+. Esther's daughter was born without proper medical attention and also has HIV, something which Esther feels incredibly guilty about. Eventually Esther managed to flee from the DRC and arrived in the UK as an asylum seeker. Her native language is French and she speaks little English. She recently had her application for asylum status denied and is in the process of appealing. She attends her appointments regularly but her CD4 count and viral load often fluctuate. She is sometimes very quiet and hard to engage in clinic, especially when there is a male consultant. She has told you that she feels very angry and ashamed about how she contracted HIV, and that having to take medicine reminds her of what happened. Sometimes she has flashbacks to sexual violence she suffered as well as nightmares. You notice she is often very quiet during appointments and home visits, and she has told you she does very little out of the house as she does not know many people. Her face lights up whenever she plays with or talks about her daughter, Grace. Grace is doing really well, her HIV is well controlled and she is flourishing at nursery.

- What relevant biological factors can you identify?
- What relevant psychological factors can you identify?
- What relevant social factors can you identify?
- How might these factors impact on each other, and as a consequence, affect Esther's healthcare?

Widening the lens even further, this also highlights the need for healthcare professionals to have an active voice and role in social reforms that may impact on the health of the nation. Government policies can have an effect on people's health (positive or negative), either directly through things such as changes to healthcare provisions or indirectly through things that impact on people's psychological and social wellbeing, such as the standards of social housing, the benefits system, and funding provided to various third sector charities and community projects that offer indispensable support to many people in need.

In summary, modern healthcare must address physical health issues within the context of the wider psychological and social factors at play. The reasons for this can be summed up by the '3 Es':

Effectiveness

Biological treatments may effectively ameliorate physical symptoms, but only if treatments are adhered to as necessary. As such, it is imperative to address any psychological or social barriers to adherence to enable biological treatments to work. Moreover, unitary biological treatments are unlikely to result in long-lasting change as symptoms are likely to reoccur over time if ongoing psychological or social contributors to ill-health are not addressed.

Economics

Following on from the above point, the implicated economical cost of repeated ill-health can be high both in terms of direct treatment costs, but also wider societal costs such as lost working days. Therefore an approach that aims to bring about long-lasting change by addressing the wider psychological or social factors causing and/or maintaining ill-health will prove more cost-effective in the long term.

Ethics

As mentioned already, the WHO defines health as physical, psychological, and social wellbeing, and as such healthcare services have a duty of care to address all these factors. It seems fair to say that it is not enough to keep someone physically healthy if they are suffering socially and psychologically.

This biopsychosocial model therefore has two big implications for clinical practice: (1) assessments needs to be holistic to ensure all relevant information is gathered to make an informed diagnosis; and (2) health outcomes and goals need to go further than reducing ill-health; they must strive for improving general wellbeing and quality of life. To do this well, we must consider how we work in unity with our colleagues in other disciplines, and inclusively with service users, to conduct thorough assessments of need and develop comprehensive care plans. The next section focuses on how this might play out in HIV care; ideas will be introduced to encourage a holistic approach to care provision.

Living with HIV: attending to the whole person

There is no doubt that HIV is a very complex and complicated condition and, like all long-term physical health problems, it is routinely accompanied by medical complications, adjustment issues, social isolation, and interpersonal conflict. It is well documented that there exists a bidirectional link between physical illness and mental health difficulties, and this is immediately apparent when working with people living with HIV. Mental health problems are both a risk factor and a consequence of HIV (Gonzalez et al., 2011; refer to Chapter 4). We know that individuals are more susceptible to HIV if they are from a vulnerable group, have low self-esteem, and if they have a mental health problem like depression. For those living with HIV, there is a high prevalence of depression, with some figures suggesting prevalence as high as 72% (Gonzalez et al., 2011). This figure is unsurprising when we consider the challenges HIV brings to an individual: the demands of a strict medication regime; fears associated with health complications; concerns about relationships; and worries about the negative judgement from family and friends and the potential of being rejected for the condition.

Depression undoubtedly adversely impacts on everyday functioning, patient well-being, healthcare engagement, and treatment adherence. This is understandable when we consider the impact of low mood on an individual's motivation and self-belief. When depressed, a person can feel helpless and powerless; they may feel more pessimistic about their situation and have a distorted view of their future. Classic characteristics of depression are lethargy, tiredness, and lack of energy. Given that treatment adherence relies on a routine – particularly with some antiretrovirals that should be taken at the same time daily – we can appreciate how a person soon slips in terms of consistent adherence. A feeling of failure and concerns about letting people down, together with a 'what's the point?' attitude, can often lead to disengagement from healthcare – which we see frequently in HIV services with missed appointments. As seen in other long-term conditions like diabetes (Ali et al., 2006; Barnard et al., 2012, 2006; Ciechanowski et al., 2000) and coronary heart disease (Barefoot et al., 1996; Carney et al., 2003; Wells et al., 1989), depression among people with HIV is associated with poor outcomes and greater mortality (Sherr et al., 2011). Untreated depression is associated with reduced access to appropriate HIV care and non-adherence to HIV treatment. Research suggests that people living with HIV and chronic depression have a two-fold greater risk of dying than people living with HIV who are not depressed (Ciesla & Roberts, 2001; Cook et al., 2004; Sherr et al., 2011).

This highlights the need for early detection and, as most practitioners would agree, there is rarely one known cause for depression, so it is fitting that it is viewed from a biopsychosocial perspective. Responding to the psychosocial needs of people living with HIV will undeniably improve health outcomes. This relatively new favoured approach to health is reflected in the government white paper *Healthy Lives, Healthy People* (DoH, 2010), which provides a framework and a vision for mental health to become an integral part of physical healthcare. The paper acknowledges the bidirectional relationship between mental and physical health and highlights the necessity of routine assessment of the psychosocial needs in people with long-term conditions.

Reflection point 3

Let's take a few minutes to think about bidirectional relationships. First, consider how living with mental health problems may bring about physical health problems. To get you started: consider how depression can lead to poor motivation and reduced activity, which in turn may lead to health complications like increased risk of heart and respiratory problems. Now consider other issues faced by people with mental health problems that might increase the likelihood of physical health complaints. Don't forget to consider the social milieu and the impact of social deprivation.

Now consider how living with chronic physical health problems might increase the likelihood of developing mental health problems. Again, to get you started, think about chronic pain; living in pain is restrictive and associated with significant losses and undeniably impacts on a person's self-identity, which can lead to anxiety and depression. Have a think about other challenges that physical health problems bring and reflect on how this might change a person's mood and impact on their relationships.

Multifaceted impact on wellbeing

Among the many issues faced by people living with HIV are fears of death, dependency, relationship issues, physical and emotional isolation, issues relating to telling people about their HIV, secrecy, changes in lifestyle, financial responsibility, stigma/discrimination, and burnout. It affects the entire person – physical, psychological, social, and spiritual. As a health professional working in HIV care, it is imperative that you are mindful of, and address when possible, the wider effects of HIV. In the current economic state of the NHS, we are all far too familiar with the external demands that impose greater restrictions on our roles: time pressures, services being cut, overbooked clinics, staff shortages, additional role expectations, increasing documentation and record-keeping, expanding waiting lists, and financial restraints. Sadly, it is these strains and stresses that can cause us to strip back the care we provide for the patient to what feels like the primary, most important focus in the moment and the most effective use of our skills in the time we have available. Consequently, for people with a chronic health condition, care in the hospital setting often becomes centred primarily on the physical aspects of the disease. An understandable outcome is that clinic visits with doctors and nurses tend to concentrate on physical examinations, blood tests, diagnostic procedures, liver function tests, and medication adherence, with a medical-focused dialogue being established between patient and health professional: health of immune system, complete blood count, HIV viral load, CD4 count. There is no disputing the importance and necessity of these health checks and medical conversations; obviously the goal of HIV care is to stay as medically healthy as possible. However, the lived experience of a person with HIV is so much more than the physical aspects of the disease and failure to address these other equally important areas is like a jigsaw with missing pieces: the picture will never be fully apparent.

An integrated approach

There is a need to view a person holistically to fully understand the true 'health' of a patient. An integrated approach to physical and mental health entails taking a biopsychosocial perspective. This often leaves health professionals feeling uncomfortable when they consider themselves to not have the 'right' training to delve into mental health issues. This is when effective interdisciplinary working comes to your aid. We are not implying that you should feel like the 'experts in everything', and by no means are you going to be expected to 'fix' the problems identified; however, we encourage a willingness to explore the wider needs for a person living with HIV, and this may sometimes require you working beyond what feels like the boundaries of your role. Integrated care relies on multidisciplinary teams, with good professional relationships, effective clinical leadership, and a collaborative culture. Improved communication during consultations (refer to Chapter 5) is paramount to supporting an integrated approach; a patient's early conversations with a health professional can begin to model the biopsychosocial perspective and support a whole-person approach to care. It is hoped that from reading this chapter, you will feel encouraged to shift to proactive, not reactive, care provision – anticipating the impact of mental health on physical health and vice versa.

Biopsychosocial care planning

So in what ways can health professionals help mitigate the impact of these issues and improve the quality of life for people living with HIV? Hopefully your thoughts are now taking you to considering ideas of action from a biopsychosocial perspective. Only when we have an understanding of the lived experience of an individual can we begin to work together as teams and tailor the care we provide so it is holistic and person-centred. A biopsychosocial intervention may involve correcting misinformation that patients and caregivers may have, improving the coordination of community services and support groups, encouraging patients to maintain control over their lives and establish a network of support contacts, being alert to mood disorders, and encouraging conversations about distressing emotions such as grief, guilt, shame, fear, and anger.

We believe a way of conceptualising the biopsychosocial stance to health is by drawing parallels to the magic eye pictures we were once mesmerised by as a child. At first glance we simply see a 2D flat pattern, but if we look closer and adjust the way we view the image, a 3D picture presents itself. We consider the 2D pattern to reflect the restricted biomedical model stance; although it gives enough to draw inferences about the picture, it is perhaps lacking in depth, features, and detail. Whereas a holistic approach informed by the biopsychosocial model is the search for this 3D hidden picture – a representation with very fine detail, an image that provides the perception of depth that allows various dimensions to be represented. The 3D image is akin to a biopsychosocial formulation and enables us to attend to the whole person.

Reflection point 4: case study

Read the case study of Paul below. See if you can answer the questions by thinking about what we have discussed in this chapter so far.

Paul is a 42-year-old, white, heterosexual male who has been living with HIV for over five years. When he was originally diagnosed with HIV he was extremely unwell in hospital and was incredibly shocked by it. He then found out that he had a 21-year-old son, Leon, who was born after a brief relationship with a woman he had not seen since. The medical team estimated he had contracted HIV around ten years earlier based on his blood markers and Paul realised that he had probably become infected by sharing needles when he was younger. Paul's friends had very strong, prejudiced views about certain groups in society, particularly those who might be associated with HIV. He worried that if he told them about his diagnosis they would reject, or even attack, him. Paul found it very difficult to accept his diagnosis and tried to deny that he had it. As a result, he had great difficulty taking the antiretroviral medication needed to treat the HIV, as taking the treatment was 'like admitting that I have it'. As a result, Paul's health began to decline significantly. He is very keen to try and build a relationship with Leon, and they have begun to communicate through texts and social media.

- What relevant biological factors can you identify?
- What relevant psychological factors can you identify?
- What relevant social factors can you identify?
- How might these factors impact on each other and, as a consequence, affect Paul's healthcare?

The impact of HIV on sense of self

Self-identity is integral to our sense of self – that is, the representation we hold that defines who we are. Our sense of self may be defined by the role we have: that of a mother, a teacher, a gymnast, a son. It is also a reflection of our identity: our morals, beliefs, emotions, and aspirations. Let us think again about the social milieu in which a person exists; sense of self is heavily influenced by different environments, cultures, genders, and sexuality. A person's attitude is shaped by their experience, and for this reason it is important to understand how a person contracted HIV. Intersectionality is a word you may be familiar with; it relates to structural oppression experienced by minority groups. A significant number of our patients presenting to HIV services are African women who have contracted HIV as a consequence of sexual abuse. The reason we draw your attention to this is to encourage reflection on the impact of HIV on an individual's attitude towards self. Sense of self also relates to a person's self-esteem and their self-image. Sense of self is a complex concept, not only because it covers both the way the person views themselves and the world around them, but also because it is a dynamic concept. As we grow, our sense of self transforms (see Chapter 2).

Reflection point 5

Think back to when you were 10 years old: are you the same person? Some aspects may be the same, for example hobbies and certain personality traits, but undoubtedly some factors will have changed.

Now if we are to consider this concept in relation to HIV, already it is hoped you are beginning to think about the impact that living with HIV has on a person's sense of self. Initially, for most but not all, at time of diagnosis a person's sense of self is thrown into disarray. Diagnosis of any long-term condition can threaten a person's sense of self – both their internal image of who they are and their outward appraisals of how they now interact with the systems they exist in are altered. For a lot of people living with HIV, the condition dominates their thoughts and there is a tendency for the HIV to overshadow other aspects of self-identity. Added to this are factors relating to HIV acceptance and status-sharing; it is very common for many people living with HIV to keep their HIV status secret due to the very real existence of stigma in society. Living in secrecy may be motivated by fear of losing social status or image, to avoid rejection by family and friends, in order not to feel dependent or inferior, or due to fear or depression. Consider the subtle difference between the label of a 'person living with HIV' and an 'HIV person' – the first defines the person as a sum of parts, with HIV being just a part, but the second label defines the person by the HIV. Medical appointments can sometimes, unintentionally, collude with this mindset and reinforce the second label, which can be destructive for a patient's quality of life. The biopsychosocial perspective encourages clinicians to notice and respond to the psychosocial aspects and to highlight the other defining parts of self, independent of the HIV.

Reflection point 6

Read the case study of Fredrick below. See if you can answer the questions by thinking about what we have discussed in this chapter so far.

Fredrick is a 35-year-old, white, single, homosexual male who has been living with HIV for just over a year. He is a well-educated businessman and holds a senior position at his place of work in the city. When he was originally diagnosed he seemed unaffected and took a very pragmatic stance; he wanted the facts and figures and seemed compliant immediately with the treatment recommendations. He always requested that his appointments were at quiet times at the clinic and was never seen sitting with other patients in the waiting room. He always appeared well kempt and often arrived to the medical appointments smartly dressed in a suit. The medical team had been satisfied with his HIV-related health checks, and initially remained undetectable.

However, he missed his two last scheduled appointments with the clinical nurse specialist. Frederick had been struggling. He did not tell anyone about his HIV status; he worried that being gay and having HIV would ruin his career. He was finding it difficult to take his medication at the regular time each day due to work demands, which resulted in him sporadically taking his antiretroviral medication. He was struggling to be the same confident, self-assured, and respected man he considered himself. He was introduced to GHB on a night out in London a few months ago and now regularly engages in chemsex; he no longer feels alone. As a result, Frederick's health began to decline.

- What relevant biological factors can you identify?
- What relevant psychological factors can you identify?
- What relevant social factors can you identify?
- How might these factors impact on each other and, as a consequence, affect Fredrick's healthcare?

It may be helpful to present this idea to patients in a pictorial way (as depicted in Figure 3.5) to encourage conversations relating to personal strengths, interests, values, and aspirations – parts of self that sometimes become overshadowed and temporarily lost from sight

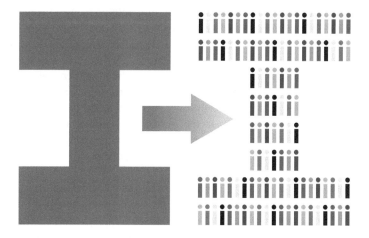

Figure 3.5 Conceptualisation of what defines sense of self

for people living with long-term conditions. For some people living with HIV, the condition becomes central to their identity, swallowing up and overshadowing all other aspects of self that they once knew. This is represented by the solid capital 'I' in Figure 3.5. Early conversations may acknowledge that the HIV is currently dominating the picture; but the role of the clinician is to help the patient to recognise that, yes, they now have a lifelong condition, but this condition does not have to define their self-identity. I refer you back to Figure 3.5 – a shift towards seeing the whole person is a process of genial inquisition, helping the patient to understand and accept that HIV can be a small 'i' in reality, and a person has many more defining parts that are worth connecting to. Through reflective listening, a clinician can identify these parts of self, which enables them to see more than the HIV and work with the whole person. Patients can be positively supported to reconnect with all manner of skills and ideas about how to live with, and negotiate the challenges of living with, HIV.

Reflection point 7

Perhaps take some time to now consider what little 'i's might make up your own big 'I'.
What are your likes and dislikes?
What are your values and aspirations?
Do you show different qualities in different settings, for example at home compared with at work?
How would a close friend describe you?

Narrative explorations and systemic practice in HIV

The narrative of a patient's story is invaluable. It is beyond the scope of this chapter to discuss at breadth narrative practices (White, 2007; White & Epston, 1992); however, it is perhaps fitting to discuss briefly the general ethos of narrative approaches that regard people as affected by problems rather than as the problem, as the medical model would imply. A narrative position to care provision adopts a non-pathologising stance, and therefore is aligned with the biopsychosocial model. We must all too often witness in clinical practice the labelling of 'good' and 'bad' patients, the latter being those that perhaps do not comply with treatment or pose a challenge to the service (see Chapter 6). The dominant problem-saturated story for them tends to be about not engaging with treatment, not practising safe sex, and not attending healthcare appointments. When a person *living with* HIV *becomes* a 'patient', they may feel imperilled to the power of medicine; and it is easy to unintentionally erase the person. It is important to hold in mind that people have a host of stories that map the effects of HIV on their lives. Being curious and hearing and attending to individual stories can prevent us from making unhelpful assumptions.

So if we think of what constitutes a 'story', there needs to be characters, a setting, and a plot. The setting, or the social milieu, is paramount to the lived experience of HIV. Let us now consider how the condition impacts on the individual and the system in which they exist. What do we mean when we talk about systems? We all live within a system in which we interact; this could be our family, school, college, university, religious affiliation, workplace, social group, sporting team, political alliance, cultural group. Each system contains expectations about roles, norms, and rules. Let us consider a person recently diagnosed with HIV: if we hold in mind the system theory, we can immediately begin to consider the psychosocial effects for that individual in the context of the immediate and wider systems in which they interact. For example, disclosing their HIV status to a partner or family members, thinking about the implications of the condition on employment, considering how HIV is regarded within their religious group and/or culture. It is the interaction with these systems which may shape psychological adjustment, both at the time of diagnosis and throughout the life course of the condition (see Chapter 10). Remember, the systems in which we exist are constantly evolving; as humans we are actively involved with our environment in a reciprocal and interactive manner. And therefore a person living with HIV will be continually reassessing their position in the system and renegotiating new rules for living which may be specific to the HIV status.

Successful interventions can come from considering these social and relational determinants – for example, interventions focused on building self-efficacy, assertiveness, stigma reduction (Kaufman et al., 2014) (see Chapter 8). The biopsychosocial perspective recognises the existence of multiple-causal pathways which reflect complex interactions of between and within these identified systems. Treatment is not single-system-dominant, but interdisciplinary, often involving a combination aimed at restoring the functioning of the whole person within the context. Human functioning, and the broadly defined 'health' of a person living with HIV, can be comprehensively understood only by incorporating a systems approach to clinical practice (see Figure 3.6).

The importance of considering the impact of personal values

When considering the whole person, we need also to consider 'values', which represent what is important to us and guide how we want to live our lives. The reason we introduce this concept is to again encourage a shift in focus to the 'psychological' and 'social' aspects of the model. Sometimes we innocently operate from our own values and passively assume that they are shared by others. The danger of this is when goals are set from the agenda of the health professional – driven by their values, and not the patient (see Chapters 2 and 5). It is important to ensure that

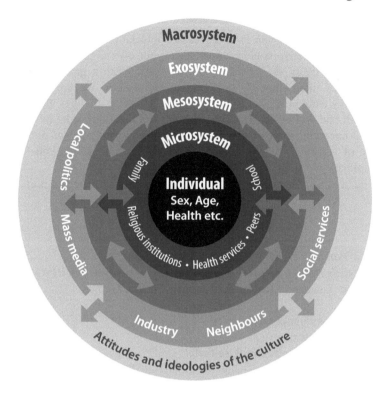

Figure 3.6 Bronfenbrenner's ecological systems theory (adapted from Bronfenbrenner, 1992)

goals being set are aligned with the individual values of the patient. You can never feel truly confident and motivated if the things you do, or those being asked of you, do not reflect your own values. Our values and beliefs are important components of our attitudes, and our attitudes subsequently govern our behaviour. Simply providing a patient with facts about an illness and their condition will not automatically change their behaviour; a person's motivation to change behaviour is heavily influenced by their values and aspirations.

Thinking about the determinants of health behaviour, we need rounded, robust knowledge of the biological, psychological, and social processes (Ajzen, 1991) that include the person's understanding of the health risks, denial and avoidant behaviours, interpersonal processes (e.g. relationship breakdowns), organisational and cultural effects (e.g. normative pressures, stigma, and discrimination in society). It is imperative to consider the social and relational context that may influence opinions of a person living with HIV. Again, we encourage reflective listening and the use of appropriate questions to uncover beliefs and attitudes that may be maintaining risk behaviours. For example, pressures from peers or partners may encourage activities that place them at risk (Rosenstock, 1974; Rosenstock et al., 1996). NICE guidance and Department of Health guidelines may set the targets for behavioural change, but as a health professional supporting people with HIV, it is only from identifying personal values that are important to a patient that allows you as a clinician to reflect on the discrepant behaviours, and from there build motivation for change.

Summary

Hopefully after reading this chapter you have a greater appreciation of the biopsychosocial model and how the perspective could be applied to your own clinical practice, and inform how you work effectively as a multidisciplinary team. With a growing recognition of the importance of integrating physical and mental health, we are witnessing a shift on the ground in care provision to support this transition in how we support people with their health and wellbeing. We hope that this introduction to the biopsychosocial perspective will encourage you to be more mindful of the whole person and adopt a more holistic way of working. To optimise this approach and to enable you to feel supported, interdisciplinary working is even more paramount.

Resource box

Books
Living with HIV: A Patient's Guide (2009) by Mark Cichocki.
Living Confidently with HIV: A Self-Help Book for People Living with HIV (2009) by Liz Shaw, Erasmo Tacconelli, Robert Watson, and Claudia Herbert.
Websites
George House Trust https://ght.org.uk/
Terrance Higgins Trust www.tht.org.uk
Self-help materials https://web.ntw.nhs.uk/selfhelp/
HIV standards of care www.bhiva.org/standards-of-care-2018

References

Ajzen, I. (1991). The theory of planned behaviour. *Organisational Behaviour and Human Decision Processes*, 50, 179–211.

Alexander, F. (1950). *Psychosomatic medicine*. New York: Norton.

Ali, S., Stone, M., Peters, J., Davies, M., & Khunti, K. (2006). The prevalence of co-morbid depression in adults with Type 2 diabetes; a systematic review and meta-analysis. *Diabetic Medicine*, 23, 1165–1173.

Barefoot, J. C., Helms, M. J., Mark, D. B., Blumenthal, J., Califf, R., & Hanley, T. (1996). Depression and long-term mortality risk in patients with coronary artery disease. *American Journal of Cardiology*, 78, 613–617.

Barnard, K., Lloyd, C., & Holt, R. (2012). Psychological burden of diabetes and what it means to people with diabetes. In K. Barnard & C. Lloyd (Eds.), *Psychology and diabetes care: A practical guide* (pp. 1–22). London: Springer-Verlag.

Barnard, K., Skinner, T., & Peveler, R. (2006). The prevalence of co-morbid depression in adults with Type 1 diabetes: Systematic literature review. *Diabetic Medicine*, 23, 445–448.

Bronfenbrenner, U. (1992). Ecological systems theory. In R. Vasta (Ed.), *Six theories of child development: Revised formulations and current issues* (pp. 187–249). London: Jessica Kingsley Publishers.

Carney, R. M., Blumenthal, J. A., Catellier, D., Freelans, E., Berkman, L., & Watkin, L. (2003). Depression as a risk factor for mortality after acute myocardial infarction. *American Journal of Cardiology*, 92, 1277–1281.

Ciechanowski, P. S., Katon, W. J., & Russon, J. E. (2000). Depression and diabetes: Impact of depressive symptoms on adherence, function, and costs. *Archives of Internal Medicine*, 160, 3278–3285.

Ciesla, J. A., & Roberts, J. E. (2001). Meta-analysis of the relationship between HIV Infection and risk for depressive disorders. *American Journal of Psychiatry*, May; 158(5), 725–730.

Constitution of the World Health Organization. Geneva: World Health Organization; 1948. World Health Organization. Poliomyelitis factsheet. Retrieved from www.who.int/mediacentre/factsheets/fs114/en/ Updated April 2017.

Cook, J. A., Grey, D., Burke, J., Cohen, M. H., Gurtman, A. C., Richardson, J. L., Young, M. A., & Hessoal, N. A. (2004). Depressive symptoms and AIDS-related mortality among a multisite cohort of HIV-positive women. *American Journal of Public Health*, July; 94(7), 1133–1140.

Department of Health. (2010). Healthy lives, healthy people: Our strategy for public health in England.

Diener, E., & Chan, M. Y. (2011). Happy people live longer: Subjective well-being contributes to health and longevity. *Applied Psychology: Health and Well-Being*, 3, 1–43. doi:10.1111/j.1758-0854.2010.01045.x.

Dunbar, H. F. (1947). *Mind and body: Psychosomatic medicine*. New York: Random House.

Engels, G. (1977). The need for a new medical model a challenge for biomedical science. *Science*, 196, 126–129.

Engels, G. (1980). The clinical application of the biopsychosocial model. *The American Journal of Psychiatry*, 137, 535–544.

Freud, S. (1953). *A general introduction to psychoanalysis*. New York: Permabook Edition.

Gonzalez, J. S., Batchelder, A. W., Psaros, C., & Safren, S. A. (2011). Depression and HIV/AIDS treatment non adherence: A review and meta-analysis. *Journal of Acquired Immune Deficiency Syndromes*, Oct 1; 58(2), 181–187.

Kaufman, M. R., Cornish, F., Zimmerman, R. S., & Johnson, B. T. (2014). Health behavior change models for HIV prevention and AIDS care: Practical recommendations for a multi-level approach. *Journal of Acquired Immune Deficiency Syndromes (1999)*, 66(Suppl 3), S250–S258. doi: doi:10.1097/QAI.0000000000000236.

Keyes, C. L. M., & Magyar-Moe, J. L. (2003). The measurement and utility of adult subjective well-being. In S. J. Lopez & C. R. Snyder (Eds.), *Positive psychological assessment: Handbook of models and measures* (pp. 411–425). Washington, DC: American Psychological Association.

Musselman, D. L., & Nemeroff, C. B. (2000). Depression really does hurt your heart: Stress, depression, and cardiovascular disease. *Progress in Brain Research*, 122, 43–59.

Ogden, J. (2012). *Health psychology* (5th ed.). Maidenhead: McGraw-Hill Education.

Rosenstock, I. M. (1974). Historical origins of the health belief model. *Health Education Monographs*, 2, 328–335.

Rosenstock, I. M., Stretcher, V., & Becker, M. (1996). The health belief model and HIV risk behaviour change. In R. J. DiClemente & J. L. Peterson (Eds.), *Preventing AIDS: Theories and models of behavioural interventions* (pp. 5–24). New York: Plenum Press.

Sherr, L., Clucas, C., Harding, R., Sibley, E., & Catalan, J. (2011). HIV and depression – a systematic review of interventions. *Psychology, Health and Medicine*, Oct; 16(5), 493–527.

Wade, D. T., & Halligan, P. W. (2004). Do biomedical models of illness make for good healthcare systems? *BMJ*, 329(7479), 1398–1401. doi:10.1136/bmj.329.7479.1398.

Wells, K. B., Stewart, A., Hays, R. D., Burnam, A., Rodgers, W., & Daniels, M. (1989). The functioning and well-being of depressed patients: Results from the medical outcomes study. *Journal of American Medical Association*, 262, 914–919.

White, M. (2007). *Maps of narrative practice*. New York: Norton.

White, M., & Epston, D. (1992). A conversation about AIDS and dying. In D. Epston & M. White *Experience, contradiction, narrative and imagination* (pp. 27–36). Adelaide: Dulwich Centre Publications.

4 HIV diagnosis

The impact on mental health and wellbeing

James Meeks and Emma Jones

Chapter description

This chapter will outline the impact of a diagnosis of HIV on a person's mental health and wellbeing. It will consider helpful ways to inform a person of their diagnosis, the stages of acceptance and how this might affect people on an individual level. Mental health and wellbeing will be explored specifically focusing on illness-related post-traumatic stress disorder. Furthermore, it will encourage reflection on the specific links between mental health and HIV and the intertwining nature of the two areas. By the end of the chapter, the reader will be able to identify, understand and consider the complexities of the impact of diagnosis on a person's mental health and wellbeing, which is likely to aid and enhance holistic support skills. This chapter will be supported by appropriate and contemporary research. Within each section case examples, questions, thinking points or exercises are included to enhance the reader's development

---

As previously explored in Chapter 1 by India Amos and Roland Chesters, the giving of an HIV test result can have a significant impact on the person receiving the news. Therefore, the impact of giving an HIV diagnosis should not be underestimated. We have already heard through the participants' accounts in Chapter 1 that the giving of a positive test result requires time and skill to provide the emotional support needed for the information to be processed by the person receiving the positive result. Building on the first chapter, we will explore ways in which healthcare professionals (HCPs) inform a person of their diagnosis, whilst acknowledging the complexities of the impact of a diagnosis on a person's mental health and wellbeing.

Telling someone they've got HIV: the sooner the better

Informing someone of their recent test results for HIV can be a real challenge for clinicians. This section will assist clinicians to consider the practicality of telling someone they have a diagnosis of HIV. Breaking bad news has been studied extensively and is often learnt through experience of trial and error rather than through direct teaching. Observing colleagues may be beneficial to aid learning, although conversely, it may also demonstrate how clinicians do not wish to practise (Colletti,

Gruppen, Barclay, & Stern, 2001). Breaking bad news has been defined as 'any information which adversely and seriously affects an individual's view of his or her future' (Buckman, 1992). How the news is delivered to the service user is important to ensure the level of distress is managed and minimised.

Task

Think about a time when you told someone some bad news. This could be a friend, a colleague or a service user.

Spend 5 minutes reflecting on the answers to these questions:

- How did you tell that person?
- Do you think you did this in a sensitive way?
- How did that person react to the news?
- Would you change the way you told that person following their reactions?
- How did you support that person?

There are models used for informing someone they have a life-limiting condition, which include the ABCDE model (Rabow & Mcphee, 1999), the SPIKES model (Baile et al., 2000) and the BREAKS model (Narayanan, Bista, & Koshy, 2010). However, many points in these models are not appropriate for breaking the news to people with HIV. This is because these models focus very much on a medicalised approach, discussing cancer and death, whereas an HIV diagnosis is much more about life adjustments, as it is a life-changing diagnosis and not necessarily life-limiting (Flowers, Davis, Larkin, Church, & Marriott, 2011). The model below is designed specifically for informing someone they have HIV, although it can be adapted for use with other conditions.

The 5S model

The 5S model is a framework for supporting clinicians in informing a service user that they are HIV positive. The model includes the following areas:

Setting the scene
Subject broaching
Staff and service user reflection
Signposting
Sensitive, supportive and informal approach

Setting the scene

Advanced preparation is needed for informing a service user that they are living with HIV. First, ensure the room is appropriate for the diagnosis to take place. The environment can play a large part in how comfortable a person feels. If a room is 'clinical', it can feel scary or frightening, and possibly remind people of negative hospital experiences in the past. Whilst it may not always be practical to change the physical appearance of a room, small adjustments may be possible. A further point to consider is interruptions, as it is essential that during the appointment with the service user that you are not disturbed. The service user may understandably become emotional and distressed and not want others to observe this (Brook et al., 2014); it is therefore important you are in a private environment that provides a safe space.

Reflection point

Finally, ensure you are prepped and prepared. Do you know enough about the condition you are going to be diagnosing? Would it be useful to work with a colleague the first time you do it? If you were a service user, what questions would you ask the clinician?

Below are some questions you can ask yourself before the appointment. Use these questions as prompts to help you consider the environment in which you are going to conduct the consultation:

- Is the room confidential? Can anyone else hear what is going to be said?
- Are there windows? Are they closed?
- Is it the right temperature?
- Is the lighting right?
- Are there comfortable seats available?
- Is there access to tissues?
- Is literature nearby to give to the service user?
- Is the room reasonably tidy?
- Can you make sure you will not be disturbed? Is your mobile phone switched off?
- Has there been enough time allocated for the appointment?

Subject broaching

It can be difficult to decide how to start the conversation. However, you need to be clear, direct and tell the patient within the first couple of sentences. Interestingly, this is different from breaking bad news in cancer care. Clinicians who work in cancer care approach informing the service user in an explorative way, asking them what they know and what the result may mean for them (Narayanan et al., 2010). In HIV care, evidence indicates that service users need to be informed clearly, honestly and within the first couple of sentences of the consultation. You may need to repeat what you have said or 'check in' to ensure the person has understood, as receiving an HIV diagnosis can be traumatic and some people can 'opt out' of hearing as a coping response (see Chapter 1). It is helpful to give people their results as this allows them to make links between the test results and the information they are given. This can be facilitated easily by showing them the laboratory report and/or providing a copy of it to take away with them if they wish to.

Staff and service user reflection

Immediately after a person has been informed that they have HIV, they need time to reflect and think about what the diagnosis means to them. Allowing the person time to sit back, soak it in and think about what being HIV positive means for their life is vitally important. Adequate space and time for the free flow of emotions that may appear is required (Narayanan et al., 2010). People often want to think about the potential source of the transmission, which can come with difficult feelings. Having a moment or two of silence also gives the clinician time to reflect on how the service user is coping having just been informed they are HIV positive. This two-way reflection allows the clinician to observe the service user and follow any cues that indicate they may be ready to continue the consultation (Baile et al., 2000).

Signposting

During the consultation, it is good practice to offer supporting literature to service users about the condition diagnosed. It gives the service user a chance to read and understand the diagnosis in their own time, following the consultation. Multiple studies have highlighted the importance of supporting literature; Sustersic, Gauchet, Foote, and Bosson's (2016) review highlighted that leaflets can be extremely useful in acute episodes of care and can also improve adherence to treatment. Furthermore, specific to sexual and reproductive health, Varma, Chung, Townsend, and Power's (2016) findings support the provision of patient leaflets, although in conjunction with access to online materials. Offering support from local and national HIV organisations may also be beneficial. Service users may get support and advice from non-clinical professionals and have the opportunity to attend support groups for peer-on-peer advice (such as Project 100 from Positively UK http://positivelyuk.org/project-100/).

Task

Spend 5 minutes finding the answers to these questions:

- Who provides your local HIV community support group?
- Where is this service provided and when can service users access it?
- What national websites can I direct service users to?

Finally, ensure the next appointment for the service user is planned and they know when and where they need to attend to make sure they do not feel alone and know they have support.

Sensitive, supportive and informal approach

The therapeutic relationship clinicians have with their service users is of vital importance in practice (Peplau, 1998; Rogers, 1951). Building this relationship is likely to be helped by the use of good communication skills (Arnold & Boggs, 2015) (see Chapters 5 and 6). This is particularly important when telling a service user that they are living with HIV. The use of open-ended questions allows the service user to open up and talk rather than provide yes or no responses to more closed questions.

Example

'You are okay with that, yes?'
Instead, you could use:
'How do you feel about that? Tell me a bit more about that? What do you think about that? What are your thoughts about that?'

Thinking point

Think about some regular questions that you ask service users in practice. Can you change it into a more open-ended question?

One of the most important features of the consultation is how the practitioner and the service user interact. It is vital that there is a good rapport between them. Using the SOLER acronym (Egan, 1986) may help you think about the importance of non-verbal communication when undertaking consultations with service users.

SOLER

S = squarely face the person. This is showing you are ready to engage with them.
O = open your posture. This is a non-defensive position – it shows you are open to the consultation and what they are going to say. Try to avoid crossing your legs or arms.
L = lean forward to the other person. Leaning shows you are listening to them.
E = eye contact maintained. Your eyes are important to show you are listening and engaging with the person.
R = relax while attending. It is entirely possible to be both focused and relaxed and will help the service user relax too.
(Egan, 1986)

However, regarding the first point in the model, it is important to remember that each service user is individual, and as Stickley (2011) states, sitting squarely can be intimidating for some people, so a seated position slightly turned may be useful. Also, for some people, intensive eye contact can be uncomfortable. So small glances away from time to time might be helpful (but be careful not to appear distracted). Finally, think about the language that you choose to use. Avoid patronising and insensitive words that might build up a barrier between you and the service user. Address any emotions with empathy and provide supportive and caring suggestions to the consultation. This is discussed in further detail in Chapter 5.

Reflection point

Have you ever observed a clinical interaction where patronising or insensitive language was used?
What was said that was unhelpful?
How did the service user respond to this?

Stages of accepting an HIV diagnosis

Reaction to the diagnosis and coming to terms with or accepting the diagnosis can be more debilitating than the actual physical symptoms of HIV. It may take some time for a person to adjust. The diagnosis of HIV is likened to experiencing loss or grief due to the life-changing nature of the issues associated with the condition. One of the most well-known models of grief was developed by Elizabeth Kübler-Ross, who discussed the five stages of grief in her famous book *On Death and Dying* (Kübler-Ross, 1969, 2009). The stages of grief are commonly known by the acronym DABDA (Denial, Anger, Bargaining, Depression and Acceptance) and this model has been used in a range of settings and situations.

The model was focused on the journey of dying and accepting 'the end', which was perhaps more relevant when HIV was considered life-limiting rather than life-changing. However, permanent change relating to a diagnosis could be received by some service users as an end to the previous 'self' or previous way of life. Therefore, this model still continues to be relevant today and can be a useful tool when working with people who have recently been diagnosed with HIV or other chronic conditions. The model assists healthcare professionals to understand the stages the service user may experience.

The healthcare professional should listen to the language the service user uses to identify where they may be in the differing stages. Using Kübler's (1969) model can highlight the way forward in your approach to the consultation and assist in identifying appropriate interventions. For instance, if a service user is experiencing anger, the healthcare professional should be sensitive in their approach and not become defensive in the consultation or take any comments personally. Listed below are some examples of statements that service users could say about living with HIV and how they might be explained by the model.

DENIAL: 'When I was first diagnosed with HIV, I did not believe the nurse telling me. I thought it was a joke and it was not my result.'

ANGER: 'I was cross with the nurse. I knew it wasn't his fault but I wanted to blame him for telling me this. Why did he have to tell me?'

BARGAINING: 'If only I could go back in time, I would have done this differently, I would have been more careful to avoid HIV. I want to go back in time.'

DEPRESSION: 'Life is bad. I don't want to think about or do anything. I miss my life living without HIV. I feel empty and useless.'

ACCEPTANCE: 'It's okay, I will win this battle. I know I can learn to live with this. This is a part of me now.'

It is important to acknowledge that people living with HIV may experience their diagnosis outside of these stages. Studies have found other responses which may or may not be part of the stages above. Anderson et al. (2010) found that people who are diagnosed with HIV are potentially faced with a multi-layered loss of themselves, their life, their future and a partner. The diagnosis can cause shock and distress because of the historical association with death and the reality of stigma (Anderson et al., 2010; Leyva-Moral, de Dios Sanchez, Lluva-Castario, & Mestres-Camps, 2015). Furthermore, Anderson et al.'s (2010) study highlights the importance of giving service users time to absorb the information. The study highlights several cases where service users acknowledge that the healthcare professional seemed oblivious to the impact of the diagnosis to their mental health and wellbeing. Another viewpoint illuminated in Anderson et al.'s study is that some service users may have a differing reaction to the diagnosis, which does not align with Kübler-Ross's model. Some people receiving their diagnosis may be relieved that they finally know their results, that they do not have to worry any longer about contracting HIV or that they just accept it because they know they had taken a risk.

People who see HIV as a chronic illness can be encouraged to be proactive in seeking care (Moskowitz, Wrubel, Hult, Maurer, & Acree, 2013). However, people whose initial reaction is influenced by their belief that HIV is terminal need reassurance and education about interventions, as this is potentially very traumatising (which will be discussed below). It is important to be aware of the service user's understanding of their diagnosis, which may be influenced by their socio-cultural context, in order to meet their individual needs (see Chapter 3).

Identity

A diagnosis of HIV can be a threat to the person's identity and this can have a negative impact on their motivation to access services (Moskowitz et al., 2013). They could be embarrassed about how they came to be living with HIV. Part of coming to terms with a new identity of living with HIV may be seen as part of the acceptance process. This may take a short or considerable amount of time for service users, and healthcare professionals need to be adaptive to individual needs. As part of the acceptance stage, people with HIV may choose to embrace their diagnosis into their identity (Moskowitz et al., 2013) and becoming a peer support mentor for others who are living with HIV is one example of how they might do this.

Reflection point

Think about a time when you received bad news. Write your experiences of the five stages:
Denial
Anger
Bargaining
Depression
Acceptance

Containing concerns and worries

Reflection point

What is being 'mentally healthy' to you? Do you think you are mentally healthy? Why? How do you know this?
What would be 'mentally unhealthy' to you? What would you notice? How would you feel? What would others notice?

'Mental health' is a very broad term which is difficult to define (Barker, 2009; Ryrie & Norman, 2013b). It is unique to all of us, in that what might be 'mentally healthy' for one person may not be for another. It is a completely individual concept and is influenced by surrounding environmental and societal systems that we develop and live in. Being mentally healthy might mean having a good sleep pattern, eating well, having positive and supportive relationships, having hobbies and interests, having hope, leading fulfilling lives, giving back to the community and/or doing regular exercise. It can mean being 'stable' in your mood, your thoughts, your reactions, being able to fluctuate in mood 'appropriately' in reaction to events or situations and/or having resilience to cope with changes (World Health Organization, 2007). It can mean being able to 'function' day to day in the society or culture you are in (Ryrie & Norman, 2013b).

Activity

Container
Imagine you are holding a container. Add a little bit of water into your container – this is your vulnerability to adverse experiences. Now, add in more water. Over time we experience stress, trauma and negative experiences (often from very early in life) that all pour into our container. What is happening? The water is going to overflow. This is when someone may experience a mental health crisis. Now, pop holes in your container – what is that doing? Draining the water. These holes are your coping mechanisms/strategies – things you do to cope, things that help you when you are stressed/upset/struggling. They help drain the water to stop it from overflowing.

Everyone has a different-sized container, a different amount of water already in the container, the additional water added is different in amount, the holes in the container are different in terms of number and size. Essentially everyone is different. We all cope differently and experience things differently; therefore, if two people experience the same thing, they will experience it uniquely.

How big is your container?
How much water is already in? Why?
What water is added to your container? Why?
What are the holes in your container?
Has your container ever overflowed or come close to overflowing?
How would you know if your container overflowed?
How can you drain the water?
Based on Zubin and Spring (1977)

Mental health problems

There are various terms used to describe 'mental ill health'. These include but are not limited to: 'mental illness', 'mental health problem', 'mental disorder' and 'mental health difficulties'. We will use the term 'mental health problem' in this chapter. Anyone can develop a mental health problem at any point in their lives. One in four people experience a mental health crisis over a lifetime (Ryrie & Norman, 2013a; The Health & Social Care Information Centre, 2009). There are many reasons why someone may develop a mental health problem, which can be due to biological, psychological or social reasons (Barker, 2009), and more often than not a combination of these factors (refer to Chapter 3). If someone is unable to function on their own or are a risk to themselves or others, because of their mental health problem, they may come into contact with mental health services.

Some common mental health problems include: depression, anxiety, dementia, personality disorder, schizophrenia, bipolar, post-traumatic stress disorder, to name a few. There are two diagnostic manuals used to diagnose people with a mental health problem: the International Classification of Mental and Behavioural Disorders [ICD] (World Health Organization, 1992) and Diagnostic and Statistical Manual of Mental Disorders [DSM] (American Psychiatric Association, 2013). There are many who criticise these categorical classification systems due to the stigma attached to the labels they give (Ryrie & Norman, 2013a), and also the flawed nature of such systems, particularly personality disorder (Tyrer, Crawford, & Reed, 2015). The classification systems (ICD 10 and DSM 5) for diagnosing mental health problems have been referred to as outdated and inaccurate (Gaebel, Zielasek, & Reed, 2017). This is because people do not 'fit in' to set categories (Bach et al., 2017). Clinicians, academics and researchers are promoting that mental health problems are viewed on a continuum and seen as a 'normal' response to adverse experiences such as trauma (Boullier & Blair, 2018; DeLisi et al., 2017) (refer to Chapters 3 and 6).

Our role as healthcare professionals is to work with the person, their strengths and needs rather than focus on a label, which may not tell you very much. It is important to focus on a person's quality of life and recovery. Many challenge the diagnosis of mental health problems due to the flawed nature of diagnosis itself, as discussed above (Hyman, 2010). Often a person's diagnosis can change and co-morbidity is commonplace, bringing into question the validity of diagnosis itself (Weaver et al., 2003). However, it is important to know some of the common terms you may hear within healthcare services, whilst being mindful of the criticisms of diagnosis.

Resources

These are a number of useful websites that include links to support groups and information leaflets. There are many more.
Rethink: www.rethink.org/
Mind: www.mind.org.uk/
Mental Health Foundation: www.mentalhealth.org.uk/
Time to Change: www.time-to-change.org.uk/
Sane: www.sane.org.uk/

Illness-related post-traumatic stress disorder

The diagnosis of a life-threatening or significantly life-altering physical health problem can considerably affect the mental health and wellbeing of the individual. There are increased rates of PTSD following a diagnosis of a life-threatening illness (Delahanty, Bogart, & Figler, 2004). In relation to HIV, the person can feel in shock, anxious, fearful, paranoid and distressed (Flowers et al., 2011). In the study the service users identified a change in their identity that occurred once they received the diagnosis of HIV and described the negative links this had with their mental wellbeing.

For people living with HIV, there is an increased risk of developing illness-related or HIV-related post-traumatic stress disorder (PTSD) (Boarts, Buckley-Fischer, Armelie, Bogart, & Delahanty, 2009; Nightingale, Sher, & Hansen, 2010). People living with HIV report disproportionately high rates of post-traumatic stress disorder (PTSD) (Boarts et al., 2009), and it has been reported that 30% of people diagnosed with the condition develop PTSD as a result of being informed they have HIV (Kelly et al., 1998). It appears that PTSD is more prevalent than other conditions for people living with HIV (Kanga & Henry, 2002).

'PTSD may either precede an HIV diagnosis due to previously experienced traumatic events, or may emerge post-HIV diagnosis as a result of the stress of being diagnosed with a life-threatening illness' (Martin & Kagee, 2011). Many service users report that being informed of their diagnosis was the index trauma causing PTSD (Olley, Seedat, & Stein, 2006; Olley, Zeier, Seedat, & Stein, 2005). HIV-related PTSD has a similar impact on a person's life as non-HIV-related PTSD (Boarts et al., 2009). This can include such experiences as flashbacks, nightmares, overwhelming emotions, distressing thoughts and difficulties in functioning with daily living. Service users with HIV-related PTSD are more likely to also experience depression than services users without PTSD (Boarts et al., 2009). In addition to the impact of PTSD experiences, this could also be related to the additional psychosocial stressors of living with the condition.

Task

Spend 5 minutes finding the answers to these questions:

- Where are the local mental health services based and how can service users access them? How can you access them?
- What useful websites can you direct service users to?
- In a crisis situation, what mental health support is available in your area?
- Where can you get support from? Are there any established care pathways in place?

How intertwined are HIV and mental health?

Service users with a mental health problem are at an increased risk of contracting HIV – Chapter 6 explores the reason why people can be at increased risk of being vulnerable to this. Service users with HIV are at an increased risk of developing mental health problems, demonstrating the interlinked nature of the two areas. This is depicted in the 'mental health and HIV circle' shown in Figure 4.1. It shows that having a diagnosis of

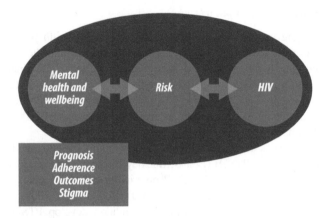

Figure 4.1 Mental health and HIV circle

HIV and a mental health problem can increase the risk of developing either and can then have implications for adherence, outcomes, prognosis and stigma, which the chapter will go on to explore.

Bucket and water analogy

HIV and mental health problems are water pouring into the bucket. If you have a higher severity of these conditions, it can add in even more water and increase the risk of the bucket overflowing. If you have both HIV and a mental health problem, the bucket will fill up more quickly and overflow, causing each condition to worsen.

Risk

People living with HIV can have poorer mental health than the general public (Bogart et al., 2011). Over one in three people with HIV screen positive for major depression (Bing et al., 2001). People living with HIV are twice as likely to be diagnosed with major depression in comparison with those not living with HIV (Ciesla & Roberts, 2001). The lifetime prevalence of PTSD is much higher in people who have HIV as compared with the general population, which has been found to be as high as 60% (Bogart et al., 2011). The high prevalence of depression of people living with HIV can not only affect a person's general wellbeing; it also has implications for adherence, outcomes and prognosis (Wagner, Ghosh-Dastidar, Garnett, Kityo, & Mugyenyi, 2012). Psychiatric co-morbidity for people with HIV is associated with increased rates of hospitalisation for both physical and mental health complications (Mijch et al., 2006).

Adherence

Service users with HIV and mental health problems are less likely to adhere to medication regimes and treatment for either their mental health problem or HIV (Schadé, Van

Grootheest, & Smit, 2013). This can be due to the person struggling with motivation, experiencing decreased memory function and/or struggling to adapt to a change in routine. Poor adherence to treatment can cause significant negative effects on a person's recovery and quality of life (Schadé et al., 2013). Wagner et al. (2012) found that the service users in their study that were concordant with antiretroviral medication experienced benefits not only in terms of the impact of HIV but also in relation to their mental health. This shows that adherence to treatment can have positive effects not only on a person's HIV symptomology but also their general wellbeing. Experiencing PTSD symptoms is especially linked to poor adherence, due to the constant reminder of the diagnosis of HIV when taking medication (Boarts et al., 2009). Furthermore, lower levels of adherence have been associated with higher risk of depression (Boarts et al., 2009). However, it is important to note that this may be a correlation rather than causation. Chapters 6, 7, 10 and 11 explore a range of reasons why people living with HIV might find it difficult to adhere to medication.

Life outcomes

Life outcomes related to the diagnosis of HIV is an important area to consider, as HIV is no longer a life-limiting condition, rather it is life-altering (Flowers et al., 2011). Therefore, the quality of life of the person should be key to clinical assessments and care plans. A diagnosis of HIV can impact on a person's wellbeing, their relationships, life in general, employment and daytime activities and hobbies, as explored throughout this chapter.

Sleep disturbance is a difficult resultant impact of having HIV. Not only does poor sleep have negative effects on a person's mental health, but it can also cause poor adherence to medication due to missing or forgetting doses (Crum-Cianflone et al., 2012). Furthermore, sleep disturbance is associated with an increase in mental health problems, including depression, and is a major negative factor for service users with HIV (Crum-Cianflone et al., 2012). Regardless of what causes insomnia, it impacts on adherence to medication, general cognition and quality of life (Crum-Cianflone et al., 2012).

Another issue highlighted between HIV and mental health is increased drug usage. People who have HIV and mental health problems are more likely to use illicit substances to cope (Zanjani, Saboe, & Oslin, 2007). Substance misuse is a risk factor for contracting HIV (Schadé et al., 2013). Substance misuse is discussed in more detail in Chapters 6 and 7.

Prognosis

Having both a mental health problem and HIV can impact heavily on prognosis of both conditions (Schadé et al., 2013). However, Mijch et al. (2006) conclude that although utilisation of health systems increases in those with HIV and a mental health problem, the person's survival is not reduced.

Stigma

A further area that is relevant to both service users with HIV and service users with a mental health problem is the impact of stigma, which can significantly impact on their quality of life (Bogart et al., 2011), especially if a service user experiences both of these conditions (Flowers et al., 2011). This potential 'double layer' of stigma can be further added to if a person belongs to other minority groups. This is particularly relevant to the HIV population as the condition is concentrated in already marginalised populations, in relation to factors including ethnicity, sexuality and social status (refer to Chapters 6, 7 and 8 for further explanations).

Positive relationships

A key element when working with people in healthcare services is the therapeutic relationship and developing trust (Arnold & Boggs, 2015; Meek, Jones, Kennedy, & Jones, 2016; Reynolds, 2009). By being open and transparent, professionals can effectively build good relationships with their service users and support them (Reynolds, 2009). It is essential we foster positive and supportive relationships with our service users in order to support them through difficult experiences. It is important to recognise service users with HIV and mental health problems are so much more than their diagnoses. There is a person, a friend, a family member, as well as a whole range of aspects of their identity. It is vital that healthcare professionals work with the person, not the diagnosis, with a focus on their needs and strengths. As healthcare professionals we often have long-standing relationships with people living with HIV. We can therefore have a unique and privileged role where we can help reduce suffering by providing support, understanding and person-centred care, in order to ensure our service users have the best quality of life they can. As HIV is a lifelong condition, this can lead to lifelong care relationships. Open and consistent caring relationships can lead to more effective care and ultimately better outcomes for the service users.

Reflection point

Reflect on a time when you had what you believe was a positive relationship with a service user and consider these questions:

- What would you call this 'relationship'?
- What did this relationship mean to you?
- What did the relationship feel like?
- How do you think the service user experienced this relationship?
- How do you know it was helpful/therapeutic/positive? What showed you that it was?
- What can you do to ensure you build positive relationships in the future?

Conclusion

In this chapter we have outlined the impact of the diagnosis of HIV on a person's mental health and wellbeing. We have considered how to inform someone they have HIV, utilising the 5S model, reviewed the stages of acceptance, and explored mental health and wellbeing with a focus on illness-related post-traumatic stress disorder. We finished by considering the intertwining nature of HIV and mental health. We hope this chapter has enabled the reader to identify, understand and consider the complexities of the impact of a diagnosis on a person's mental health and wellbeing, in order to enhance a supportive approach.

Task

Now you have read this chapter, list three things that you might do differently in your practice.
List three things that you have learned.

References

American Psychiatric Association. (2013) *Diagnostic and statistical manual of mental disorders: DSM 5* (5th ed). Washington, DC: American Psychiatric Publish.

Anderson, M., Elam, D., Gerver, S., Solarin, I., Fention, K., & Easterbrook, P. (2010) 'It took a piece of me': Initial response to a positive HIV diagnosis by Caribbean people in the UK. *AIDS Care, 22, 12*, 1493–1498. doi:10.1080/09540121.2010.482125.

Arnold, E. C., & Boggs, K. U. (2015) *Interpersonal relationship: Professional communication skills for nurses*, Elsevier Health Sciences.

Bach, B., Sellborn, M., Kongerslev, M., Simonsen, E., Krueger, R. F., & Mulder, R. (2017) Deriving ICD-11 personality disorder domains from DSM-5 traits: Initial attempts to harmonize two diagnostic systems. *Acta Psychiatrica Scandinavica, 136, 1*, 108–117. doi:10.111/ecps/12748.

Baile, W. F., Buckman, R., Lenzi, R., Glober, G., Beale, E. A., & Kudelka, A. P. (2000) SPIKES-a six step protocol for delivering bad news: Application to the patient with cancer. *The Oncologist, 5, 4*, 302–311.

Barker, P. (2009) Psychiatric diagnosis. In P. Barker (ed.) *Psychiatric and mental health nursing* (2nd ed, pp. 123–132) London: Arnold Edwards.

Bing, E. G., Burnam, M. A., Longshore, D., Fleishman, J. A., Sherbourne, C. D., London, A. S., & Vitiello, B. (2001) Psychiatric disorders and drug use among human immunodeficiency virus-infected adults in the United States. *Archives of General Psychiatry, 58, 8*, 721–728.

Boarts, J. M., Buckley-Fischer, B. A., Armelie, A. P., Bogart, L. M., & Delahanty, D. L. (2009) The impact of HIV diagnosis related Vs non-diagnosis related trauma on PTSD, depression, medication adherence, and HIV markers. *Journal of Evidence Based Social Work, 6, 1*, 4–16. doi:1080/15433710802633247.

Bogart, L. M., Wagner, G. L., Galvan, F. H., Landrine, H., Klein, D. J., & Sticklor, L. A. (2011) Perceived discrimination and mental health symptoms among black men with HIV. *Cultural Diversity and Ethnic Minority Psychology, 17, 3*, 295–302. doi:10.1037/a0024056.

Boullier, M., & Blair, M. (2018) Adverse childhood experiences. *Paediatrics and Child Health, 28, 3*, 132–137.

Brook, G., Bacon, L., Evans, C., McClean, H., Roberts, C., Tipple, C., & Sullivan, A. K. (2014) 2013 UK national guideline for consultations requiring sexual history taking, clinical effectiveness group British association for sexual health and HIV. *International Journal of STD and AIDS, 25, 6*, 391–404.

Buckman, R. (1992) *How to break bad news: A guide for healthcare professionals*. Baltimore, MD: Johns Hopkins University Press.

Ciesla, J. A., & Roberts, J. E. (2001) Meta-analysis of the relationships between HIV infection and risk of depressive disorder. *American Journal of Psychiatry, 158, 5*, 725–730.

Colletti, L., Gruppen, L., Barclay, M., & Stern, D. (2001) Teaching students to break bad news. *The American Journal of Surgery, 182, 1*, 20–23.

Crum-Cianflone, N. F., Roediger, Mp., Moore, D. J., Hale, B., Weintrob, A., Ganesan, A., & Letendre, S. (2012) Prevalence and factors associated with sleep disturbances among early-treated HIV-infected persons. *Clinical Infectious Diseases, 54, 10*, 1485–1494.

Delahanty, D., Bogart, L., & Figler, J. (2004) Post-traumatic stress disorder symptoms, salivary cortisol, medication adherence, and CD4 levels in HIV-positive individuals. *AIDS Care*, *16*, *2*, 247–260.

DeLisi, M., Alcala, J., Kusow, A., Hochstetler, A., Heirigs, M. H., Caudil, J. W., & Baglivio, M. T. (2017) Adverse childhood experiences, commitment offense, and race/ethnicity: Are the effects crime- race- and ethnicity specific? *International Journal of Environmental Research and Public Health*, *14*, *3*, 331.

Egan, G. (1986) *The skilled helper: A systematic approach to effective helping*. Pacific Grove, CA, Brooks: Cole Publishing Company.

Flowers, P., Davis, M. M., Larkin, M., Church, S., & Marriott, C. (2011) Understanding the impact of HIV diagnosis amongst gay men in Scotland: An interpretative phenomenological Analysis. *Psychology and Health*, *26*, *10*, 1378–1391. doi:10.1080/08870446.2010.551213.

Gaebel, W., Zielasek, J., & Reed, G. M. (2017) Mental and behavioural disorders in the ICD-11: Concepts, methodologies, and current status. *Psychiatria Polska*, *51*, *2*, 169–195.

Hyman, S. E. (2010) The diagnosis of mental disorders: The problem of reification. *Annual Review of Clinical Psychology*, *6*, 155–179.

Kanga, M., & Henry, J. L. (2002) Post traumatic stress disorder following cancer: A conceptual and empirical review. *Clinical Psychological Review*, *22*, *4*, 499–524.

Kelly, B., Raphael, B., Judd, F., Perdices, M., Kernutt, G., Burnett, P., & Burrows, G. (1998) Post-traumatic stress disorder in response to HIV infection. *General Hospital Psychiatry*, *20*, *6*, 345–352.

Kübler-Ross, E. (1969) *On death and dying*. New York, NY: Macmillian.

Kübler-Ross, E. (2009) *On death and dying: What the dying have to teach doctors, nurses, clergy and their own family*. London: Taylor & Francis.

Leyva-Moral, J. M., De Dois Sanchez, R., Lluva- Castario, A., & Mestres-Camps, L. (2015) Living with constant suffering: A different life following the diagnosis of HIV. *The Journal of the Association of Nurses in AIDS Care: JANAC*, *26*, *5*, 613–624. doi:10.1016/j.jana.2015.006.

Martin, L., & Kagee, A. (2011) Lifetime and HIV- related PTSD among persons recently diagnosed with HIV. *AIDS and Behaviour*, *15*, *1*, 125–131. doi:10.1007/s10461-008-9498-6.

Meek, J., Jones, E., Kennedy, N., & Jones, M. (2016) An exploration of student mental health nurses' narrative about working with service users living with HIV. *HIV Nursing*, *16*, *1*, 10–13.

Mijch, A., Burgess, P., Judd, F., Grech, P., KOmiti, A., Hoy, J., & Street, A. (2006) Increased health-care utilization and increased antiretroviral use in HIV infected individuals with mental health disorders. *HIV Medicine*, *7*, *4*, 205–212.

Moskowitz, J. T., Wrubel, J., Hult, J. R., Maurer, S., & Acree, M. (2013) Illness appraisals and depression in the first year after HIV diagnosis. *PLos ONE*, *8*, *10*, doi:10.1371/journal.pone.0078904.

Narayanan, V., Bista, B., & Koshy, C. (2010) 'BREAKS' protocol for breaking bad news. *Indian Journal of Palliative Care*, *16*, *2*, 61.

Nightingale, V. R., Sher, T. G., & Hansen, N. B. (2010) The impact of receiving an HIV diagnosis and cognitive processing on psychological distress and post-traumatic growth. *Journal of Traumatic Stress*, *23*, *4*, 452–460.

Olley, B., Seedat, S., & Stein, D. (2006) Persistence of psychiatric disorders in a cohort of HIV/AIDS patients in South Africa: A 6-months follow-up study. *Journal of Psychosomatic Research*, *61*, *4*, 479–484.

Olley, B., Zeier, M., Seedat, S., & Stein, D. (2005) Post-traumatic stress disorders among recently diagnosed patients with HIV/AIDS in South Africa. *AIDS Care*, *17*, *5*, 550–557.

Peplau, H. E. (1998) *Interpersonal relations in nursing: A conceptual frame of reference for psychodynamic nursing*. New York, NY: Springer Publishing Company.

Rabow, M. W., & Mcphee, S. J. (1999) Beyond breaking bad news; how to help patients who suffer. *Western Journal of Medicine*, *171*, *4*, 260.

Reynolds, B. (2009) Developing therapeutic one to one relationships. In P. Barker (Ed.) *Psychiatric and mental health nursing: The craft of caring* (2nd ed, pp. 313–321) London: Arnold.

Rogers, C. R. (1951) *Client-centred therapy*. London: Constable and Robinson.

Ryrie, I., & Norman, I. (2013a) Mental disorder. In I. Norman & I. Ryrie (Eds.) *The art and science of mental health nursing: Principles and practice* (pp. 17–31) Berkshire: Open University Press.

Ryrie, I., & Norman, I. (2013b) Mental disorder. In I. Norman & I. Ryrie (Eds.) *The art and science of mental health nursing: Principles and practice* (pp. 17–31) Berkshire: Open University Press.

Schadé, A., Van Grootheest, G., & Smit, J. H. (2013) HIV-Infected mental health patients: Characteristics and comparison with HIV-infected patients from the general population and non-infected mental health patients. *BMC Psychiatry, 13*. doi:10.1186/1471-244X-13-35.

Stickley, T. (2011) From SOLER to SURETY for effective non-verbal communication. *Nurse Education in Practice, 11*, 6, 395–398.

Sustersic, M., Gauchet, A., Foote, A., & Bosson, J. L. (2016) How best to use and evaluate patient information leaflets given during a consultation: A systematic review of literature reviews. *Health Expectations, 20*, 4, 531–542.

The Health and Social Care Information Centre (2009) National statistics: Adult psychiatric morbidity in England – 2007 – results of a household survey. *Retrieved from Northampton, United Kingdom*.

Tyrer, P., Crawford, M. J., & Reed, G. M. (2015) Classification, assessment, prevalence, and effects of personality disorder. *The Lancet, 385*, 9969, 717–726. doi:10.1016/S0140-6736(14)61995-4.

Varma, R., Chung, C., Townsend, A., & Power, M. (2016) Sexual health-related information -delivery – are patient information leaflets still relevant? *Sexual Health (Online), 13*, 2, 289–291.

Wagner, G. J., Ghost-Dastidar, B., Garnett, J., Kityo, C., & Mugyenyi, P. (2012) Impact of HIV antiretroviral therapy on depression and mental health among clients with HIV in Uganda. *Psychosomatic Medicine, 74*, 9, 883–890. doi:10.1097/PSY.ob013e31826629bd.

Weaver, T., Madden, P., Charles, V., Stimson, G., Renton, A., Tyrer, P., & Wright, N. (2003) Comorbidity of substance misuse and mental illness in community mental health and substance misuse services. *The British Journal of Psychiatry, 183*, 4, 302–313.

World Health Organization. (1992) *The ICD-10 classification of mental and behavioural disorders: Clinical descriptions and diagnostic guidelines*. Geneva: World Health Organisation.

World Health Organization. (2007) Mental health: Strengthening mental health promotion. retrieved from: www.google.co.uk/url?sa=t&rct=j&q=&esrc=s&source=web&cd=5&ved=0ahUKEwjXtZa ZofnRAhVJJcAKHfa4CK0QFghFMAQ&url=http%3A%2F%2Fmindyourmindproject.org% 2Fwp-content%2Fuploads%2F2014%2F11%2FWHO-Statement-on-Mental-Health-Promotion. pdf&usg=AFQjCNEDe2oDv1OZ58aDEWHDmzZ2kyg6XA&sig2=JALw9FAyDEzvGuim3mqO FA&cad=rja.

Zanjani, F., Saboe, K., & Oslin, D. (2007) Age differences in rates of mental health/substance abuse and behavioural care in HIV positive adults. *AIDS Patient Care and STDs, 21*, 5, 347–355.

Zubin, J., & Spring, B. (1977) Vulnerability: A new view of Schizophrenia. *Journal of Abnormal Psychology, 86*, 2, 103.

5 Navigating stormy waters

Difficult conversations in HIV care

Michelle Croston and Stuart Gibson

Chapter description

Working with people living with HIV can be both rewarding and satisfying, yet it can be challenging at both professional and personal levels. Establishing and maintaining effective therapeutic relationships with patients is paramount. Good communication is an essential aspect in creating such professional relationships, and they can have a positive impact on a variety of health outcomes for patients, including increased longevity (Schneider et al., 2004). This chapter provides an overview of what factors can influence professional relationships between patients and their healthcare providers in an HIV setting. A discussion of a variety of factors that can promote good communication in a clinical encounter is provided, in addition to an overview of what can hinder it. These discussions will be illuminated by case discussions and opportunities for self-reflection.

The emergence of successful antiretroviral therapy treatments has significantly contributed to the improvements in HIV care of the last 20 years. As a result of these medical advances, HIV has been redefined as a chronic manageable condition (WHO, 2017), of which the medical management of HIV may seem quite straightforward. Despite the advances within the disease area, significant challenges remain to achieving successful engagement in care, adherence to treatment and enjoyment of a good quality of life (BHIVA, 2018). Therefore, it is important for healthcare professionals to explore how they provide care over a prolonged period of time with patients. Establishing and maintaining therapeutic relationships are essential to ensuring long-term health outcomes and facilitating engagement in care.

Person-centred communication – Rogers' core conditions

In 1961, Carl Rogers published a book on counselling that has remained instrumental to this day in understanding how a therapeutic relationship is key to creating conditions for change for patients. In this book, Rogers described three 'core conditions' for creating a therapeutic space: unconditional positive regard, congruence or authenticity, and empathy (Rogers, 1961). Unconditional positive regard is often defined as the ability to accept another person's perspective or opinion, regardless of how much it may differ from one's own. Each patient's response to illness reflects how they respond to life's challenges. There are multiple different factors that can affect a person's response to life events. For example, cultural issues, societal factors, religion, gender and sexuality are just a few that can be interrelated and shape a person's response to illness. Within HIV care there are a wide range of subcultures that exist that are on the increase as diversity in society in general also continues to develop. This requires nurses to be curious, open, accepting and non-judgemental in working with patients who may hold beliefs or positions that are fundamentally different from their own.

Task – consider the following case

Jane has been taking the same antiretroviral medications since her diagnosis nearly 10 years ago. She reports she is beginning to struggle with dizziness and is experiencing sleeping difficulties. After a lengthy discussion about her life at the moment, it appears that Jane's medication may be playing a role in her symptoms. You suggest she may want to consider changing her antiretroviral medications. You describe what the new treatment may be, how she could take it and the potential side effects. Despite the medications being very similar to Jane's current regime, she seems very reluctant to change her treatment. In the end, she says that 'if it ain't broken, then I don't want to fix it.'

*   What questions can you ask to gain a better understanding of her perspective without sounding judgemental?
*   How do you convey your understanding of her opinion but share your own in a respectful way?

Like anyone else in the world, patients need to be treated with respect and accepted for their choices. In the end, acceptance does not necessarily mean agreement. However, it is acceptance that needs to be conveyed to patients so they can feel honoured and respected – and it is under these conditions when patients may start to take action to improve their wellbeing. However, they may choose to not take action for reasons unclear, unknown or even disagreed with – and this position needs to be accepted by healthcare professionals if they want to maintain an effective and helpful relationship with their patients. For example, patients may choose not to take medication for a variety of different reasons, and whilst this is often a source of great anxiety for practitioners in HIV care, it is important to respect the patient's wishes (see Chapter 6, 7 and 8). This is likely to help maintain the therapeutic relationship, meaning that the provision of client-centred healthcare can continue.

Congruence in a therapeutic relationship requires healthcare providers to be authentic and genuine with their patients. Being congruent is sometimes described as when actions and words match each other (Rogers, 1961). Healthcare providers (HCPs) who demonstrate openness and transparency by not hiding behind a professional façade are often described as being genuine or authentic – and this helps in promote their trustworthiness and credibility for patients (see Chapter 1). When such positive interpersonal qualities are conveyed, their communications will be more influential in promoting behaviour change. As previously mentioned, providing care for people living with HIV will occur over a prolonged period of time; therefore, the need for genuine and authentic care from the HCP is paramount when considering long-term outcomes and encouraging patients to remain engaged in care.

According to Rogers (1961), being aware of one's own feelings and attitudes that are flowing within the moment is essential for being genuine. When being congruent, there is a close matching between what is being experienced at the gut level, what is present in awareness and what is expressed to the patient. If there is a persistent feeling that is not shifting or changing, it needs to be acknowledged and possibly used in the moment therapeutically with the patient.

Displaying happiness to a patient when they are discussing their hard efforts and success in changing something is being authentic, genuine or congruent. However, it can be more challenging in circumstances when feeling frustrated, stuck or even annoyed when a patient refuses to adopt your perspective on the importance of changing their behaviour. In such circumstances, simply acknowledging the opposing views and proposing to discuss it again at a later point in time may be the best way forward.

Task – consider the following case

David's engagement with the HIV clinic has been sporadic over the past three years since he was first diagnosed. Today he is giving a blood sample, as this is the first time in eight months that he has been in to the clinic. When asked about how life is going for him, he breaks down in tears as he tells you about a recent job loss and his relationship of five years falling apart with his recent return to drug-fuelled sexual activity. He says that he doesn't really know if life is worth the continued struggle at the moment. You suggest that maybe he could benefit from meeting the clinic's psychologist. However, he declines your offer as he doesn't believe talking about his problems can lead to any change.

- What would be an authentic or genuine response to David?
- What could interfere with you being open and transparent about your feelings in this moment?
- How important is it in this moment to change his opinion about seeing a psychologist?

The importance of empathy

Empathy refers to being able to understand and appreciate another person's experience and then communicating this understanding to this person (Ancel, 2006). According to Rogers (1984), an empathetic person strives to enter another person's 'private perceptual world' and, in doing so, becomes thoroughly 'at home within it' (p142). Empathy facilitates the development of mutual trust and shared understandings, which are fundamental features of an effective therapeutic relationship (Herdman, 2004).

The terms 'sympathy' and 'empathy' are often used interchangeably with good intentions. However, they do refer to different emotive and interpersonal processes. Sympathy is an emotional reaction of pity and showing concern for another's welfare when feeling sorry for their loss or misfortune. All across the UK, many cups of tea are offered in response to learning of another's troubles and difficulties. Empathy, on the other hand, refers to under-standing and acknowledging the experience of another person, in the pursuit of fostering a working therapeutic relationship (Sinclair et al., 2017). The metaphor of 'putting yourself in the shoes of the other' is often used to describe what it feels like to truly understand another's experience of suffering. When this personal connection is established, a therapeutic relationship will become more effective in ameliorating suffering and promoting wellbeing.

Task – consider the following case

Juliet is a 43-year-old woman who has been a patient in your HIV clinic for nearly 20 years. Her 19-year-old daughter Rebecca, who is also living with HIV, is just about to leave for university. She will be more than 150 miles away from home, so she does not anticipate visiting her mother very often, except for school holidays. Juliet's husband died of HIV-related causes nearly 12 years ago, and they do not have any other family in your local area. Over the past year or so, your colleagues have often commented on how Juliet may struggle in adjusting to her 'empty nest' when Rebecca leaves home.

Juliet comes into the clinic to get her bloods drawn for her annual visit. She doesn't look herself, in that she's not dressed up and her hair is not in good shape. When alone with her, you ask how she is doing. Juliet whispers that she is 'okay' and that everything is 'fine' – but her eyes well up with tears and she avoids eye contact by looking down at the floor. You then ask how Rebecca is getting along and if she is excited about Rebecca going off to uni. At that point, Juliet starts to cry.

- At this moment, how do you feel? What if you were also a single parent and you have your own daughter who is already away at university?
- What empathetic response could you give to Juliet?
- How would that be different from displaying sympathy to her?

Creating an effective clinical encounter

Each clinical contact with a patient is considered an opportunity to promote their health and wellbeing. The Four Habits Model is a method or guide for delivering patient-centred care that is based on 'mutually beneficial partnerships' between patients and their healthcare providers (Hart, 2009). This model of care is based on four basic principles of dignity and respect, infor-mation-sharing, participation and collaboration (Frankel and Stein, 2001). These core concepts require active listening on the part of the healthcare provider in a non-judgemental and respect-ful manner. By structuring a clinical encounter with these steps, the potential for collaboration increases and patients will be more likely to engage in self-care. Additionally, a clinical contact with these features may lead to positive health outcomes that are promoted by a patient's improved adherence to treatment recommendations (see Table 5.1).

There is an old proverb about first impressions being the most lasting impressions – and can certainly apply to your clinical encounters with patients. This may be of particular importance in HIV care, where a person may have experienced previous rejections, either based on their HIV status or previous life story (see Chapters 6, 7 and 8). A warm welcome, with appropriate informal conversation and body language, can help put patients at ease. Set-ting an agenda and seeking their input into planning the visit helps to improve your

Table 5.1 Habit/skills table

Habit	Skills	
1. Invest in the beginning	a.	Create rapport
	b.	Elicit patient's concerns
	c.	Plan the visit with the patient
2. Elicit patient's perspective	a.	Ask for the patient's ideas
	b.	Elicit specific request
	c.	Explore the impact on the patient's life
3. Demonstrate empathy	a.	Be open to the patient's emotions
	b.	Make an empathic statement
	c.	Convey empathy non-verbally
	d.	Be aware of your own reactions
4. Invest in the end	a.	Deliver diagnostic information
	b.	Provide education
	c.	Involve patient in making decisions
	d.	Complete the visit

assessment of their needs for a more accurate diagnosis. Asking for their own ideas about what is causing their problems or what most concerns them helps to convey respect and dignity. By using open-ended questions to gather information, patients will be more likely to believe that you are interested in them.

Demonstrating empathy is vital, as it helps to shape positive clinical encounters and build therapeutic alliances. Communicating interest, conveying compassion and naming feelings can help develop trust. This helps patients to feel cared about. Bringing such positive therapeutic qualities to a helping relationship will not only make your clinical encounters more pleasant, but it will also help to make them more effective in promoting behaviour change and fostering good health and wellbeing.

Explaining the rationale for various tests and specific treatments is paramount, as well as involving patients in making decisions in how they might carry out these treatments. Identifying and exploring possible barriers to implementing treatments or behaviour change to promote health are also essential aspects of a clinical encounter. A collaborative working relationship is also promoted by expressing interest and respect towards alternative healing practices and complementary therapies. In doing so, you help to celebrate your patient's own initiative and creativity in caring for themselves and promoting their wellbeing.

Paying attention to and focusing on a good ending in a clinical encounter is just as important as how you begin one. Summarising your visit, reviewing your next steps, seeking additional questions and assessing satisfaction are ways to ensure a good outcome for that specific clinical encounter. In the end, promoting self-care is maximised when a clinical encounter is ended on a productive, pleasant and encouraging note.

Task – assessing your own clinical encounters

Think about your most recent clinical encounters with patients in your clinic. Which *habit* are you best at? Which one can you improve upon? What practical barriers may interfere with your efforts to improve upon them? What personal challenges may do the same?

Barriers to effective communication

Effective communication is central to the provision of effective, high-quality care in HIV. Health outcomes and patient satisfaction can be enhanced when communication involves compassion, empathy and active listening. Communication is improved when healthcare providers can feel confident in managing potentially tricky communication situations, such as breaking bad news, handling difficult questions and responding helpfully to strong emotions (Bramhall, 2014). However, there are a variety of factors that can hinder and even interfere with effective communication. Some of these factors are within a healthcare provider's control to modify and improve, whereas others are not. However, becoming aware of these potential barriers to effective communication can become the first step to managing and possibly improving them (Wilkinson, 1991). Maintaining effective communication in a busy and pressurised clinic where patients might feel vulnerable in some way and healthcare providers are frequently stressed requires good interpersonal skills as well as an awareness of self and others (Chapter 2). Effective communication is a core skill for healthcare providers. Every contact with a patient provides an opportunity to improve patient care.

However, barriers to good communication are not uncommon. Research over the past 20 years with various patient groups suggests that patients do not always share their concerns with their healthcare providers, and not all healthcare providers follow up on everything that is shared by their patients (Farrell et al., 2005; Heaven and Maguire, 1998; Heaven et al., 2006; Mullan and Koffe, 2010). There are numerous reasons for such missed opportunities for effective communication, most of which can be related to patient and/or professional factors. The following Task Box highlights these barriers to effective communication.

Task – how many of these barriers can apply to your patient encounters?

Patient barriers:

- Environment – noise, lack of privacy, no control over who is present or not present (staff or relatives).
- Fear and anxiety – related to being judged, being weak, or breaking down and crying.
- Other barriers – difficulty explaining feelings (no emotional language to explain feelings), being strong for someone else, or communication cues being blocked by healthcare professionals.

Healthcare professional barriers:

- Environment – high workload, lack of time, lack of support, staff conflict, lack of privacy or lack of referral pathway.
- Fear and anxiety – related to making the patient more distressed by talking and/or asking difficult questions.
- Other barriers – not having the skills or strategies to cope with difficult reactions, questions and/or emotions. Thinking 'it is not my role', and 'the patient is bound to be upset'.

Source: Bramhall (2014)

Behaviours that block communication

Blocking behaviours have been identified as barriers that can inhibit a patient's ability to disclose feelings and concerns (Del Piccolo et al., 2011; Maguire et al., 1996; Wilkinson et al., 2008). We all have the potential to engage in blocking behaviours for a variety of reasons, some of which are unintentional. Many of us are often unaware of the impact that these blocking behaviours can have on our patients. These blocking behaviours in HIV care can reinforce a patient's sense of shame, create feelings of rejection and/or cause patients to disengage from care, particularly if there is a difficult relationship history (refer to Chapter 6 for more information on this).

An example of an overt blocking behaviour in a consultation might be when a healthcare provider changes the topic of conversation. For example, when a patient discloses that he was really upset about being unwell recently, a healthcare provider might respond by changing the topic to asking about his family. More subtle blocking behaviours could be when a healthcare provider changes the time frame (*but are you upset now?*); or changes the person of interest (*and was your partner upset too?*); or ignores the emotion (*how long were you unwell?*).

In all these examples, the healthcare provider's blocking responses prevent the patient from talking about their concerns. If this happens, this patient might not feel listened to or cared about (Booth et al., 1996). This is particularly important in HIV care, as the healthcare team may be the only people who are aware of the patient's diagnosis and therefore the only people they can speak to about their concerns. Patient satisfaction, adherence to treatment recommendations and other forms of positive health outcomes will probably not happen when these kinds of blocking behaviours dominate our consultations.

Examples of blocking behaviours that prevent the facilitation of patients' concerns

- Physical questions
- Giving inappropriate information
- Using closed questions
- Using multiple questions
- Using leading questions
- Defending or justifying the patient's reactions
- Giving premature information
- Minimising patient's concerns
- Passing the buck: 'This is not my job'

Identifying and responding to cues

Cues can be anything you see or hear when you are interacting with patients. They can be relatively obvious, such as crying, or subtle, such as when patients look away when disappointing blood results are being talked about. People living with HIV can experience high levels of shame and therefore may not feel confident expressing themselves (Chapter 8). By recognising and acting on cues, HCPs can gain insight into patient difficulties and concerns (Bramhall, 2014; Levinson et al., 2000). By using facilitative, open-ended questions in response to cues, patients will be more likely to speak about more personal details and relevant information, which can be helpful to the clinical encounter. Ignoring or even missing cues by rigidly following a pro forma or scripted protocols only serves to close down the conversation, with the possibility of missing vital diagnostic information.

Some HCPs fear that responding to cues might take too much time and/or open up emotionally laden conversations that will be difficult to respond to (see barriers to communication discussed in the above box). However, research demonstrates that recognising and responding to cues can actually improve time management (Butow et al., 2002; Zimmerman et al., 2003). Cue-based consultations are not only shorter in duration; they can also be more effective in eliciting important diagnostic information and improve the clinical relationship (Bramhall, 2014).

Responding to patients in distress

Emotions enrich the human experience, sometimes in ways that mystify or even confuse others and ourselves. We don't always express our emotions or feelings, even when we feel them poignantly and deeply. And sometimes we can experience emotional reactions, yet be confused by not knowing the reasons for them or what purpose they serve. However, we experience them anyway, as emotions are a natural response to something that has happened, be it real or perceived.

How many different emotions are there? How long is a piece of string? Some say there are five fundamental emotions: anger, happiness, fear, sadness and disgust. However, others might say that shame is another distinctly unique emotional response (Grant and Bach, 2009). The sense of shame is particularly prevalent in people living with HIV due to stigma and this affects multiple aspects of their quality of life and experiences. Whatever the case may be, emotional reactions are inevitable, useful and important. HCPs need to be attuned to emotional reactions in their patients if they want to be able to provide effective and compassionate care to them.

An HCPs ability to help patients manage their emotional distress is essential. However, nurses can sometimes experience difficulties in assisting their patients in coping with their emotions for a variety of reasons. Sometimes they may not recognise distress or may not know what to do when negative emotions are exhibited. Sometimes they may think helping with emotions is someone else's job or believe discussing the distress could possibly harm the patient rather than help them (Dean and Street, 2014). However, there are ways for the healthcare provider to effectively identify and respond to patients' emotions as they assist them in improving their health and wellbeing. In reviewing the literature on how best to respond to emotional distress in a clinical encounter, Dean and Street (2014) have proposed a three-stage model of recognition, exploration and therapeutic action.

Recognising emotional distress – Patients are sometimes reluctant to express their feelings during clinical encounters, as they may not want to burden their healthcare provider with their distress. They may believe it is unimportant or inappropriate to their care or they may assume that their nurses are too busy for such things.

However, there is ample evidence that it is actually healthcare providers who are not attending and responding to emotions during their clinical encounters with patients (Dean and Street, 2014). Sometimes healthcare providers may purposely ignore emotions such as distress, because they believe addressing it will take too much time or that their primary goal at that particular moment is to focus on something else more practical. However, sometimes healthcare professionals may be fully aware of the need for responding to difficult feelings, but they may believe they do not possess the appropriate skills for dealing with such distress.

In the end, not identifying and recognising emotional distress during clinical encounters can become problematic as patients may be unwilling or uncertain about discussing their feelings, and healthcare professionals are either poor at recognising their distress or are reluctant to address it (Dean and Street, 2014).

Exploring emotional distress – Attending to the emotional aspects of a patient's presentation during a clinical encounter is an essential aspect of compassionate care. Engaging in active listening and facilitative communication by asking open-ended questions, displaying curiosity and acknowledging feelings can assist healthcare providers in attending to the emotional needs of their patients. Inviting patients to talk a little bit more about their feelings can go a long way in assisting them to understand and manage them. But in the end, not all patients will accept such invitations to discuss their feelings, and this needs to be noted and respected. The invitation, by itself, is sometimes more than enough to convey empathy, acceptance and respect – all vital ingredients for effective and compassionate care.

Therapeutic action – Acknowledging, exploring and providing empathic responses to difficult emotions can help to decrease and alleviate distress during a clinical encounter. Sometimes anxiety and fear are natural responses to uncertainty and not understanding or knowing what is about to happen to one's health and wellbeing. If this is the case, healthcare providers can offer clear and detailed explanations about their patients' current health situation and their possible treatment options. Such information can assist patients to manage their uncertainty, gain some control and increase hopefulness (Dean and Street, 2014).

However, sometimes providing a safe space for emotional expression followed by clear information to help foster certainty, control and hope for a patient is not enough to alleviate their emotional distress. There are times when making an onward referral for professional support is sometimes warranted. How that referral is discussed plays a pivotal role in what happens afterwards. When making such a referral, healthcare providers should express willingness to continue assisting their patients by following up with them, review their next steps, invite additional questions and summarise everything that has just happened. Healthcare providers need to be mindful that patients could feel dismissed, passed on or even rejected by their well-intended offer of a referral to a counsellor or mental health professional. People living with HIV may have experienced multiple rejections from family, peers, lovers, etc, and therefore could be very sensitive to feelings of rejection. As a result HCPs need to be extremely mindful not to trigger these painful feelings for patients. In the end, great care and attention need to be provided to alleviate any misgivings, which could ultimately *hinder patient care and wellbeing.*

Tips for fostering communication

Effective communication skills can help keep the focus on the patient when they are in distress, therefore it is important to remember the following:

- Look and listen for cues (either verbal or non-verbal).
- Ask open questions: 'how are you feeling?'
- Ask open and direct questions: 'Are you able to share with me why you are crying?'

- Ask open questions about feelings: 'Are you feeling ...?'
- Explore cues: 'You said you had a difficult conversation with the doctor?'
- Use pause and silence to enable the patient to think, reflect and process information.
- Use minimal prompts to encourage the patient to disclose concerns before continuing with discussions.
- Use screening question to ensure you have identified all the patient's concerns: 'Is there something else?'
- Clarify what you understand with the patient: 'You said that you are crying because you are upset about starting treatment. From what you have said, this sounds like it is very hard for you?'

Therapeutic use of self

Therapeutic relationships between patients and their HCPs are human relationships. Like everybody else, HCPs bring their personalities or 'real selves' into the consultation room. Therefore, it is important that we understand ourselves in order to improve upon our therapeutic relationship with our patients. When we can do this, we maximise the chances of our interventions having a positive impact on the health and wellbeing of our patients (refer to Chapter 2).

Using oneself as a therapeutic tool has been a concept in the helping professions for more than 50 years. According to Jerome Frank (1958), the therapeutic use of self helps to identify and reinforce our patients' positive and adaptive potential while helping them to understand and manage their own distressing and difficult experiences. In doing so, healthcare providers use their own intrapersonal and interpersonal skills by being aware of their own strengths and limitations they bring into the therapeutic relationship (Currid and Pennington, 2010). Therapeutic use of the self requires healthcare providers to use their own personalities, insights, perceptions and judgements as part of the therapeutic process (Punwar and Peloquin, 2000). The therapeutic use of self is to enable the therapeutic relationship to develop by sharing common ground. However, it does not mean that the HCP should disclose personal information or give the HCP permission to say whatever they want, as ultimately the relationship, albeit therapeutic, should remain professional. Professional boundaries are important in ensuring that the patient feels secure, as they provide a framework for the relationship and what the HCP can and cannot provide. This will be explored further in Chapter 6.

Dewane (2006) cites five components or aspects of the therapeutic use of self:

1. Use of belief system
2. Use of personality
3. Use of relational dynamics
4. Use of anxiety
5. Use of self-disclosure.

Most broadly, the use of our own personality in the therapeutic relationship is integral. However, this requires self-awareness of our own self-limitations and strengths. The potential for self-healing is realised when one can develop and foster self-awareness and self-acceptance. When this becomes possible, one becomes capable of helping others.

Other aspects of the therapeutic use of self include the use of our belief systems and awareness of relational dynamics. We must become aware and responsive to how our values, judgements and beliefs can influence the therapeutic process, both in helpful and unhelpful ways. A therapeutic relationship will become undermined if we impose our views of the world on our patients. We must also develop awareness of how our therapeutic relationships will grow and evolve over time. A sense of closeness, intimacy and trust has the potential to naturally develop, especially if we share our own personal responses during these encounters in a helpful, affirming and appropriate manner.

All therapeutic relationships will have moments of emotional intensity at some point, which can become anxiety-provoking for both patients and healthcare providers. These moments are inevitable and they can provide opportunities for developing self-awareness and self-acceptance. For HCPs, experiencing anxiety within a therapeutic encounter can become a moment for self-reflection, which can generate insights that can be used in helpful ways for our patients. They are not moments to be avoided; rather they can be acknowledged and used therapeutically.

These aspects of the therapeutic use of self share a common fifth factor: self-disclosure. The appropriate use of self-disclosure has generated considerable support as well as concern amongst the helping professions over the years. Objections are generally based on the fear that inappropriate and unhelpful self-disclosure changes the focus from the patient to the healthcare provider. But on a positive note, it can generate a positive therapeutic effect when it is judiciously used at the appropriate time. According to Currid and Pennington (2010), one needs to ask, 'for whose benefit am I disclosing this?', if they want self-disclosure to have an appropriate therapeutic impact. If the disclosure is not patient-centred, there will be an undesired effect of changing the focus of the consultation from the patient.

So how can healthcare practitioners develop this *therapeutic use of self*?

Broadly speaking, developing self-awareness is the essential task at hand if healthcare providers want to be able to use their own experience in a therapeutic manner.

Self-awareness involves knowing one's own strengths and limitations. It involves identifying, exploring and understanding one's own thoughts, feelings and values, with a view towards understanding and appreciating how they can impact on others. This journey of self-discovery is purposeful, with a focus on self-growth and self-determination (Freshwater, 2002).

Reflective task

One of your patients has come into the clinic today because he is in a distressed state. Apparently he may be charged for reckless transmission of HIV to a sexual partner who was unaware of his HIV status. You have known this patient for many years, and this is not the first time he has experienced difficulties with not sharing his HIV status to sexual partners.

- What thoughts, beliefs and values come to mind with this situation?
- Where do these thoughts come from?
- How could you develop a better understanding or self-awareness of your beliefs on this?

Self-awareness is also connected to a concept known as emotional intelligence (EI). EI is instrumental in helping us to identify, understand and manage emotions in ourselves and others (Mayer and Salovey, 1997). Our ability to regulate emotions helps us to foster and maintain relationships, in all domains of life. EI involves empathy, compassion and motivation to alleviate suffering, in addition to self-control and adeptness in relationships. These are all essential features in the therapeutic use of self (Robertson and Flint-Taylor, 2010).

Supervision and reflective practice

Working in a healthcare setting such as an HIV clinic can be challenging as well as rewarding, sometimes involving considerable stress. If these difficult experiences are not managed well, it can have a negative impact on caregiving. Maintaining warmth, empathy and genuine compassion towards others requires adept skills in identifying stress, strain and burnout, particularly through the history of HIV care. For many healthcare providers, clinical supervision is a fundamental aspect of good practice, as it provides the structured and safe space to identify and work through these challenging experiences. Clinical supervision provides the means for supporting, developing and promoting competence. According to Gibbs et al. (2010), clinical supervision is essential for developing the art and skill of therapeutic use of self. It provides a structured, in-depth reflection, with the aim of identifying and examining how thoughts, feelings, values and behaviours can impact on therapeutic practice. It can also provide the opportunity to explore how caring for oneself is also essential. When working with complex issues, clinical supervision enables the responsibilities, stress and concerns to be shared to ensure the most effective outcomes for the patient. Clinical supervision also provides an opportunity for interdisciplinary working. It can facilitate the ability to gain a holistic understanding of the patient's needs and assist when planning care.

Reflection, self-awareness and teamwork

When working in areas such as HIV where patients may be living with complex psychological and emotional issues, to which HCPs understandably respond, it can also be helpful to explore self-awareness and emotional intelligence across the multidisciplinary team (MDT). This can be facilitated by reflective practice meetings for MDT members, run by a clinician with appropriate training for this type of activity. Group reflection allows professionals from all disciplines within HIV care to make sense of experiences from their perspective and also to find common themes within the narratives of co-workers. This can offer an opportunity for mutual support within the team, potentially improving team cohesion and reducing the risk of burnout. Importantly, it also provides a space for shared understanding of patient issues and needs, which can inform collaborative care planning and the delivery of healthcare that is consistent across team members. Consistency of care is particularly salient for people living with HIV who have a complicated history and complex psychosocial needs (see Chapter 6). For patients with particularly complex and inter-relating physical and mental health issues, it may be beneficial for professionals from different disciplines to work in an interdisciplinary fashion. Examples of interdisciplinary working could be running joint clinics or joint visits to a patient at home. Working together, alongside a patient, can facilitate shared decision-making from a holistic perspective, meaning that inter-relating problems can be addressed at once, with patients and relevant HCPs all bringing their unique perspective. This may help patients experience a cohesive sense of care.

Working together as a team and sharing reflections can help manage the impact of difficult emotions; looking after one's own wellbeing is vital for providing compassionate care for others. This is especially the case when working with a chronic health condition that is ultimately life-threatening for patients, many of whom are already vulnerable, marginalised and living in anticipated shame with fear of rejection. All of these are very difficult and sometimes heart-wrenching circumstances. Without a doubt, working in HIV can be challenging and at times distressing. However, the therapeutic relationships that we develop with our patients are unique and special. This can help to make care rewarding, meaningful and satisfying, which will sustain us during difficult, stressful and busy times in the clinic.

Reflective task

Our lives are moulded and shaped by our personal experiences, some of which can be profoundly sad and others fantastic and delightful. These experiences help to form our beliefs and values, which we bring into our therapeutic encounters with our patients.

*   What experiences have led you to become a healthcare provider?
*   How have they helped to shape you as a caring and compassionate person?
*   What were your reasons for choosing your healthcare specialty?
*   How do these reasons influence your clinical practice?
*   What future developments will sustain you in this challenging field of work?
*   What might threaten your desire to continue in this work?

Summary

In summary, within this chapter we have explored the significance of good communication when establishing and maintaining therapeutic relationships. We have discussed the importance of creating an effective clinical encounter and the role of authentic, genuine and empathetic responses, when reacting to and eliciting patients' concerns. Exploring emotional distress and patients' emotional needs is an essential aspect of compassionate care. We hope that this chapter has highlighted ways in which the healthcare provider can acknowledge, explore and provide empathetic responses to the emotions that are being expressed within the clinical encounter. It has also been highlighted that utilising an interdisciplinary approach to patient care has increased benefits for both HCPs and patients. Interdisciplinary working enables complexity to be shared and holistic care plans to be developed.

References

Ancel, G. (2006) Developing empathy in nurses: An inservice training program. *Archives of Psychiatric Nursing*, 20, 6, 249–257.
Booth, K., Maguire, P.M., Butterworth, T., and Hillier, V. (1996) Perceived professional support and the use of blocking behaviours by hospice nurses. *Journal of Advanced Nursing*, 24, 3, 522–527.

Bramhall, E. (2014) Effective communication skills in nursing practice. *Nursing Standard*, 29, 14, 53–59.

British HIV Association. (2018) Standards of care for people living with HIV. Available at: www.bhiva.org/documents/Standard-of-care/BHIVAStandadsA4.pdf

Butow, P.N. et al. (2002) Oncologist reactions to cancer patients verbal cues. *Psyco-oncology*, 11, 1, 47–58.

Currid, T., and Pennington, J. (2010) Therapeutic use of self. *British Journal of Wellbeing*, 1, 3, 35–42.

Dean, M., and Street, R.L. (2014) A 3-stage model or patient-centred communication for addressing cancer patient's emotional distress. *Patient Education Counselling*, 94, 2, 143–148.

Del Piccolo, L. (2012) People-centered care: New research needs and methods in doctor–patient communication. *Challenges in Mental Health*, 21, 2, 145–149.

Dewane, C.J. (2006) Use of self: A primer revisited. *Clinical Social Work Journal*, 34, 4, 543–558.

Farrell, G., and Cubit, K. (2005) Nurses under threat: A comparison of content of 28 aggression management programmes. *Journal of Mental Health Nursing*, 14, 1, 44–53.

Frank, J. (1958) The therapeutic use of self. *American Journal of Occupational Therapy*, 12, 4, 215–225.

Frankel, R.M., and Stein, T. (2001) Getting the most out of a clinical encounter: The four habits model. *Journal of Medical Practice Management*, 16, 4, 184–191.

Freshwater, D. (2002) *Therapeutic Nursing: Improving Patient Care Through Self-awareness and Reflection*, London, Sage.

Grant, A., and Bach, S. (2009) *Communication and Interpersonal Skills for Nurses*, London, Sage.

Gibbs, J., Cameron, I. M., and Hamiton, E. (2010) Mental health nurses' and allied health professionals' perceptions of the role of the Occupational Health Service in the management of work-related stress: How do they self-care? *Journal of Psychiatric and Mental Health Nursing*, 17, 9, 838–845.

Hart, B. (2009) *Patient-Provider Communications: Caring to Listen*, London, Jones & Bartlett.

Heaven, C.M. (2006) Transfer of communication skills in training from workshop to workplace: The impact of clinical supervision. *Patient Education and Counselling*, 60, 3, 313–325.

Heaven, C.M., and Maguire, P. (1998) The relationship between patients' concerns and psychological distress in a hospice setting. *Psycho-oncology*, 7, 6, 502–507.

Herdman, E. (2004) Nursing in a postemotional society. *Nursing Philosophy*, 5, 2, 95–103.

Levinson, W., Gorawara-Bhat, R., and Lamb, J. (2000) A study of patient clues and physician responses in primary care and surgical settings. *Journal of American Medical Association*, 284, 8, 1021–1028.

Maguire, P., Booth, K., Eilliot, C., and Jones, B. (1996) Helping healthcare professionals involved in cancer care acquire key interviewing skills the impact of workshops. *European Journal of Cancer*, 32, 9, 1486–1489.

Mayer, J.D., and Salovey, P. (1997) What is Emotional Intelligence? In Salovey, P., and Sluyter, D.J. eds., *Emotional Development and Emotional Intelligence: Implications for Educators* (pp. 237–248), New York: Basic Books.

Mullan, D., and Koffe, E. (2010) Evaluating a nursing communication skills training course. The relationships between self-related ability, satisfaction and actual performance. *Nurse Education in Practice*, 10, 6, 374–378.

Punwar, J., and Peloquin, M. (2000) *Occupational Therapy: Principles and Practice*, Philadelphia, Lippincott.

Robertson, I., and Flint-Taylor, J. (2010) Wellbeing in healthcare organizations: Key issues. *British Journal of Healthcare Management*, 16, 1, 18–25.

Rogers, C.R. (1961) *On Becoming a Person*, Boston, Wiley Publishers.

Rogers, C.R. (1984) Person-Centered Approach Foundations. In Corsini, R., ed., *Encyclopedia of Psychology* (pp. 200–220), New York: John Wiley.

Schneider, J. et al (2004) Better physician patient relationships are associated with higher reported adherence to antiretroviral therapy in patients with HIV infection. *Journal of General Internal Medicine*, *19*, *11*, 1096–1103.

Sinclair, S., Raffin-Boucha, L.S., Venturato, L., et al. (2017) Compassion fatigue: A meta-narrative review of the healthcare literature. *International Journal of Nursing Studies*, *69*, 9–24.

Wilkinson, S. (1991) Factors which influence how nurses communicate with cancer patients. *Journal of Advanced Nursing*, *16*, *6*, 677–688.

Wilkinson, S., Perry, R., Blanchard, K., and Linsell, L. (2008) Effectiveness of a three-day communication skills course in changing nurses' communication skills with cancer/palliative care patients: A randomised controlled trial. *Palliative Medicine*, *22*, *4*, 365–375.

World Health Organization. (2017). HIV/AIDS: Fact sheet. Available at: www.who.int/news-room/fact-sheets/detail/hiv-aids.

Zimmerman, C., Del Piccolo, L., and Mazzi, M.A. (2003) Patient Cues and medical interviewing in general practice: Examples of the application of sequential analysis. *Epidemmiologia e Psichiatria Socilae*, *12*, *2*, 115–123.

6 Traumatic beginnings, complicated lives

Attachment styles, relationships and HIV care

Sam Warner and Sarah Rutter

Chapter description

This chapter explores how trauma in early attachment experiences can impact physical health outcomes for people living with HIV. Key theoretical perspectives, reflective points and case studies are used to enhance understanding of the impact of different attachment styles on service users' ability to manage their health condition and engage in healthcare relationships. Attention is paid to sociocultural factors relevant to the HIV population and the context of healthcare delivery. The importance of healthcare professionals' own attachment styles is also considered in understanding clinical relationships. The case is made for person-centred clinical responses that are tailored to attachment needs, supported by strong interdisciplinary relationships which underpin supportive, consistent and cohesive interventions.

Attachment theory and mental health

Experiences in early caregiver relationships provide the foundations for emotional and cognitive development and are highly salient in later mental health. Attachment theory (Ainsworth & Bowlby, 1991; Bowlby, 1969, 1973, 1980; Fonagy & Target, 1997; Rutter, 1979, 1981) offers an explanation of how the characteristic ways that people develop their sense of self, their relationships and the worlds in which they live develop through childhood experiences. This view asserts that babies are evolutionarily primed to be social beings that are biologically driven to seek protection from safe adults. From birth, able-bodied babies demonstrate 'attachment behaviours', such as making eye contact, vocalising and attempting to mirror those around them, which in turn invite caregivers to stay close and meet the baby's need for care and comfort. How, and indeed if, these needs are met has implications for whether secure or insecure attachment bonds are created. The particular attachment style that people adopt will not only impact on how they approach intimate relationships and engage in sexual behaviour, but also on their mental health in general and how they engage in help-seeking behaviour thereafter.

Secure attachment

If caregivers respond fairly consistently to attachment behaviours and the infant's (physical) needs are generally met, their internal emotional arousal decreases. This results in mutually reinforcing bonds between the baby and primary caregivers. When expressed needs are met, the baby learns that they are worth caring for and deserving of love, whilst the caregivers experience themselves as competent and loved in return. Through this process of consistent care, the infant develops an enduring sense of safety and security (see Figure 6.1). Children whose parents respond consistently with love and care learn to accept that people will care about them and be responsive to their needs. This helps build a sense of self-worth. Emotionally attuned carers are able to recognise, understand and anticipate the infant's needs. By providing a 'running commentary' about the infant's external behavioural needs (e.g. to be fed, cuddled, changed, etc) and their internal emotional arousal/states (e.g. hungry, sad, scared, uncomfortable vs full-up, happy, calm, etc), such carers help their infant to understand and put labels to their needs and feelings. Thus, they develop an internal working model or template for making sense of their physiological and emotional states, as well as themselves and their relationships. Being helped to label, differentiate and grade the intensity of their feelings enables the developing child to understand different emotional states and to understand the emotional responses of others. Safe, secure and consistent parenting also enables children to internalise their parents' strategies for soothing them when they are distressed. Eventually children will adopt the strategies independently and develop ways to 'self-soothe' when in distress. These internal working models are thought to be stored in neural pathways in the brain, reinforced through repetition, and the template tends to be carried forward into adulthood (Crittenden, 2017; Fisher, 2000).

Insecure attachment

When children have not experienced safe and consistent care, they develop insecure relationship styles. There have been numerous attempts to name and differentiate insecure

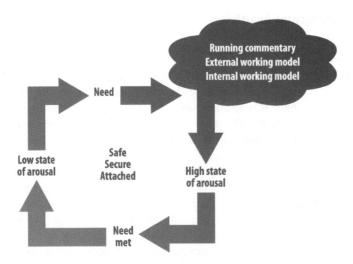

Figure 6.1 Arousal/relaxation cycle
(Warner, adapted from Bowlby)

attachment styles, with ever increasing complexity (e.g. Crittenden, 2017). In simple terms, there are thought to be three main patterns: anxious/ambivalent, avoidant and disorganised/fearful. Of course, in real terms, children can have a range of attachment experiences; however, we will consider the impact of each separately for ease of explanation.

Anxious/ambivalent attachment

The anxious/ambivalently attached person is likely to have received highly inconsistent care as a child. This means that they were never certain whether or not their needs were going to be met, and therefore attachment behaviours are escalated to try to draw more attention to the needs. As caregivers do not always respond to the needs expressed, the child perceives that they are not worth taking care of and becomes constantly fearful of rejection. This can lead to clinginess coupled with anger as proximity does not bring the desired sense of security (they do not trust that person to stay with them). There is also limited opportunity to learn how to self-soothe, as the caregiver has not sufficiently helped the child understand and name their distress and has not demonstrated strategies to manage distress (that would eventually be internalised by the child).

Avoidant attachment

The avoidantly attached person is likely to have experienced a more consistent level of rejection from an emotionally shut-down primary carer. The child's expression of needs is often met with unwanted (e.g. cold, dismissive, blaming) responses. This can result in children learning to avoid all emotional connection and to becoming overly independent and self-reliant. However, although they learn to stay 'under the radar' to avoid negative reactions, internally they continue to experience distress. Again, there has been minimal caregiver support to develop a framework of coping to aid self-soothing.

Disorganised attachment

The disorganised/fearful person has usually experienced highly inconsistent and frightening/frightened carer behaviours. When caregivers are frightening (e.g. abusive), children are too scared to approach them to seek comfort. Where caregivers are frightened, and therefore unavailable (e.g. significant substance use, neglect and/or victimised themselves), the child's needs are not responded to at all or the carer is too disempowered to provide safety and protection. Whether carers are frightened or frightening, the child still wishes to find comfort and feel safe; however, this is not an option as the caregivers are the source of the fear and distress. With absolutely no framework for self-soothing in a situation that brings persistent threat, these children are unable to either escape or resolve the trauma. They therefore adopt survival strategies that best offer some sense of safety, such as dissociation (mentally cutting off from emotional and physical pain) or becoming aggressive to try to fend off threats. As a result the person develops an incoherent and erratic relationship style: they desire connection, but close relationships terrify them. It is these types of experience that tend to lead to severe and enduring mental health problems (Mikulincer & Shaver, 2012; Read, van Os, Morrison, & Ross, 2005)

It is important to note that the impact of care, and the neuro-biological correlates, is influenced by other environmental factors (e.g. Verhage et al., 2016). This points to the need to understand the value of relationship style in the specific sociocultural context in which children and adults live. This is particularly important when thinking about these issues for people living with HIV, as the population is very diverse.

The impact of traumatic stress

Trauma is understood as the experience and/or witnessing of events that elicit a sense of horror, coupled with a feeling of helplessness within that situation. When a person is facing a traumatic event, the body releases a range of stress hormones, which result in physiological changes meant to equip the person with the bodily and mental recourses to engage in either fight or flight behaviour. Additionally, if neither fight nor flight are options, people can freeze, and when people have no way out of a traumatic situation this might lead to a dissociative coping response (the automatic process of cutting off from emotional/physical pain).

During these processes, memories are laid down in a different way and it is these 'unprocessed memories' that later return as flashbacks and nightmares.

If a person does not receive sensitive support after a trauma, meaning that these experiences are not expressed (and therefore not processed), they may begin to experience intrusive recollections of what happened, coupled with overwhelming experiences of the emotions that were present at the time of the event. This is clearly a very distressing experience, where the person feels completely out of control, and often they begin to adopt avoidant coping responses (e.g. avoiding triggers/reminders of the event or trying to suppress trauma-related thoughts and feelings). However, unfortunately, the more a person avoids trauma triggers, the less likely they are to process the experience. Traumatic stress can then increase its power over the person. The resulting sense of helplessness can further fuel fear, which, in turn, exacerbates emotional anxiety and uncomfortable physiological arousal. Without sensitive support, feeling out of control and experiencing the world as a threatening place is likely to have a negative influence on cognitions (the person's view of the world, self and others) and may further lower mood. Additionally, trauma is known to have cumulative impact, in that the more traumas a person experiences, the more intense the impact on their internal state, and their ability to function in the world. For further detail regarding trauma processes, see Brewin, Gregory, Lipton and Burgess (2010), Ehlers and Clarke (2000), Foa, Steketee and Olasov-Rothbaum (1989) and Van der Kolk (2007).

Reflection point

Think about children with disorganised attachments and the amount of trauma they are likely to have lived through (including experiences of severe abuse and neglect).

How will a constant state of fear have affected their emotions and their body at the time?

If they were having to cope by 'cutting off' mentally or adopting aggressive behaviours, how might this have impacted their ability to engage with relationships and the world?

Resilience: why are some people less affected by trauma?

When we are thinking about trauma, it is important to consider how this impacts resilience (see Felitti et al., 1998). Of course, not all people who experience trauma in their early life will develop problems in managing relationships, as some will have supportive factors in place to protect them from this. Resilience can be understood as

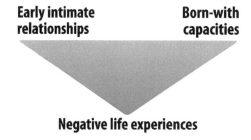

Early intimate relationships

Born-with capacities

Negative life experiences

Figure 6.2 Interactive factors relating to resilience
(Warner, adapted from Bowlby)

being an interactive process influenced by born-with biological capacities, early intimate relationship experiences, environmental factors and negative life events (Warner, 2020, and see Figure 6.2). Each of the factors identified interacts with the other ones. It is in adversity that people learn how to survive: without any trauma, people have no reason to develop a coping repertoire. Yet 'too much' trauma will be too debilitating. A person with a high level of cognitive function (born-with capacity) may be more equipped to make sense of traumatic events (negative life experiences), which can aid resilience. People who have good family support may also be more quickly able to learn coping responses that are modelled and supported by the people around them (early relationships). Hence resilience is not static, but a developing skill, that is impacted by biology, relationships and life.

Adverse experiences: the influence on physical health

Direct impact on health

Trauma and post-trauma stress responses can have a direct impact on physical health, and associations have been found with health problems such as cardiovascular, respiratory, musculoskeletal, genitourinary and gastrointestinal conditions (Banyard, Edwards & Kendall-Tackett, 2009; Robles & Kane, 2014). Regarding HIV specifically, in a review of global literature, stress was found to be associated with disease progression, lower CD4 counts and higher viral loads (Weinsten & Li, 2016). It is also generally accepted that being diagnosed with HIV can count as a traumatic incident in itself (due to the fear of death and stigma) and can therefore have an additive impact on existing post-trauma stress. Biological models point to physiological processes resulting from psychological trauma and anxiety (e.g. sympathetic over-activity, endocrinologic changes (e.g. cortisol levels), chronic inflammation and altered immune system function) that can directly impact health (Brandt, Zvolensky, Woods, Gonzalez & O'Cleirigh, 2017; Nightingale, Sher & Hansen, 2010; Nightingale, Sher, Mattson, Thilges & Hansen, 2011). It is known that stress impacts the hypothalamic pituitary adrenal axis (HPA) and the autonomic nervous system, and repeated exposure to traumatic stress can result in allostatic load (wear and tear on the body). Therefore, people who have lived through repeated and persistent childhood trauma may be at considerable risk of poor health outcomes in comparison with the general population (Felitti et al., 1998). Poor health can then add to existing stressors and thus these reciprocal processes can lead to a downward spiral of physical and mental health.

Indirect impact on health

As well as the direct physiological impact on physical health from trauma experienced in early relationships, there can be an ongoing effect through indirect processes (Norman et al., 2012). A history of abuse, neglect and loss creates problems, and then the strategies that people develop to cope add another layer of difficulty. As noted above, we all learn to take care of ourselves within the context of early relationships, in that carers teach us the skills to cope with distress and manage our well-being. However, if neglect and trauma are present in these relationships, these skills are not learnt. There are also behaviours that children will adopt in situations where carers are the source of trauma and neglect, such as playing down distress (avoidant) or elevating distress signals (ambivalent). These behaviours can be considered adaptive when used in the past, as they help children who are in difficult situations to survive. However, they can become unhelpful in later life and, in the context of healthcare, they can prevent people from accessing required care and treatment (Randhawa et al., 2018). People may decline treatment through denial or opt not to engage in healthcare relationships for fear of reprisal/negative judgement (avoidant); be inconsistent and show high distress in engagement because they never had a consistent care relationship (ambivalent); or be actively self-destructive (disorganised).

In HIV this can be particularly pertinent, as diagnosis and treatment are essential to survival. Antiretroviral treatment (ART) must be taken daily to keep the virus under control in the body so that it cannot attack the immune system. It must also be taken consistently, or resistance is developed, meaning that a particular regime is no longer effective. Although a range of regimes are available, continual adherence issues will lead to more and more resistance and eventually options will run out. Early adversity, perhaps exacerbated by a trauma response to HIV diagnosis, can impact service users' ability to consistently manage their healthcare (Boarts, Buckley-Fishcher, Armelie, Bogart & Delahanty, 2017; Hutchinson & Dhairyawan, 2017). Here, the attachment model outlined above will be applied in terms of understanding the difficulties that people living with HIV, who have complex histories, might have in managing this long-term condition.

Lack of self-care (not worth taking care of)

If a person experiences neglect as a child from their main caregivers, and many needs are left unmet, the inherent message they are likely to receive is that they are not worth caring for. If somebody's physical and emotional needs are left neglected for long enough, they are likely to begin to believe they do not deserve to be cared for, internalising this message and seeing themselves as worthless. Thinking about this in the context of HIV, it then follows that a person who feels worthless may view themselves as unworthy of taking treatment. Feelings of worthlessness, stemming from a history of feeling unloved, are understandably related to low mood and hopelessness (Gilbert, 2002; Howe, 2005). People living with HIV who are experiencing these issues may not be motivated to take life-prolonging medication when they are unable to see a future for themselves. It is also possible that people living with HIV who have been neglected in childhood have not actually learned the skills to take care of themselves in the first place. Without a framework for self-care, the management of a long-term condition like HIV, which requires regimented adherence to antiretroviral therapy and regular health monitoring, can be challenging. Additionally, the experience of being looked after by a healthcare team may be unfamiliar and therefore uncomfortable for a person not accustomed to their needs being met (Berry, Roberts, Danquah & Davies, 2014; Klest, Tamaian & Boughner, 2019; Morris et al., 2009). This is likely to be the most marked for those with disorganised attachments, who hold the framework that people who are meant to care for them, abuse them.

Neglect can often be accompanied by the experience of abuse from caregivers. This can take the form of children being punished for expressing their needs, which can reinforce the idea that they are not worth caring for, and may also lead to the development of thoughts that they are inherently bad in some way and deserve punishment (Horowitz & Stermac, 2018). This framework for thinking is then likely to inform how they approach self-care in adult life (Hutchinson & Dhairyawan, 2017). It may be that when feelings of distress (unmet needs) arise, there is an automatic shame response, as shame is often experienced by people who have lived through abuse because of the nature of what abusers have said in order to silence them, such as 'you are dirty'; 'you are stupid'; 'you deserve this' (Warner, 2000). Longstanding feelings of shame can also be associated with an assumption of deserving punishment (Gilbert, 2002). This can perhaps be even more prevalent for people living with HIV, as the diagnosis is often associated with high levels of shame due to the stigma experienced by this population (see Chapter 8 for more on stigma) . Therefore, not adhering to essential medication can sometimes be interpreted as a form of self-punishment, and this non-adherence can lead to significant health problems.

Self-harm: using self-injury, alcohol and/or drugs (can't self-soothe)

Whatever the attachment style, individuals who are high in attachment anxiety (see Yerkes & Dodson, 1908) can have difficulty regulating strong, often overwhelming emotions that are related to the experience of early trauma (Robles & Kane, 2014). As stated above, those who have been neglected and abused are unlikely to have a framework for self-care, which would include coping with difficult feelings (self-soothing). If caregivers did not teach a child how to manage distress, they will not have internalised these skills and are likely to struggle with this in adulthood. There is a strong chance then of learning to rely on external methods of soothing distress, which can include coping behaviours such as using self-injury, alcohol and/or drugs to regulate their feelings (Norman et al., 2012). Self-injury can be used to distract from otherwise overwhelming emotions (ambivalent attachment style) or to provoke feelings when emotionally numb (avoidant attachment style). Self-injury also enables control over and punishment of the body, which, in terms of HIV, can be experienced in terms of betrayal (of health) and being the 'cause' of feelings of helplessness and hopelessness (about the future) (see Warner & Spandler, 2012).

In terms of alcohol and drug use, people with avoidant attachment styles tend to become cut off and depressed, and are therefore more likely to use stimulants to alter this state. Those with more ambivalent attachment styles, who may be highly emotional, are more likely to use 'downers' to provide relief from overwhelming feelings. Of course, attachment histories can be complex, and in reality people may switch between states and engage in multiple types of substance use to manage hypo- and hyper-emotional states. Using external methods to cope with emotional distress is, of course, not limited to people who have experienced trauma, and we can all engage in 'unhealthy' coping strategies from time to time. Perhaps then it is easy to understand how someone with persistent overwhelming emotional experiences stemming from a complex trauma history may use self-injury, alcohol and drugs to escape these high levels of overwhelming emotion (Warner & Shaw, 2016).

Reflection point

Think about the things we all might do after a stressful experience that might not be good for your health?
Does being aware they are not good for you always stop you doing it?

It is known that there are higher levels of emotional distress within the HIV population (British HIV Association, 2018; World Health Organization, 2008), and within some sub-sections of the HIV population, alcohol/substance use is high, presumably (to some degree) related to coping with living with the condition (e.g. Flentroy, Young, Blue & Gilbert, 2015; Maxwell, Shahmanesh & Gafos, 2019; Van Tieu & Koblin, 2009; Warner & Shaw, 2016). Alcohol and drug misuse can lead to people having chaotic lifestyles, and for people living with HIV this can make it difficult to manage medication regimes and attend health appointments. Alcohol and drug use affects thinking and memory, meaning medication doses may be missed, or taken repetitively. ART adherence issues, along with the inherent additional health risks of alcohol and drug use (e.g. chronic obstructive pulmonary disease, cardiac, vascular) and other risks such as (further) exposure to sexually transmitted infections, can lead to poor health outcomes (Vagenas et al., 2015). For those people who have an attachment history where they had to please others in order to keep themselves safe, this can impact their ability to negotiate safe sex and also means they easily follow the influence of others, which can lead to a variety of risk situations. Furthermore, attachment anxiety has been found to affect glucose levels, which is in turn related to self-control (Robles & Kane, 2014), and this could add to the risks described above through further increased risks of disinhibited and impulsive behaviours.

Stigma and shame (reliving previous abuse)

For many people who have experienced abuse in their early life, strong feelings of shame are carried into adulthood (Gilbert, 2002). A diagnosis of HIV can add to a sense of shame, due to the societal stigma attached to the condition (see Chapter 8 on stigma for further detail). In addition, HIV is more concentrated in already marginalised groups in society (Watkins-Hayes, 2014), for example men who have sex with men (MSM), asylum seekers and people with mental health issues, which can increase the experience of stigma and therefore the likelihood of shame. The fear of stigma and the resulting discrimination may prevent someone (particularly disorganised and avoidant copers) being tested for and/or seeking healthcare support after HIV diagnosis (Hutchinson & Dhairyawan, 2017). Without testing and treatment, the condition is likely to lead to serious health deterioration, even death, as well as risk of onward transmission of HIV.

Stigma and shame can be issues for many living with HIV, but for those who had adverse early experiences, this is likely to be heightened. The deeply held expectation of negative judgement from others may sensitise a person to more intense emotional responses when they are faced with stigma and discrimination. This can lead to people living with HIV to conceal their condition from others, which can pose problems for healthcare engagement, such as taking treatment and attending appointments (Hutchinson & Dhairyawan, 2017). Keeping HIV a secret can also, inadvertently, reinforce feelings of shame – the secrecy giving it validation. Shame is a very powerful feeling that brings considerable emotional distress, and as already discussed, people with complex histories can find difficulty managing strong feelings. This means that defensive coping styles are likely to be adopted, such as avoidance of shame-triggering situations or engagement in external distress reduction (e.g. substance use). Medication adherence can be impacted by avoiding healthcare, or through inability to engage due to a chaotic lifestyle (e.g. drug or alcohol use). Additionally, the daily requirements of ART act as a reminder of HIV and can reactivate current feelings of shame, which are underpinned by longstanding issues. People may, therefore, opt not to take medication to avoid reminders of HIV and associated negative emotional responses (Ehlers & Clarke, 2000).

It is also important to think about the influence of different environments and subcultures on people's responses to a diagnosis of HIV. Some MSM enter into sexualised drug use (chemsex) to escape the persistent psychological adversity/trauma associated with societal homophobia and HIV stigma (Pollard, Nadarzynski & Llewellyn, 2018) (see Chapter 7). This can lead to a range of physical, relational and emotional harms (Morris, 2019). In communities where there are intolerant social and/or religious frameworks, lack of knowledge and understanding relating to HIV or where prejudices against certain groups are openly expressed, people living with HIV may struggle to access support (Addo-Atuah & Lundmark, 2015). This adds to concealment and can worsen adjustment to and coping with the condition. These factors can also affect access to treatment. For example, some people living with HIV decline to use interpreters where there is a language barrier, due to fears about breaches of confidentiality that would mean their HIV status may become known in their local community. This impacts care via limitations to clear communication of HIV-related information, lack of understanding of treatment and choices and may be a further barrier to seeking out medical care when required. Conversely, people who are otherwise privileged (e.g. straight white men) may feel they are not catered for within the HIV community. Alongside struggling with a sense of dislocation, they may feel shame engendered by their HIV status and their now felt rejection from dominant normative society (ibid.).

Reflection point

Think about how it would feel if people in your life found out a secret of yours that you felt very ashamed of? How do you think you would cope with this?

Relationships and sexual choices/not choices

Our understanding of relationships and how we expect to be treated within them is rooted in our early experiences. If we have had relatively secure attachments to important people in our lives, we are more likely to be able to make choices regarding sex and relationships that are non-damaging and fulfilling. This is because people who have been loved and cared for will probably be equipped with adequate levels of self-esteem and therefore are more able to negotiate within relationships to have needs met, are less likely to tolerate mistreatment or to mistreat others (as this is not what they expect/are familiar with).

For those who have had insecure or disorganised attachments, expectations within relationships will also be skewed toward what they have already experienced. This may include exposure to neglect, persistent criticism, punishment and various forms of abusive behaviours. With the accompanying low self-esteem, it may be difficult for the person to challenge these patterns or leave the relationship, as there is often the belief that they are worthless and may not, therefore, attract another partner. This may be exacerbated in situations where people feel an extra layer of shame in association with issues relating to sexuality, gender or cultural expectations. The fear of being alone may outweigh the fear experienced in the relationship. This points to the issue of inter-partner violence, which has a high prevalence in the HIV population (UNAIDS, 2019). It is important to note that both survivors and perpetrators of inter-partner violence are likely to have difficult histories that influence their relational behaviours. People will learn how to be afraid, self-critical, etc, and will adapt how they behave in order to survive, which unfortunately often perpetuates the cycle and keeps them trapped in adverse situations (ibid.).

People living with these issues may not always be able to negotiate safe sex practices to protect either themselves or others. For those in abusive relationships, threats and fear may dictate whether or not protection is used (ibid.). Those engaging in more casual sexual encounters may not feel confident (due to low self-esteem) to insist on protected sex as they fear rejection. These issues will similarly affect confidence to tell people that they are living with HIV, particularly when coupled with deep-rooted feelings of shame stemming from childhood, which may have been reinforced by acquiring a condition where stigma/discrimination is a reality. Again, we can think about engagement in chemsex, which is often in order to avoid persistent shame and low self-esteem of MSM, and how this can lead to a wide range of relational encounters, where problems relating to consent can arise (Ward, McQuillan & Evans, 2017). Therefore, they may be at increased risk of contracting (further) sexually transmitted conditions themselves, or could be conceived as putting others at risk if they are living with HIV/STIs (ibid.).

These risks are likely to be enhanced for those with disorganised attachment styles that have resulted in extreme victimhood, where issues such as inter-partner violence/abuse, considerable substance abuse and limited ability to self-care might be present. People with considerable mental health difficulties may be powerless to keep themselves safe in many aspects of their life, including choices around safe sex (Boni-Saenz, 2016). Additionally, some people who were victimised in childhood can present as perpetrators in adulthood: people learn by modelling and some people can adopt the abusive or neglectful behaviour themselves, as a defence against further victimisation and as a learned strategy for getting their needs met. This may explain why some people living with HIV deliberately transmit the condition to others, perhaps in an attempt to attain a sense of power to push away the pain and fear of victimhood. Thankfully, this is extremely rare, as most survivors of abuse become protectors, rather than perpetrators. This is evidenced by those HIV positive persons who draw on their lived experience to inform their work in healthcare settings and service user groups.

Attachment and marginalised groups

The HIV population is made up of people from all backgrounds, as anybody can acquire the condition; however, there are certain populations who are at greater risk than others. Risks can be increased for some groups based on factors including, but not limited to, gender, ethnicity, sexuality, religion, age, physical ability and learning ability (Watkins-Hayes, 2014). As mentioned above, psychosocial factors relating to homophobic societal attitudes have been found to underpin the practice of 'chemsex' by MSM, placing them at greater risk of acquiring HIV (Pollard et al., 2018; Ward et al., 2017). We have also discussed risk pertaining to inter-partner violence, perhaps especially vulnerable women and gay men (UNAIDS, 2019) and to people belonging to ethnic groups where there is a strong religious influence and inaccurate information about HIV is promoted (Addo-Atuah & Lundmark, 2015). Heightened risk of HIV transmission is generally due to structural inequalities, although physical risk factors can also play a part. For example, certain sexual practices of MSM, sexual assault or female genital mutilation carried out by subsections of African, Middle Eastern and Asian communities increase the likelihood of HIV transmission/acquisition (UNAIDS, 2019). Additionally, structural inequalities intersect with each other. Individuals from groups that are multiply marginalised in society through discrimination can find their ability to keep themselves safe severely compromised.

However, there are of course many individuals who overcome oppressive forces and develop strong resilience. These are likely to be people, as indicated earlier, who have born-with adaptation skills coupled with secure attachment experiences that have allowed the development of sufficient self-worth and esteem and whose early experiences of adversity have provoked the development of survival skills and considerable post-trauma growth (Jay, 2018). The case study below provides an example of how the intersection of a range of social identities can render someone vulnerable to acquiring HIV.

Case example

Melanie is a black transgender woman who moved from Africa to the UK when she was 5 years old and grew up in a small town. Her family was very religious and had fixed ideas based on traditional values. She was an only child and the atmosphere of the home was one characterised by an emphasis on 'good behaviour' and not bringing embarrassment to the family. Although she was well looked after in terms of her physical and material needs, Melanie often felt controlled in terms of expression of her psychological needs due to her experience of punitive responses from her parents should she become 'overly emotional'. Melanie knew from a young age that her body did not fit with her gender; however, she was fearful of discussing this due to worries that she would be punished and/or rejected.

During her school years Melanie did not have many friends. As she was perceived by others to be male at this point, she was teased by other boys who called her 'soft' and 'gay'. The majority of students were white and it was difficult for her to fit in, as she also sometimes experienced prejudicial comments related to race. She tried to remain under the radar by keeping herself to herself and concentrating on her studies, at which she did very well. However, she recalled feeling different from other children, due to her African heritage and gender dysphoria. She spent a lot of her social time at home in her room.

In adulthood, Melanie began to transition to the gender with which she identified, which eased her internal distress, and she made a couple of friends through supportive online networks who she met up with occasionally. However, she had worries about pursuing relationships as her self-esteem was low, underpinned by feelings of shame. She thought that she would not find anyone to love her, as she was 'weird'. Although Melanie worked, she avoided social contact outside of this for several years after her transition. However, her sense of loneliness was becoming overwhelming. She accepted an invitation to go out one evening; feeling extremely anxious, she drank alcohol to cope with these feelings. Melanie adopted this as a strategy whenever she went out, and although she found it easier to make intimate connections, this often resulted in vague memories about what had happened. Due to her low self-esteem and need to feel accepted/loved, Melanie found herself participating in sexual acts that she did not really enjoy in order to please the other person. She also lacked the confidence to negotiate safe sex and so was often placed in a position of risk. After unsafe sexual encounters, Melanie tended to feel ashamed and withdrew socially for a while. However, such was her need to feel emotionally connected, she would use alcohol, and eventually other substances, in order to engage on an intimate level.

- What type of attachment style do you think Melanie developed and why?
- What early events underpinned her unmet needs and emotional issues in adulthood?
- Reflecting on how people had treated Melanie in her earlier life, why do you think she avoided social contact? Used alcohol to socialise? Participated in unpleasurable acts to please others?

Attachment styles are thus shaped not only by within-family experiences, but also through wider structural discrimination and oppression that can instigate further traumatic experiences, increase relationship anxiety and negatively impact self-worth. Whilst this is not inevitable, for those individuals who cope with both family *and* societal rejection/ oppression, this can further undermine their resilience.

The context of care

When the HIV epidemic initially began and there were no effective treatments, this meant that end of life was expected and somewhat inevitable for those diagnosed with the condition. This, in combination with the huge stigma attached to HIV, resulted in services providing a wraparound care approach. It may have been that many healthcare professionals working in the area felt strongly protective over their patients and historical documentation of this time indicates an 'over and above' approach to care. This was perfectly understandable and appropriate to the circumstance where there was no hope, and healthcare professionals did all that they could to help those who were dying. However, this will no doubt have come at some personal cost, evidenced by the history of burnout in HIV staff (Ginossar et al., 2014).

With the vast improvements in medication, HIV is thankfully now a manageable long-term condition. However, alongside this, there has been an accompanying change to health service delivery, which advocates a self-management approach. This has been underpinned by NHS structural changes resulting from the implementation of the Health and Social Care Act (2012), including the establishment of local clinical commissioning groups that affect how care is delivered. Within HIV services, this meant that service users could no longer get their non-HIV-related healthcare needs met by the HIV team. For many people living with

HIV, this has not caused significant issue, specifically those who are resilient – that is, emotionally and cognitively equipped to get on with their lives and look after their health. However, for some (particularly long-term survivors) this shift from what could be understood as 'ideal care' can feel like a form of abandonment. This is most likely to be the case for people with adverse histories, whose insecure attachment style and template for relationships predicts they will be rejected or abandoned.

HIV teams as a 'pseudo family'

Although there have been vast improvements in HIV treatment, there is no cure, which means people living with the condition require lifelong care. Service users are generally able to choose where they receive this care (not postcode dependent) and can therefore move around services at will. However, quite often people choose to remain under the same service for many years, perhaps due to a wish to share the diagnosis with as few services as possible, or because the team may be the only people in the person's life who are aware of the diagnosis. This means that the relationships that form are not transient, as they can be in other healthcare situations. The attachments that are formed can be experienced as an extended support network, perhaps mimicking a type of family unit if we relate this to attachment theory. If the team can resemble a family/support network, it is easy to see how issues from early relationships can play out.

This can be a challenge to delivering optimum care, as service users with experiences of insecure attachments, together with experiences of trauma, can have difficulties accurately interpreting the thoughts, feelings and behaviours of others (Howe, 2005). This can lead to problems managing relationships and to the triggering of strong emotions. Where there has been a significant history of abuse and/or neglect, without sufficiently protective relationships/experiences, it is understandable that there may be historically based unmet needs, which can then manifest in healthcare relationships. Service users from marginalised communities may also fear that healthcare providers will replicate the rejecting, dismissing or aggressive behaviour they have experienced within wider society and sometimes from within their own specific communities. This is why all services must be mindful of the Equality Act (2010) and the need to work fairly with people who have 'protected characteristics'. It may be helpful, therefore, to consider how different attachment styles require different approaches by the healthcare team.

Styling services to specific attachment needs

Easing high distress: proactive and consistent approaches

In terms of how relational issues can play out, people presenting with an ambivalent attachment style may require frequent reassurance around healthcare, and make regular contact with services to try to feel adequately cared for (Berry et al., 2014). This is because, in their experience, there was no guarantee that carers would respond to needs, which results in underlying anxieties that essential care will not always be provided. To begin to counteract these assumptions, it may be helpful for the team to adopt a proactive and consistent approach to care delivery. This will include drawing up care plans agreed in collaboration with the person that clearly define health needs and how they will be addressed, paying attention to how and how often contact will be made. So for example, it may be agreed that a designated professional will proactively contact the person once a month to check in on their general needs. Times may also be set around regularity of care such as monitoring HIV-related bloods (dependent on the person's health circumstances) and the provision of prescriptions. It will be important to set out a concise framework relating to the boundaries of care: including what the service can provide and what it cannot. This may help to avoid a situation where a person, who remains anxious about their needs not being met, feels rejected or abandoned when a service is unable to respond to a certain request.

In order for this to be helpful over time, boundaries set out must be adhered to consistently across all involved in the care. The ultimate aim would be to support the person to build their coping repertoire to empower them to self-manage. However, for those with disorganised attachment styles and severe mental health issues, a certain level of support is likely to be an ongoing need. Additionally, if clients have experienced highly inconsistent care as children, they are likely to be inconsistent themselves. As noted, this can lead to inconsistent adherence to medical regimes and/or clients being experienced as argumentative, difficult or challenging. When this happens, professionals need to remain calm and consistent, and not be drawn into 'telling off' the client, as this can re-invoke feelings for the client of being threatened and frightened. Paradoxically this can lead to a greater chance of the undesired behaviour through trigger of the distress system and employment of historical 'unhelpful' coping.

Sometimes less is more

On the other hand, where people have more of an avoidant attachment style, there may be fears relating to the receipt of care. This is because historical expressions of need were usually unmet or responses were routinely hostile, punishing and/or abusive. The person would then have learned not to rely on others and/or to remain 'under the radar' to avoid hostility and aggression. Here we might see people avoiding contact with healthcare professionals and disengaging from services, as this feels safer than risking rejection (reject first, before being rejected) or facing potentially punitive responses again (Morris et al., 2009). This is likely to be heightened in the context of HIV, where there may be associated feelings of shame and anticipated negative judgement. In terms of a team response, this might contrast somewhat with one offered to people who will benefit from one that explores their needs in detail. This would be likely to feel too intense and result in the person retreating even further. Teams would fare better to find a plan of care that has minimal intrusion, whilst meeting the basic needs that require care. For example, arranging clinical contact only when necessary (based on health situation) and not pressing on matters of sensitivity that may result in the person feeling they are being backed into a corner.

It is likely to be helpful to take time to build the relationship, perhaps by discussing matters within the person's comfort zone, until a 'safe base' begins to form. This may then be a basis to begin to explore deeper matters, if the person initiates or consents to this. Again, a collaboratively agreed care plan and a consistent approach will still be of upmost importance, so that the person can feel informed and in control of their care. People who are highly anxious about intimacy will benefit from reassurance, open dialogue, clear explanations and understandings about the extent and limits of care. This type of approach, in which the professional provides a 'running commentary' about care, mimics the behaviour of attuned parents with infants and can help promote healthy attachments in care-based relationships.

Recognising the complexity: interdisciplinary responses

To aid thinking about attachment styles, the above paragraphs approached these relational patterns in terms of a person having one style or another. However, in reality, it is often more complex than this, with a person deriving different attachment styles from various relationships in their life. Additionally, attachment styles can shift over a lifetime, with different coping styles being triggered by significant life events. For example, when relationships end in adulthood (perhaps through breakdown or a bereavement), this can cause considerable distress. Previously securely attached people might then temporarily withdraw from relationships, or seek intimacy with multiple partners (Muller, 2014), the latter perhaps increasing risks relating to unsafe sex.

This ever-shifting complexity can create challenges for the team to meet needs in the context of healthcare relationships. A thorough assessment of a person's presentation would be required to ascertain how they would prefer their care to be managed. Additionally, although the overall aim of care plans would be to empower to the person to eventually manage their healthcare with increasing independence, there may be some people who will always require a full package of support. These are likely to be people who have experienced extreme levels of abuse and neglect in their childhood and have therefore developed disorganised attachment styles. An interdisciplinary approach may be the optimum way to support people with such complex issues, as medical and psychosocial problems are likely to be inter-related. Therefore, addressing intertwined aspects of care together as a team, with MDT members combining knowledge and skills to work alongside the person, could offer the most coherent and effective healthcare approach. This approach has been found to be helpful within other medical settings (Crawford, Espie, Bartlett & Gunstein, 2014; Erskine et al., 2013). Joint working can be useful where there are inter-related physical and mental health issues. Being in a room together with the service user and sharing decisions, rather than professionals discussing care plans just with each other, can help avoid a person feeling 'done to' (unintentionally re-enacting dynamics from the past). It is also important to remember that, developmentally, dependence comes before independence and that inter-dependence is the usual state for human beings. As such, it is okay for clients to express feelings of dependency, particularly in the early stages following diagnosis, as this is a highly anxious time, whatever the attachment style. Securely attached clients may move through the high dependency stage more quickly than insecure clients. Some insecure clients, as noted, may always need a greater level of ancillary support.

The attachment style of healthcare professionals: why this matters

When delivering care, the personal characteristics and interpersonal style of the healthcare professional are, of course, highly pertinent (Mimura & Norman, 2018). We all have our own stories, which contain a range of different experiences that have shaped who we are and how we interact with the world (see Chapter 2, which explores self-awareness). The early experiences of all healthcare professionals will have led to the development of particular attachment styles, just as they have for service users. Individual attachment styles will guide the care delivered in the context of relational interactions with those receiving care, and when there are insecure templates (for service user, healthcare professional or both), this can create a complex clinical situation (Khodabakhsh,

2012). It is also important to note that healthcare professionals are in an unavoidable position of power as a care provider (Bullock, Gergel, & Kingma, 2015; Johnstone, 2012). This can clearly exacerbate issues in interpersonal relationships where there is a history of abuse and carers withholding care.

As outlined above, where there has been childhood trauma, the template a person has for relationships has been developed with the aim of keeping safe. However, these strategies that are formed in childhood, such as escalating attachment behaviours to ensure care, or withdrawal to avoid aggression, can begin to cause relationship issues in adulthood. This can bring complications when a person living with HIV, who has an adverse history of parenting, is then in a position of having to receive lifelong care. The expectations of poor care (e.g. abuse, neglect, etc) can be, unconsciously, placed onto the care providers. This can result in the service user been experienced as difficult to care for, as they might either place high demands on service resources (ambivalent), withdraw/disengage from service contact (avoidant) or present with an erratic combination of both (disorganised). This can feel stressful for those providing care and experiences of distress can trigger the healthcare professional's own attachment system.

As such, it is important for healthcare providers to reflect on their own attachment styles and developmental history/life experiences (which are not static, but ongoing) and how these impact their relationships with clients (the ones we like *and* the ones that 'push our buttons'). We should also be mindful of the local, legal and professional contexts in which we work and which also shape our interpersonal relationships with our clients and our colleagues. For example, a stressful, under-resourced work environment, where staff may not feel 'looked after', can trigger healthcare workers' own attachment systems and lead to potentially 'unhelpful' coping behaviours rooted in their own developmental history. Figure 6.3 sets out how these implicit factors may all interact (which mirror the client's explicit issues).

Reflection point

Think about a time when you have had a stressful interaction with a patient. What kind of feelings did you experience? Where did these come from (something about you and/or the client)? And how did you cope with them?

Were any healthcare system stressors playing a part?

Did this affect how you provided care?

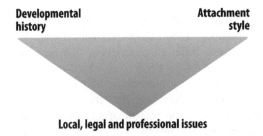

Figure 6.3 Implicit factors in assessment: professional issues

Given that most people can have elements of ambivalent or avoidant attachment style (albeit, not as marked as those who have experienced significant trauma), situations and relationships experienced as challenging in a work context may elicit strong responses. For instance, a staff member with a slightly avoidant attachment style might avoid contact with a service user (with a more ambivalent attachment style) who has called to complain about receiving what they perceive as being poor care, e.g. they have not been contacted with their HIV blood results as was agreed. This avoidance of addressing the issue with the service user might then reinforce the idea that adequate care is not being provided, thus intensifying the service user's distress. This distress may build up, and if the service user is unable to self-soothe, it could eventually erupt in an aggressive outburst. An avoidant staff member may then try to further retreat from involvement in their care, thus perpetuating the problem. Alternatively, a healthcare professional with a more ambivalent attachment style, who is primed to experience their own needs as unacknowledged, with a resulting build-up of stress, might respond to the service user in a similarly aggressive manner. This would clearly also have a negative impact on the healthcare relationship, no doubt adding to problems for the service user trusting others with their care and perhaps leading to service disengagement. The situation might exacerbate underlying feelings of worthlessness for the service user if there has been considerable trauma and neglect (not worth taking care of). For the healthcare professional, underlying worries about job capability may be triggered, particularly if the reason for their ambivalent attachment style was a background that was shaped by critical parenting. There are endless ways in which these complicated historical dynamics can play out in the here and now, with different scenarios triggering different aspects of our attachment style and coping systems. The following case study gives a further example.

Case study

Elizabeth is from Eastern Europe and experienced significant neglect and abuse in her childhood. Her father was an aggressive and punitive man and her mother had been too frightened to protect her from this. Elizabeth was an only child and spent much of her early life alone in her room, as the atmosphere in the family home was volatile. She had also experienced persistent sexual abuse as a child from an uncle. The abuser had used threats to silence her; however, when she reached her teenage years she told her parents what had happened. Her father beat her when she spoke of this and her mother told her not to mention it again as it would bring shame on the family.

As she entered adulthood, Elizabeth formed a relationship with a man who was initially supportive and promised to look after her. However, over time he became more and more controlling and began to use her history to convince her that nobody else would want to be with her. Whenever she tried to leave him he became violent. Throughout their relationship she was aware he was engaging in sexual contact outside of their relationship but was powerless to address this. He insisted on unprotected sex and became threatening if she tried to suggest otherwise.

Elizabeth was very unwell on the run up to receiving the diagnosis, and she was referred to an HIV team. She met with her consultant and a specialist nurse,

Jeanette, and for some time was consistent in attending appointments and main-taining her treatment regimen. However, she began to struggle to take treatment and started to miss appointments. Jeanette was understandably anxious about this and would contact her regularly. Whenever she was able to meet with Elizabeth, she asked her a lot of questions, trying to understand her situation. She also reiter-ated how serious her health condition was and reminded her of the negative conse-quences of not taking ART. Jeanette was constantly worried that she would not adhere to her regime. Elizabeth would agree to treatment plans, but then would 'go off the radar' and not take her ART. This irritated Jeanette as she felt she was not being listened to or respected. They would make plans to meet to monitor Eli-zabeth's blood results, and she would often text her in between appointments to check her intentions about attending, expressing the importance of this.

- What does Elizabeth's behaviour suggest about her attachment style?
- What does Jeanette's behaviour suggest about her attachment style?
- How do you think the styles are interacting in the situation?
- What might have helped?

Although Jeanette's anxiety and urge to gain further details was understandable, this may have made Elizabeth feel backed into a corner. It may also have led to her feeling criticised regarding not taking her ART. Therefore these interactions, although based in good intentions, could have unintentionally re-activated early dynamics of feeling controlled and threatened. In this case, it may have felt safer for Elizabeth to be supported whatever her choices at that time, and for Jeanette to continue regular, planned contact that did not necessarily push to explore adher-ence issues. This way they may have been able to begin to build a relationship ('safe base') where eventually Elizabeth may have felt safe/comfortable to begin discussing sensitive issues.

Complicated healthcare interactions and shifting roles

In light of the complex interpersonal interactions that occur between service users and healthcare professionals, particularly when the former have had severely adverse life experiences, it can be helpful to use a framework to understand the complex and shifting dynamics. If we are better able to understand what is happening, we are better able to address complex issues and less likely to be pulled into unhelpful dynamics that can negatively affect service user care. The 'drama triangle' (Karpman, 1968) (Figure 6.4) can be a useful tool when thinking about how past trauma can affect present interactions (see Figure 6.4) based on the idea that the states are fluid, and we can all shift between them dependent on the situation and the personal responses triggered.

The framework works on the assumption that when a person has experienced abuse (including neglect) in childhood, that person understands what it feels like to be a victim of this abuse, which forms part of their identity. The victim state can be triggered by conditions where the person feels under threat, or that their needs are not being met. However, as well as understanding how it feels to be a victim of abuse, it is proposed that the person has also learned by modelling – observing what it is like to be an

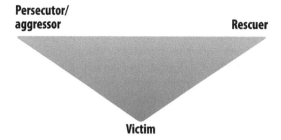

**Persecutor/
aggressor**   **Rescuer**

Victim

Figure 6.4 The 'drama triangle' (Karpman, 1968)

aggressor/abuser/bully – and integrates this on some level into their repertoire of behaviours. There are then times that the person shifts into this state with the aim of self-protection. It is also hypothesised that those with histories of abuse may have experienced some kind of relationship that was protective, this being understood as someone who came in as a 'rescuer' in their situation. This could have been a grandparent, school teacher, etc, who offered relief from the intolerable situation. However, for some there was no such protection, and these people are likely to develop severe and enduring mental health difficulties (e.g. experiences of psychosis). Irrespective of whether there were protective relationships or not, the model predicts that a person in considerable distress (victim mode) is likely to draw a rescuer response from others, particularly healthcare professionals, whose job role primes them to help (rather than persecute) 'victims'. It is important to remember that at points of crisis clients may need 'rescuing'. However, if we continue to rescue, we may not be 'persecuting' the client, but it may keep them stuck in 'victim' mode. As such, as soon as the crisis is past, we should aim for negotiation: so that no one is the rescuer, persecutor or victim.

Case example

Peter is a white, heterosexual male who has been living with HIV for over ten years. He has found it difficult to accept his diagnosis and has had issues with adherence over the years. He oscillates between making frequent contact with the team and disengaging from care.

Peter's early life was characterised by domestic violence by his father toward his mother. He recalled being constantly criticised by his father, who also used physical punishments. He said that although his mother was kind to him when they were alone, she was unable to protect him when his father was present. His mother and father divorced when he was around 10 years old; however, there followed a number of 'stepfathers' who were either aggressive or dismissive of Peter. He experienced his mother as always putting the needs of her partners before his.

This history has resulted in Peter developing an expectation that his needs will not be met, a framework which he applies to his healthcare relationships. Due to him struggling to live with his diagnosis, he often feels unable to manage his condition, leaving him feeling helpless when he starts to become extremely unwell (victim state). Some of the nursing staff respond to Peter's distress by going above and beyond in terms of trying to meet his needs (rescuer state). His expression of needs tends to escalate; perhaps driven by an unconscious drive to feel ideally cared for. Other staff can become frustrated by Peter's escalating 'demands', particularly when he is not taking his treatment, and can express their annoyance by being abrupt with him, or delaying contact with him (persecutor state).

Over time, the staff who connect with Peter's distress take over his care for the most part, and continue to try to meet his needs with a view to helping him take his medication. However, there comes a point where Peter asks to be prescribed a medication that is not connected to HIV-related health issues and the staff explain they are unable to provide this. In response, Peter becomes very angry and is verbally abusive to the staff in question (persecutor state). The staff are shocked and upset by this, as they have always tried to help him as much as they can (victim state).

Why has Peter shifted to the persecutor state in his relationship with staff when they have tried their best to support him?

Although staff have had the best intentions in helping Peter and trying to meet his escalating needs, by remaining in the rescuer role for him, they have inadvertently kept Peter in the victim state. When the staff were unable to resolve a particular request, this was experienced by Peter as reinforcing his expectations that people did not care enough to support him. As Peter does not feel equipped to manage his own issues (was never taught how to), this creates a state of intense helplessness (victim state) that he is unable to tolerate. In order to protect himself from these overwhelming feelings, Peter shifts from 'victim' to 'persecutor', as it is preferable to feel like the latter than the former. However, this now leaves some of the staff feeling victimised and helpless in terms of how to go on supporting Peter. Others have had an anger response, which now places them also in the persecutor state and in conflict with Peter. This is why it is important to recognise when we are drawn into a drama triangle: step back and reflect on the process and share insights with the client in order to enable moving forward into negotiation.

As well as considering dynamics on an individual level, we can also apply the drama triangle to the history of HIV services. We can think about how in the early days of HIV treatment, healthcare professionals probably felt very helpless, as they were unable to 'save' the people they were looking after: 'victims' of an aggressive condition (persecutor) that could not be stopped. This helplessness was probably incongruent with feeling competent in a valued role, and perhaps resulted in staff shifting from the victim state to the rescuer role, which (as noted) was more in keeping with their professional identity. Although things have thankfully changed significantly since then, the complexities of living with HIV persist, and where there are histories of adverse care, complex dynamics can still play out.

Addressing complex dynamics

As indicated, the first step toward addressing unhelpful dynamics is to find a way to step back and understand what is happening. Using frameworks such as the drama triangle can help us do this and recognise when we are being pulled into certain positions. To understand unhelpful dynamics, it is important to acknowledge a service user's position (and what might underpin this), our own position (and what might underpin that) and how these positions are interacting. The idea is that if you can see it and say it, you can change it. The general aim is to resist the pull of the positions, and negotiation is a helpful strategy to achieve this. Negotiation involves hearing/validating a person's distress, working together to identify what their needs are in that situation and then having an open discussion about decisions/treatment options.

Negotiation can prevent a person feeling 'done to', which may (unintentionally) activate a feeling of being controlled (victim of the persecutor). It can also prevent the potential for the healthcare professional trying to do everything for the person, which can (unintentionally) activate a feeling of helplessness in the situation (victim of the rescuer). The very act of acknowledging a person's needs and distress and then collaboratively exploring options can also bring a service user, who may have slipped into the persecutor position (to perhaps protect them from feeling vulnerable), out of a more aggressive state. Although there is always an inherent power to the role of the healthcare professional, successful negotiation can help balance this out a little. It is also central to a patient-centred approach to healthcare and the process may also begin to empower previously disempowered service users to begin to self-manage healthcare issues.

It can also be helpful to adopt a 'visible' approach to communication (Warner, 2009). This involves healthcare professionals naming the intentions behind their actions, such as explicitly stating why they are doing what they are doing. For people who have had difficult relationship histories, there can often be (understandable) issues around trust. By naming our thinking processes, we can prevent people from having to second-guess our intentions. As we have discussed in this chapter, people with histories of abuse and neglect will often apply the expectations of this framework to current relationships, in that they anticipate that people's intentions toward them are malevolent. By making our intentions clear, we can reduce service user distress and begin to offer an alternative framework for relationships. See below for some examples of phrases that might be helpful in the process.

Hearing/validating distress

- 'I can understand why this is worrying for you.'
- 'I can see that this has annoyed you.'
- 'From what you are saying it seems this situation is quite frightening for you.'

Collaborative identification of needs

- 'What can I do to help right now?'
- 'What are the most important issues for you?'
- 'Is there something you think we should address first?'

Shared decision-making

- 'Based on the information we have discussed, what would you like to do first?'
- 'Of the different options we've explored, which feels the best fit for you?'
- 'I think this could be a helpful choice for you, but am interested in what you think.'

Visible communication

- 'I hope you don't feel backed into a corner. I just think this might be a good option for you.'
- 'I'm giving you all of this information so we can think it through together. I don't want you to feel like I am taking over.'
- 'Shall I give you some space to think about it, so you don't feel pressured? I can call you tomorrow.'

Acknowledging/apologising

- 'I am sorry that I upset you.'
- 'I am sorry that you felt like I was backing you into a corner.'
- 'I'm sorry that I wasn't very clear before.'
- 'Thank you for letting me know what didn't feel okay for you before.'

Delivering services: the provision of a secure base

Although it comes with complications, if managed well, the 'pseudo family' set-up can provide the opportunity to create a 'safe base' for those people who have difficult or traumatic histories and have never known 'good enough' care (Chen et al., 2013). There is the potential to support people who may have difficulties taking care of themselves, to begin to understand their care needs and to find healthier ways to look after themselves. Effective support can occur through a team developing care plans specific to people's needs and working alongside the service user to reliably implement them (Bennet, Fuertes, Keitel & Phillips, 2011). Such tailored care can not only provide a framework for what care can look like, but attention to individual needs can also develop a person's self-esteem ('I am worth caring for'). Working alongside people in this way may eventually empower a person to take their care into their own hands and therefore reduce anxiety about their needs not being met. Therefore, the provision of a safe base of care has the potential to improve health outcomes. Attuned healthcare workers, like attuned parents, are focused on the people they are caring for. Through careful reflection, professionals will be better able to meet their clients' health and relationship needs and to anticipate when and why ruptures in the professional–client relationship may occur. Ruptures occur in all relationships (good parents and kind professionals set limits and disagree with their children and clients sometimes). It is the ability and willingness to repair ruptures that is important and which strengthen relationships over time (Siegel, 1999)

Recommendations

On considering the information discussed in this chapter, some recommendations for service delivery can be made. However, it is recognised that this is an 'ideal' that may not be possible to fully implement without sufficient resources. The complex needs often seen in long-term physical health conditions, including HIV, often call for interdisciplinary approaches, particularly where there are mutually exacerbating physical and mental health issues (Naylor et al., 2016). In reality, many HIV teams across the UK do not have in-house psychologists or mental health professionals (National HIV Nurses Association, 2015) and, with the divisions in NHS structure, care pathways to mental health services are often limited. Medical teams, therefore, will not always be able to access the required psychological support. Nevertheless, there are still aspects of the suggested approach that can be implemented, and there is growing evidence that interdisciplinary approaches are effective within a range of medical services (Crawford et al., 2014; Erskine et al., 2013):

- **Trauma-focused care approaches**. Given the high prevalence of trauma within the HIV population, there have been calls in the literature for trauma-focused approaches to care for those with complex psychosocial issues (Damian, Gallo, Leaf & Mendelson, 2017; Sales, Swartzendruber & Phillips, 2016). This would involve responding to individual needs based on their trauma history and coping repertoire:
  - **Securely attached**. For those without a considerable trauma history, service users' abilities to manage their own health and relate to their healthcare team without any particular distress would be recognised and a standard system of appointments would be given based purely on health needs (e.g. once- to twice-yearly bloods and clinical appointments for those whose condition is stable).
  - **Ambivalent attachment style**. This would necessitate an enhanced, structured level of support for those who are anxious that people will not respond to their needs, with boundaries that all team members consistently adhere to. The aim would be to create a sense that needs will be met without the person having to escalate their distress levels. Over time the person may form trust that the service will be there if they need it, internalising new coping skills and beginning to manage their needs more independently.
  - **Avoidant attachment style**. A non-intrusive service would be required for those fearful of seeking care that is able to consistently meet basic needs without placing too many demands on the person to discuss their issues in depth. The aim would be to slowly build the relationship in the hope that the person may begin to trust the team and increase engagement with their healthcare.
  - **Disorganised attachment style**. It is likely that people with this level of need will always require some level of support that would need clear boundaries and a flexible approach that is sensitive to the shifting needs of the individual. Although the aim would always be to enable independence, gains may be small (although of great importance to the individual).

- **Boundaries and care consistency**. The sensitive establishment of care boundaries (what we can and cannot provide) can help create a secure framework for service users. This can help avoid unrealistic expectations of care provision, and therefore reduce experiences of feeling abandoned by those with a history of rejecting/abusive experiences. It is important that staff agree and stick to these boundaries, as different approaches (even if well meaning) can cause distress, and distress responses can play out across teams (e.g. splitting – some team members feeling intense empathy, others responding with frustration or anger, thus leading to conflict between team members). This may be easier to manage if small teams of care can be created around people with complex needs.

- **Psychological support training**. It would be beneficial for healthcare professionals working within HIV services to access training that assists in the understanding of the impact of trauma and develop confidence and skills regarding responding to distress and complex dynamics.
- **Reflective practice and supervision**. These interventions should be delivered by mental health professionals trained in the delivery of them. Therefore, it may not be possible for healthcare staff to access supervision or reflective practice groups within their own team. This could be considered an unmet need for staff working in HIV services (where trauma levels are high) and should be raised as a service gap. Healthcare professionals may have to think creatively about how to attain this form of support, for example by accessing local Schwartz Rounds (organised, reflective spaces for medical staff to explore emotional and social challenges of caring for patients).
- **Staff self-care**. Given the high levels of trauma and long history of burnout in HIV services, the importance of self-care cannot be overemphasised. What works for people will be highly individual; however, connecting with trusted social networks and engaging in meaningful activities are likely to be a running theme.
- **Remain mindful about power**. It is particularly important to acknowledge the inherent position of power of the healthcare professional, as for those with a trauma history, adverse dynamics can be unintentionally re-enacted within the healthcare relationship. Healthcare approaches and strategies that may help to redress the balance include patient-centred care frameworks, collaborative working and shared decision-making, and it is essential to keep service user consent at the heart of all practice.
- **Interdisciplinary working**. Where there are complex needs, there are multiple requirements for professional expertise. Working together and alongside service users to meet these needs allows all involved to share their perspectives and negotiate regarding the 'best fit' care approach. This may be within a specialist team, as well as across other relevant fields, including partnership working with the voluntary sector, to address other physical health co-morbidities, mental health issues and community support needs. Some examples of interdisciplinary ways of working follow:

  - joint working within and across teams
  - shared care plans for complex needs and a consistent approach
  - regular liaison and communication
  - relevant staff coming in and out of focus dependent on need
  - partnership working (e.g. with the voluntary/third sector)
  - working together to produce research and audits – highlighting service needs and gaps to communicating to commissioners and managers.

From dark places, some good things can grow…

If the team are able to work together and alongside service users to provide a secure, consistent framework for care (a 'safe base'), there is a real opportunity for post-trauma growth. Post-traumatic growth occurs when those who experienced adversity find a way to achieve psychological change, associated with a newfound sense of resilience and a shift in perspective that allows them to reorganise priorities, develop new goals and perhaps even begin to find ways to support others in need (Hefferon, Grealy & Mutrie, 2009). People who have benefited from effective care under HIV services may have had access to support in a way never before experienced and through this learned that some relationships are safe and some people can be trusted. Alongside trauma-informed and attachment-aware services, the importance of community support cannot be underestimated. Given the history of rejection and stigma within HIV, service user support networks and advocacy groups have been at the forefront of bringing people together to advocate for social acceptance, better treatments and equitable services. Through connecting with others with shared experiences (relating to their diagnosis, as well as other experiences of marginalisation), it is possible for people to access and build a sense of community within a mutually supportive network, as well as fighting rejection and stigma within the wider community. Such groups provide ongoing support and social connection, which extends beyond clinical relationships that are limited by necessary professional boundaries. And service users, through sharing the wisdom that comes from lived experience, enable professionals to keep learning, reflecting and growing.

Resource box

British Psychological Society, British HIV Association & Medical Foundation & Sexual Health (2011). *Standards of psychological support for adults living with HIV.* http://www.medfash.org.uk/uploads/files/p17abjjlhe7as89k45i1icg1f121.pdf
  Equality Act (2010). https://www.legislation.gov.uk/ukpga/2010/15/contents
  The Hearing Voices Network – www.hearing-voices.org/

Conclusion

This chapter has demonstrated the need to understand HIV-positive clients in their whole-life context. Adverse early experiences can undermine social and emotional development, and this can negatively impact subsequent HIV-related health outcomes. Traumatic early experiences of abuse, neglect and/or loss can directly increase physiological stress and be detrimental to immune health over the short and long term. Traumatic early relationship experiences can also lead to the development of insecure attachment styles, which have indirect negative impacts on HIV-related health outcomes. Sustained reliance on early-life trauma-based coping strategies that once ensured physical survival can thereafter lead to undesired and unhelpful consequences. Within the HIV context, this can manifest as avoidance of treatment and healthcare relationships. Additionally, over-reliance on external strategies for distress-soothing, such as the use of alcohol and drugs or engagement in sexual practices that carry risk (associated with increased HIV acquisition/transmission) also negatively impact health.

Understanding clients in their whole-life context also necessitates recognising the complex influence of sociocultural factors that further impact health outcomes and shape care relationships. Specifically, it is crucial to reflect on the impact of the healthcare system itself and for healthcare professionals to understand and acknowledge the impact of their own attachment styles within clinical interactions. In order to enable the best possible outcomes for HIV-positive clients, it is important to think beyond their physical needs to consider the their emotional relationship needs. Effective care is person-centred clinical care that is underpinned by understanding the attachment-based needs of service users. The design of care plans around this can provide a 'safe base' through consistent inter-disciplinary working. This type of approach creates the conditions for mutual learning through openness and ongoing reflection. It has the potential to support and empower people to begin to care for themselves where possible, and has the foresight, warmth and understanding to recognise how difficult this journey can be.

References

Addo-Atuah, J., & Lundmark, W. (2015). Book review: Stigma, discrimination, and living with HIV/ AIDS: A cross-cultural perspective. *Frontiers in Public Health*, *3*, 242.

Ainsworth, M. D., & Bowlby, J. (1991). An ethological approach to personality development. *American Psychologist*, *46*, 333–341.

Banyard, V. L., Edwards, V. J., & Kendall-Tackett, K. A. (2009). *Trauma and physical health: Understanding the effects of extreme stress and of its psychological harm*. Oxon: Routledge.

Bennet, J. K., Fuertes, J. N., Keitel, M., & Phillips, R. (2011). The role of patient attachment and working alliance on patient adherence, satisfaction, and health-related quality of life in lupus treatment. *Patient Education and Counseling*, *85*, 53–59.

Berry, K., Roberts, N., Danquah, A., & Davies, L. (2014). An exploratory study of associations between adult attachment, health service utilisation and health service costs. *Psychosis*, *6*, 355–358.

Boarts, J. M., Buckley-Fishcher, B. A., Armelie, A. P., Bogart, L. M., & Delahanty, D. L. (2017). The impact of HIV diagnosis related trauma on PTSD, depression, medication adherence, and HIV disease markers. *Journal of Evidence-based Social Work*, *6*, 4–16.

Boni-Saenz, A. (2016). Discussing and assessing capacity for sexual consent. *Psychiatric Times*, *33*, 7.

Bowlby, J. (1969). *Attachment and loss, Vol 1: Attachment*. London: Hogarth Press and the Institute of Psychoanalysis.

Bowlby, J. (1973). *Attachment and loss, Vol 2: Separation: Anxiety and anger*. London: Hogarth Press and the Institute of Psychoanalysis.

Bowlby, J. (1980). *Attachment and loss, Vol 3: Loss: Sadness and depression*. London: Hogarth Press and the Institute of Psychoanalysis.

Brandt, C., Zvolensky, M. J., Woods, S. P., Gonzalez, A., & O'Cleirigh, C. M. (2017). Anxiety symptoms and disorders among adults living with HIV and AIDS: A critical review and integrative synthesis of the empirical literature. *Clinical Psychology Review*, *51*, 164–184.

Brewin, C. R., Gregory, J. D., Lipton, M., & Burgess, N. (2010). Intrusive images in psychological disorders: Characteristics, neural mechanisms and treatment implications. *Psychological Review*, *117*, 210–232.

British HIV Association. (2018). Standards of care for people living with HIV. www.bhiva.org/standards-of-care-2018.

Bullock, E., Gergel, T., & Kingma, E. (2015). Conference report: Interdisciplinary workshop in the philosophy of medicine: Parentalism and trust. *Journal of Evaluation in Clinical Practice*, *21*, 542–548.

Chen, C. K., Salatas Waters, H., Hartman, M., Zimmerman, S., Miklowitz, D. J., & Waters, E. (2013). The secure base script and the task of caring for elderly parents: Implications for attachment theory and clinical practice. *Attachment & Human Development*, *15*, 332–348.

Crawford, M. R., Espie, C. A., Bartlett, D. J., & Gunstein, R. R. (2014). Integrating psychology and medicine in CPAP adherence e new concepts? *Sleep Medicine Reviews*, *18*, 123–139.

Crittenden, P. M. (2017). Gifts from Mary Ainsworth and John Bowlby. *Clinical Child Psychology and Psychiatry*, *22*, 436–442.

Damian, A. J., Gallo, J., Leaf, P., & Mendelson, T. (2017). Organizational and provider level factors in implementation of trauma-informed care after a city-wide training: An explanatory mixed methods assessment. *BMC Health Services Research*, *17*, 750.

Ehlers, A., & Clarke, D. M. (2000). A cognitive model of posttraumatic stress disorder. *Behaviour Research and Therapy*, *38*, 319–345.

Equality Act. (2010). www.legislation.gov.uk/ukpga/2010/15/contents.

Erskine, K., Griffith, E., DeGroat, N., Stolerman, M., Silverstein, L. B., Hidayatallah, N., & Walsh, C. A. (2013). An interdisciplinary approach to personalized medicine: Case studies from a cardiogenetics clinic. *Personalized Medicine, 10,* 73–80.

Felitti, V. J., Anda, R. F., Nordenberg, D., Williamson, D. F., Spitz, A. M., Edwards, V., Koss, M. P., & Marks, J. S. (1998). Relationship of childhood abuse and household dysfunction to many of the leading causes of death in adults. *American Journal of Preventive Medicine, 14,* 245–258.

Fisher, H. (2000). Lust, attraction, attachment: Biology and evolution of the three primary emotion systems for mating, reproduction, and parenting. *Journal of Sex Education and Therapy, 25,* 96–104.

Flentroy, S. L., Young, M., Blue, N., & Gilbert, D. J. (2015). Innovative assessment of childhood trauma and it's link to HIV and substance abuse in post-incarcerated women. *Journal of Creativity in Mental Health, 10,* 351–362.

Foa, E. B., Steketee, G., & Olasov-Rothbaum, B. (1989). Behavioral/cognitive conceptualizations of post-traumatic stress disorder. *Behavior Therapy, 20,* 155–176.

Fonagy, P., & Target, M. (1997). Attachment and reflective function: Their role in self-organization. *Development and Psychopathology, 9,* 679–700.

Gilbert, P. (2002). Evolutionary approaches to psychopathology and cognitive therapy. *Journal of Cognitive Psychotherapy, Suppl, 16,* 263–294.

Ginossar, T., Oetzel, J., Hill, R., Avila, M., Archipoli, A., & Wilcox, B. (2014). HIV healthcare providers' burnout: Can organizational culture make a difference? *AIDS Care, 12,* 1605–1608.

Health and Social Care Act. (2012). www.legislation.gov.uk/ukpga/2012/7/contents/enacted.

Hefferon, K., Grealy, M., & Mutrie, N. (2009). Post-traumatic growth and life threatening physical illness: A systematic review of the qualitative literature. *British Journal of Health Psychology, 14,* 343–378.

Horowitz, S., & Stermac, L. (2018). The relationship between interpersonal trauma history and the functions of non-suicidal self-injury in young adults: An experience sampling study. *Journal of Trauma and Dissociation, 19,* 232–246.

Howe, D. (2005). *Child abuse and neglect: Attachment, development and intervention.* London: Red Globe Press.

Hutchinson, P., & Dhairyawan, R. (2017). Shame, stigma, HIV: Philosophical reflections. *Medical Humanities, 43,* 225–230.

Jay, M. (2018). *Supernormal: Childhood adversity and the untold story of resilience.* Edinburgh: Canongate Books Ltd.

Johnstone, M. J. (2012). The ethics of 'nudging'. *Australian Nursing and Midwifery Journal, 24,* 27.

Karpman, S. MD. (1968). Fairy tales and script drama analysis. *Transactional Analysis Bulletin, 26,* 39–43.

Khodabakhsh, M. (2012). Attachment styles as predictors of empathy in nursing students. *Journal of Medical Ethics and History of Medicine, 5,* 8.

Klest, B., Tamaian, A., & Boughner, E. (2019). Exploring the relationship between betrayal trauma and health: The roles of mental health, attachment, trust in healthcare systems and non-adherence to treatment. *Psychological Trauma: Theory, Research, Practice and Policy,* Advance online publication. doi: 10.1037/tra0000453.

Maxwell, S., Shahmanesh, M., & Gafos, M. (2019). Chemsex behaviours among men who have sex with men: A systematic review of the literature. *International Journal of Drug Policy, 63,* 74–89.

Mikulincer, M., & Shaver, P. R. (2012). An attachment perspective on psychopathology. *World Psychiatry, 11,* 11–15.

Mimura, C., & Norman, I. J. (2018). The relationship between healthcare workers' attachment styles and patient outcomes: A systematic review. *International Journal for Quality in Healthcare, 30,* 332–343.

Morris, L., Berry, K., Wearden, A. J., Jackson, N., Dornan, T., & Davies, R. (2009). Attachment style and alliance in patients with diabetes and healthcare professionals. *Psychology, Health and Medicine, 14*, 585–590.

Morris, S. (2019). Too painful to think about: Chemsex and trauma. *Drugs and Alcohol Today*, doi: 10.1108/DAT-11-2018-0067.

Muller, R. T. (2014). Love's End: Attachment and the dissolution of a relationship: How do our early relationships affect how we deal with later breakups? *Psychology Today*. www.psycholo gytoday.com/gb/blog/talking-about-trauma/201402/loves-end-attachment-and-the-dissolution-relationship.

National HIV Nurses Association. (2015). *A national nurse-led audit of the standards of psychological support for adults living with HIV*. London: Mediscript.

Naylor, C., Das, P., Ross, S., Honeyman, M., Thompson, J., & Gilburt, H. (2016). *Bringing together physical and mental health: A new frontier for integrated care*. London: The Kings Fund.

Nightingale, V. R., Sher, T. G., & Hansen, N. B. (2010). The impact of receiving an HIV diagnosis and cognitive processing on psychological distress and posttraumatic growth. *Journal of Traumatic Stress, 23*, 452–460.

Nightingale, V. R., Sher, T. G., Mattson, M., Thilges, S., & Hansen, N. B. (2011). The effects of traumatic stressors and HIV-related trauma symptoms on health and health related quality of life. *AIDS Behaviour, 15*, 1870–1878.

Norman, R. E., Byambaa, M., De, R., Buthchart, A., Scott, J., & Vos, T. (2012). The long-term health consequences of child physical abuse, emotional abuse, and neglect: A systematic review and meta-analysis. *PLOS Medicine, 9*, 1–31.

Pollard, A., Nadarzynski, T., & Llewellyn, C. (2018). Syndemics of stigma, minority-stress, maladaptive coping, risk environments and littoral spaces among men who have sex with men using chemsex. *Culture, Health and Sexuality, 20*, 411–427.

Randhawa, G., Azarbar, A., Dong, H., Milloy, M. J., Kerr, T., & Hayashi, K. (2018). Childhood trauma and the inability to access hospital care among people who inject drugs. *Journal of Traumatic Stress, 31*, 383–390.

Read, J., van Os, J., Morrison, A. P., & Ross, C. A. (2005). Childhood trauma, psychosis and schizophrenia: A literature review with theoretical and clinical implications. *Acta Psychiatrica Scandinavica, 112*, 330–350.

Robles, T. F., & Kane, H. S. (2014). The attachment system and physiology in adulthood: Normative processes, individual differences, and implications for health. *Journal of Personality, 82*, 515–527.

Rutter, M. (1979). Maternal deprivation, 1972–1978: New findings, new concepts, new approaches. *Child Development, 50*, 283–305.

Rutter, M. (1981). Stress, coping and development: Some issues and some questions. *Journal of Child Psychology and Psychiatry, 22*, 323–356.

Sales, J. M., Swartzendruber, A., & Phillips, A. L. (2016). Trauma-informed HIV prevention and treatment. *Current HIV/AIDS Reports, 13*, 374–382.

Siegel, D. J. (1999). *The developing mind: Toward a neurobiology of interpersonal experience*. New York: Guilford Press.

UNAIDS. (2019 downloaded). The links between violence against women and HIV and AIDS. www. hivpolicy.org/Library/HPP001388.pdf.

Vagenas, P., Azar, M. M., Copenhaver, M. M., Springer, S. A., Molina, P. E., & Altice, F. L. (2015). The impact of alcohol use and related disorders on the HIV continuum of care: A systematic review. *Current HIV/AIDS Reports, 12*, 421–436.

Van der Kolk, B. A. (2007). *Traumatic stress: The effects of overwhelming experience on mind, body and society*. London: Guilford Press.

Van Tieu, H., & Koblin, B. A. (2009). HIV, alcohol and noninjection drug use. *Current Opinion in HIV and AIDS, 4*, 314–318.

Verhage, M. L., Schuengel, C., Madigan, S., Fearon, R. M., Oosterman, M., Cassibba, R., Baker-mans-Kranenburg, M. J., & van IJzendoorn, M. H. (2016). Narrowing the transmission gap: A synthesis of three decades of research on intergenerational transmission of attachment. *Psychological Bulletin, 142*, 337–366.

Ward, C., McQuillan, O., & Evans, R. Chemsex, consent and the rise in sexual assault. https://sti-bmj-com.liverpool.idm.oclc.org/content/sextrans/93/Suppl_1/A5.2.full.pdf.

Warner, S. (2000). *Understanding child sexual abuse: Making the tactics visible.* Gloucester: Handsell Publishing.

Warner, S. (2009). *Understanding the effects of child sexual abuse: Feminist revolutions in theory, reserach and practice.* London: Routledge.

Warner, S. (2020). *Understanding child sexual abuse: Making the tactics visible: Second edition.* Ross-on-Wye: PCCS Books.

Warner, S., & Shaw, C. (2016). Working with looked after children who self-harm: Understanding coping, communication and suicide, in J. Guisharde-Pine, G. Coleman-Oluwabusola, & S. McCall (eds.) *Supporting the mental health needs of children in care: Evidence for practice*, pp. 40–52. London: Jessica Kingsley Publishers.

Warner, S., & Spandler, H. (2012). New strategies for practice based evidence: A focus on self-harm. *Journal of Qualitative Research in Psychology, 9*, 13–26.

Watkins-Hayes, C. (2014). Intersectionality and the sociology of HIV/AIDS: Past, present, and future research directions. *The Annual Review of Sociology, 40*, 431–457.

Weinsten, T. L., & Li, X. (2016). The relationship between stress and clinical outcomes for persons living with HIV/AIDS: A systematic review of the global literature. *AIDS Care, 28*, 160–169.

World Health Organization. (2008). HIV/AIDS and mental health. https://apps.who.int/gb/archive/pdf_files/EB124/B124_6-en.pdf.

Yerkes, R. M., & Dodson, J. D. (1908). The relation of strength of stimulus to rapidity of habit-formation. *Journal of Comparative Neurology and Psychology, 18*, 459–482.

7 Chemsex among men who have sex with men

A social psychological approach

Rusi Jaspal

Chapter description

This chapter will explore the sexualised use of psychoactive substances within the men who have sex with men (MSM) population, referred to as 'chemsex'. The social and psychological underpinnings of chemsex among MSM and the relationship between this practice and HIV risk are explored. Recent data on the prevalence of chemsex are provided and then case studies of MSM who engage in chemsex are presented to illustrate the risk factors, the lived experience and potential mental and sexual health outcomes associated with the practice. Identity process theory from social psychology is suggested as an approach to understand the relationship between psychological adversity and engagement in chemsex behaviour. Empirical research exploring issues associated with chemsex is considered through the lens of identity process theory, case study discussions and reflective exercises. A model for supporting MSM who engage in, or who are at risk of engaging in, chemsex is outlined and thoughts given to how healthcare practitioners can offer interdisciplinary support in partnership with community services.

Introduction

In recent years, 'chemsex', the use of psychoactive drugs in sexualised settings, has emerged as an important public health concern among gay, bisexual and other men who have sex with men (MSM).[1] The practice was first observed in major cities in Western Europe and North America but is now increasing globally. It is acknowledged that drug use in sexualised settings exists in heterosexual populations, but the term 'chemsex' is most often used to refer to this practice in MSM specifically. There are several factors that make chemsex among MSM a relatively distinctive phenomenon. First, drug use in sexualised settings is more common in MSM than in heterosexual men and women (e.g. Latini et al., 2019; Lawn, Aldridge, Xia & Winstock, 2019). Second, chemsex involves the use of specific psychoactive drugs, which differ from those commonly used by heterosexuals who engage in drug use in sexualised settings (Macfarlane, 2016). Third, the prevalence of condomless sex appears to be particularly associated with chemsex among MSM and with the specific drugs commonly used in chemsex settings, but this link between condomless sex and drug use is not as strong in heterosexuals (Kenyon, Wouters, Platteau, Buyze & Florencet, 2018).

Chemsex commonly involves the use of mephedrone, crystal methamphetamine, γ-hydroxybutyrate (GHB), γ-butyrolactone (GBL) and crystallised methamphetamine, which are intended to facilitate and enhance sexual encounters – often in group settings – that can last for hours or days and with multiple partners. Physiologically, the drugs have varying effects on the individual – while mephedrone raises heart rate and blood pressure, resulting in increased sexual arousal, GHB and GBL function as potent psychological disinhibitors. These drugs are often used in combination with others, including alcohol, and in addition to physical harms, the resulting states of disinhibition and altered consciousness can lead to a range of unwanted, often traumatic outcomes (Maxwell, Shahmanesh & Gafos, 2019; Morris, 2019). However, it is important to acknowledge that not all chemsex is problematic. Some MSM engage in the practice safely and there is wide variance in approaches to participation, with some subsections of the community advocating harm reduction and supporting each other to remain safe (Bourne et al., 2015).

The prevalence of chemsex

There has been significant media attention to chemsex, which has led to the public perception that the practice is very prevalent in MSM. There is growing empirical research into the prevalence of chemsex among MSM in a number of countries. While initially observed in major Western cities, such as London and New York, chemsex is now being reported globally (e.g. Lea et al., 2019; Lim et al., 2018; Tan et al., 2018). It must be stated that the available empirical evidence suggests that chemsex is practised among a minority of MSM. It is, however, difficult to ascertain the precise prevalence of chemsex in MSM communities because many empirical studies have used convenience, rather than representative, samples. As well as sampling bias in some of the studies, there is variation in the ways in which chemsex is measured – some studies ask MSM about engagement in chemsex but some individuals do not necessarily categorise their drug use in sexualised settings as 'chemsex'. However, there have been several prevalence studies since 2014, which provide some insight into how chemsex trends appear to be changing over time.

In their re-analysis of data from the European Men Who Have Sex With Men Survey 2013, Bourne et al. (2014) found that a fifth of the 1142 gay male survey respondents living in Lambeth, Southwark and Lewisham reported having engaged in chemsex in the last five years and that a tenth had done so in the last four weeks. The MSM Internet Survey Ireland 2015 revealed that 36% of respondents had used recreational drugs and that 7% had used drugs associated with chemsex (Barrett et al., 2019). The authors found that MSM living with HIV were more likely to use drugs associated with chemsex than those who are HIV-negative. In a retrospective case notes review study in two London sexual health clinics, Hegazi et al. (2017) found that 59% of the MSM who used the clinic in the latter half of 2014 reported chemsex. Chemsex users were more likely to be HIV-positive than non-users. Crucially, the prevalence of chemsex appears to be higher in MSM living with HIV. In a study of HIV patients recruited from 30 UK HIV clinics in 2014 (Pufall et al., 2018), it was found that 29% of sexually active MSM had engaged in chemsex and that 10% had engaged in 'slamsex' (injected drug use) in the previous year.

Self-report survey data from 1484 HIV-negative or undiagnosed MSM recruited from 20 sexual health clinics in the UK demonstrated a 21.8% prevalence of chemsex in the last three months (Sewell et al., 2017). An analysis of baseline data from the PROUD study revealed that 44% of the 525 study participants reported having engaged in chemsex in the last three months (Dolling et al., 2016). However, it should be noted that eligibility criteria for the PROUD study was HIV risk behaviour and that this itself is often correlated with chemsex. In another retrospective case note review study, Pakia-nathan et al. (2018) found that 16.5% of all gay men attending two London sexual health clinics during a 12-month period reported engaging in chemsex in the past.

There is variation in the reported prevalence of chemsex in MSM, but a significant minority of MSM appear to engage in the practice, and it appears to be more prevalent in MSM living with HIV. This in turn suggests that there is a high risk of onward HIV transmission in chemsex settings.

Reflective point

Was chemsex something you had heard of or come across in your practice?
What is your response when considering this practice? How do you think this is influenced by aspects of your own identity (e.g. gender, sexuality …) and the dominant values/norms in your particular social world?

Contextualising chemsex in people's lives

In this section, two case studies of MSM involved in the chemsex scene are presented – those of James and Juan. The case studies are drawn from previous empirical research conducted by the author and some details have been changed to protect the identities of the individuals concerned.

Case study 1: James

James is a 33-year-old gay man from Leicester. He came out as gay at the age of 18 just before starting university in London. His relationship with his parents and siblings was fraught with difficulties, as he perceived them to be unsupportive of him when he came out as gay. James had always felt dissatisfied with his body and had low self-esteem – he often felt unattractive to other men. He moved to London, where he found a job and decided to move in with some gay friends. In contrast to his hometown, which had no discernible gay community, he was pleased to be living in London. All of his friends were in open relationships and most of them actually ridiculed him for being 'too straight' in his preference for monogamy. James met his boyfriend, Jack, a year ago. Despite being very fond of Jack, he never felt very comfortable around him due to his long-standing body image and self-esteem issues. He felt insecure and unattractive. This led him to acquiesce to all of Jack's demands, including that they 'open' their relation-ship to others and engage in chemsex. They now use Grindr[2] to find other men for casual sex and regularly attend gay sex parties and gay saunas, where they always use 'chems'[3] during sex with other people. Sometimes he and Jack do not use condoms when they use chems. Although he does not enjoy it much, James feels compelled to join in. Jack has told him that sober sex is boring. Yet, one advantage that James per-ceives is that the chems allow him to escape his feelings of insecurity about his body image and, at least for a short while, he feels euphoric. James is unhappy about his cur-rent situation and wishes to stop using chems. He is feeling useless and depressed and thinks he might end up losing Jack and his friends if he does give up chemsex.

Reflective point

Why does James keep returning to chemsex, even though he is unhappy with his situation?
How might this inform the support you offer James in your clinical practice?

Case study 2: Juan

Juan is a 33-year-old gay man from Spain. He was diagnosed with HIV in his hometown in 2014 and was shocked at his diagnosis. The gay men's health charity referred Juan to the local hospital. Although his CD4 count was still relatively high, Juan wanted to begin antiretroviral therapy immediately. Still shocked at his diagnosis, Juan viewed his medication as an unfortunate daily reminder of his HIV infection. Moreover, days after initiating treatment, Juan began to experience negative physical side effects. Juan raised his concerns with his doctor, who he experienced as dismissive. The doctor appeared to be suggesting that this is what life with HIV is like and that Juan should simply get used to it. He believed his doctor was discriminating against him because he was gay and HIV-positive. Juan also had a difficult relationship with his parents. He had never felt able to tell them about the sexual abuse he had faced as a child, and he also felt unable to disclose his HIV status to his family. In fact, given his strict religious upbringing, he also felt unable to come out as gay. It felt as if he was hiding a lot from his family. He moved to London but felt lonely. He disengaged from HIV care because he still felt distrustful of medical professionals. As Juan's mental health has begun to deteriorate, he is missing doses of his medication, which has increased the risk of drug resistance and of onward HIV transmission to his sexual partners. To deal with his feelings of loneliness, Juan is meeting sexual partners online and in gay bars. After facing rejection from potential sexual partners to whom he has disclosed his HIV status, he feels more ashamed and distressed about being HIV-positive. He has started to attend chemsex parties in London because nobody asks him his status there, allowing him to forget about HIV and to experience a sense of connection and intimacy with other men. Juan now has a detectable viral load but is not consistently using condoms with sexual partners at chemsex parties.

Reflective point

How might Juan's cultural background influence his perception of identity and experience? How might you explore this with him?

As a clinician, what are the main concerns that jump out to you? What kind of thoughts and emotions accompany them and how do you think these responses would influence your clinical practice?

James and Juan have faced, and continue to face, social and psychological stressors, which undermine their psychological wellbeing. It seems that chemsex could be understood partly as a means of coping with these stressors, although both men also acknowledge the adverse impact that the practice is having on their lives. In these case studies, the psychological dimension of chemsex is clearly observable – James feels pressured into the practice due to social norms but also views chemsex as a means of deflecting his negative body image and low self-esteem, while Juan uses chemsex as a form of escapism from the stigma associated with his HIV diagnosis and the rejection he habitually faces on the basis of this. These case studies are intended to illustrate the range of social psychological factors that potentially under-pin engagement in chemsex.

In the remainder of this chapter, aspects of these case studies are invoked in order to outline how clinicians can intervene to limit its adverse effects for psychological well-being among MSM who engage in the practice. In some cases, this work would be carried out in a psychological therapy context, although awareness of the complexity of the issues can assist all healthcare practitioners in the delivery of a considered, person-centred approach.

Identity process theory

The two case studies illustrate there are a range of social and psychological stressors faced by many gay men, such as homophobia, parental rejection, HIV stigma and certain coercive social norms in different subcultures of the gay scene. These events and stres-sors contribute to the social context in which gay men make sense of who they are. Iden-tity process theory (Jaspal & Breakwell, 2014) from social psychology provides an integrative model of how people construct their identities, what can plausibly 'threaten' their identities and how they subsequently cope with these threats. The theory posits that individuals construct their identity by engaging in two social psychological processes: assimilation-accommodation and evaluation:

- **Assimilation-accommodation** refers to the absorption of new information, such as new identity characteristics or social representations (values, beliefs, practices shared amongst specific groups/communities) into identity and the creation of space for it within the identity structure. For instance, an HIV diagnosis must be absorbed into existing information about the self, namely that one is HIV-positive (assimilation). Given the stigma associated with this new identity element, individuals may need to make adjustments to the existing content of identity, for example their relationships with their family members, from whom they may wish to conceal this identity elem-ent (accommodation).
- **Evaluation** refers to the process of attributing meaning and value to the components of identity. For example, a gay man diagnosed with HIV may initially attach nega-tive meaning to his infection, viewing this as a deadly virus, but subsequently come to view it as a positive turning point in his life. This demonstrates how the meanings and values appended to one's HIV status can change over time.

Reflective point

Think about an event or situation in your life that led you to assimilate and accom-modate a new identity element. How did this make you feel and why?

Clearly, social representations will in part determine which identity elements are assimilated and accommodated and how they are evaluated. Some identity elements, such as being gay or HIV-positive, are stigmatised in some social contexts and there may be difficulties in assimilating and accommodating them due to their negative evaluation. The two identity processes do not function randomly, but rather they are guided by various motivational principles, which are outlined below. These principles essentially specify the desirable end states for identity:

- **Self-esteem** refers to personal and social worth.
- **Self-efficacy** can be defined as the belief in one's competence and control.
- **Distinctiveness** refers to feelings of uniqueness and differentiation from others.
- **Continuity** is essentially the psychological thread between past, present and future.
- **Coherence** refers to the perception that relevant aspects of identity are coherent and compatible.

It could be speculated that James's dissatisfaction with his body is causing him to experience *low self-esteem* and that his inability to leave the chemsex scene might challenge his perception of *self-efficacy*, in that he lacks a sense of competence and control. Similarly, as an unexpected, undesirable life event, Juan's diagnosis of HIV could lead him to experience *distinctiveness* in an undesirable way. It could also plausibly undermine the *continuity* principle of identity as this may have changed how he views himself, perhaps influenced by how he imagines others will now view him. This, in turn, may impact a sense of *coherence*, particularly if aspects of the self relating to HIV are kept hidden or perhaps cause internalised stigma (see Chapter 8).

More generally, the multiple social and psychological stressors that MSM tend to face, such as homophobia, stigma, rejection and body image issues, can challenge all or some of the identity principles (Jaspal, 2019).

Reflective point

Think about a situation or event that compromised your own sense of self-esteem, continuity, distinctiveness and so on. How did this make you feel?

How might this apply to someone who participates in chemsex? Try to consider the identity principles when thinking about this.

When the identity principles are compromised, for instance by changes in a person's social context, identity is said to be threatened. Identity threat is generally aversive for psychological wellbeing. However, the degree to which wellbeing is compromised is determined by the nature of the threat, the number of principles curtailed by the threat and a person's ability to cope effectively. For instance, it is easy to see how an HIV diagnosis could threaten several identity principles simultaneously – self-esteem, self-efficacy and continuity – meaning it can have a detrimental impact on psychological wellbeing (Daramilas & Jaspal, 2016). Furthermore, personality traits, such as optimism and resilience, and access to high-quality social support are likely to reduce the impact of an adverse event (e.g. an HIV diagnosis, relationship breakdown) on the identity structure, leading to a decreased risk of identity threat (see Chapters 4 and 6).

Identity process theory posits that people attempt to cope in response to identity threat and describes coping strategies at three distinct levels of human interdependence: *intrapsychic*, *interpersonal* and *intergroup*:

- **Intrapsychic** refers to internal psychological processes (thoughts and associated feelings) and, thus, intrapsychic coping strategies function at a psychological level. Some can be regarded as deflection strategies in that they enable the individual to deny or think about the threat in a different way. For instance, an individual diagnosed with HIV may initially deny that they have the infection and disengage from HIV care, as Juan has. However, this can then lead to further health risks. Conversely, there are acceptance strategies that might help an individual change the way they respond to the threat – in a manner that may help facilitate behaviours that are associated with better outcomes. For instance, some individuals respond to their HIV diagnosis with acceptance by initiating medication, engaging with other people living with HIV and advocating for the rights and wellbeing of people living with the condition.

- **Interpersonal** strategies aim to change the nature of relationships with others. Some of these can have unwanted consequences and therefore may be considered 'unhelpful' in the longer term. For instance, the threatened individual may isolate himself from others or feign membership of a group or network of which they are not really a member, in order to avoid exposure to stigma. For instance, Juan has isolated himself from others to avoid stigma and, thus, threats to self-esteem. James does not actually wish to engage in chemsex but does so in order to derive a sense of belonging in the gay community and to maintain the affection of his boyfriend. An example of a proactive interpersonal strategy might be for a person to share their HIV status with trusted others. This can help access support, which both James and Juan appear to lack. However, it is important to remain mindful that stigma and discrimination are a reality for people living with HIV and that the decision to tell others must be based on a person's knowledge and experience of their own particular social context.

- **Intergroup** strategies aim to change the nature of our relationships with groups. Individuals may join groups of like-minded others who share their predicament in order to derive social support. They may create a new social group to derive support or a pressure group to influence social representations. For instance, some MSM diagnosed with HIV report benefits of joining a support group in order to manage the psychosocial challenges of their diagnosis. However, again, it is important to be aware that there is not a 'one size fits all' approach as some people may have difficult experiences if attempting to join a group does not fit with their needs.

Reflective point

How do you tend to cope with threatening events and situations? What do you do?
How do you relate to others in your life at difficult times?
Do you think changing how you tend to cope would be easy?
Think about your own clinical work. How might you work with service users to understand what is, and what is not, working for them?

Jaspal (2018) has provided an extensive overview of the coping strategies that may be used by MSM who face identity threat. In that overview, it is argued that both personality traits and the availability of coping strategies in any given social context will determine the threatened individual's choice of coping strategy. Social representations also play a crucial role because they influence the availability and the individual's evaluation of particular coping strategies. Identity threat is by no means unusual but, given the minority status and stigma experienced by MSM, threat may be more persistent and therefore be detrimental to psychological and emotional wellbeing in this population. All of the available evidence shows that effective coping is central to psychological wellbeing. However, it must always be remembered that what makes a coping strategy effective can vary for different individuals and can be specific to context. Additionally, although some coping strategies may be considered generally 'ineffective', they may be the only way that individual can find a way to cope in that particular moment. Coping strategies are based on complex factors that include the current situation and environment, wider social structures and an individual's personal history (see Chapter 6).

As highlighted in the remainder of this chapter, engagement in chemsex commonly constitutes a strategy for coping with threats to identity, but it may also be a practice that itself threatens identity. Chemsex may provide temporary respite from the adverse psychological effects of events and experiences that MSM face, but for many, in the long term, it is unlikely to be a fruitful and productive coping strategy in that it can lead to considerable harms. Crucially, engagement in chemsex appears to be associated with heightened sexual risk, as outlined next.

Chemsex and sexual risk

Empirical research into issues associated with chemsex is now emerging and is beginning to provide insight into the factors – social, psychological, economic and others – that appear to be related to both the practice of chemsex and those individuals who engage in it. This is gradually enabling us to understand the practice and, crucially, to predict who might be more likely to participate. This in turn allows policy-makers to develop more effective interventions for preventing unhelpful chemsex engagement and for providing treatment and support to those who require it.

A consistent finding in most studies is that MSM who engage in chemsex are at increased risk of HIV infection and that MSM living with HIV are more likely to report engagement in chemsex than those who are HIV-negative or undiagnosed (e.g. Maxwell et al., 2019). In their cross-sectional analysis of clinic service data, Stevens et al. (2019) found that MSM who reported chemsex were more likely to be HIV-positive and to have had more than six sexual partners in the last 90 days. Coupled with the empirical observation that condomless sex is prevalent, these data suggest that the risk of HIV transmission could be high. The available evidence shows that condomless sex is prevalent in chemsex settings (Glynn et al., 2018), and that MSM who report condomless chemsex are more likely to be HIV-positive (Kenyon et al., 2018). Data collected from a 2014 survey of people attending HIV clinics in England and Wales showed that 3 in 10 sexually active MSM living with HIV engaged in chemsex in the past 12 months (Pufall et al., 2018).

There is also evidence that MSM who engage in chemsex are more likely to test positive for bacterial STIs – in one study, the STI positivity rate was 44% (Evers, van Liere, Hoebe & Dukers-Muijrers, 2019). In that study, it was also found that those MSM who reported using three or more chemsex drugs exhibited a higher STI prevalence than those who used fewer chemsex drugs. Kohli et al. (2019) found that MSM who reported using GHB or GBL in the last 12 months were more than twice as likely as other MSM to be diagnosed with gonorrhoea and, as in Evers et al.'s (2019) study, those reporting use of all three chemsex drugs had the highest odds of infection.

The elevated HIV and STI prevalence among MSM who engage in chemsex can be attributed at least in part to the empirical observation that the practice of chemsex is associated with various sexual risk-taking behaviours. For instance, in their retrospective case notes review study of 124 MSM attending sexual health clinics in the latter part of 2014, Hegazi et al. (2017) found that 59% reported engagement in chemsex and that this practice was positively associated with transactional sex, group sex, fisting, sharing sex toys and HIV/hepatitis C serodiscordant sexual relations. Studies also show that chemsex users are more likely to engage in other high-risk sexual practices, such as fisting or having sex in exchange for money (e.g. Frankis, Flowers, McDaid & Bourne, 2018).

Reflective point

On considering James's and Juan's circumstances, and the identity principles we have explored (self-esteem, self-efficacy, distinctiveness, continuity and coherence), why do you think MSM who feel vulnerable are more likely to engage in sexual risk-taking behaviour?

In terms of sexual risk-taking, is it the sole responsibility of the person living with HIV to ensure protection is used or should everyone be responsible for their own safety?

If we place all responsibility for safe sex choices on people living with HIV, what impact do you think this has on societal attitudes towards people living with HIV?

Despite the association of chemsex with sexual risk, there is emerging evidence that chemsex users are informed about HIV risk and, thus, in a position to minimise this risk through other preventative routes. For instance, in a study of MSM in Hong Kong (Kwan & Lee, 2019), it was found that MSM who are currently using, or have recently used, drugs common in chemsex are more likely to have heard of pre-exposure prophylaxis (PrEP), which is an effective method of preventing HIV. Furthermore, a correlation between chemsex and correct use of PrEP has been observed in MSM, which suggests that this could be a viable HIV prevention option – especially in view of the fact that condomless sex is prevalent in chemsex settings (Roux et al., 2018).

Given the involvement of psychoactive drugs, it is likely that chemsex users feel disinhibited in relation to sexual exploration, which can include condomless sex and other sexual risk behaviours. Many chemsex users are already living with HIV and, thus, may be less concerned about bacterial STIs. Yet, there appears to be an opportunity for intervening to decrease the risk of HIV infection through the use of PrEP.

Reflective point

Why do some people take risks despite awareness of the hazard?

Think about a time you took a risk, knowing there could be negative consequences. What do you think made you do it?

Why engage in chemsex? Social and psychological drivers

There has been relatively little empirical research into the social psychological underpinnings of chemsex. However, qualitative research has provided some important insights. Smith and Tasker (2018) conducted a qualitative interview study of six gay men involved in the chemsex scene. Using a life course perspective, they found that engagement in chemsex was related to the development of gay identity and involvement in the gay community – chemsex was perceived to facilitate a sense of belonging. This fits with James's report of the pressure from his friends to engage in chemsex, given its consensual acceptance in his friendship circle. In their study of attitudes towards drug use among 2112 MSM in Australia, Lea et al. (2019) found that 61% reported drug use in the last six months and that gay men who were most socially engaged with other gay men were more likely to endorse drug use for social and sexual encounters. They attribute drug use in gay men at least in part to social norms within gay social networks, as illustrated by James's case. Additionally, geospatial gay social networking applications, such as Grindr, can facilitate access to chemsex in that population (Tan et al., 2018).

It can be about the sex, the confidence and the connection

In exploring the possible drivers of chemsex, it has been suggested that multiple levels of stigma, the stress associated with belonging to a minority group and coping strategies that could be considered unhelpful may be contributing factors (Pollard Nadarzynski & Llewellyn, 2017). In their qualitative research with chemsex users, Weatherburn et al. (2016) describe two distinct sets of motivations underlying the practice. On the one hand, chemsex can enable individuals to have the type of sex that they desire by increasing their sexual stamina and confidence and by decreasing inhibitions. On the other hand, chemsex drugs can enhance the quality of the sexual encounter on a relational level by increasing attraction and facilitating greater interpersonal rapport (see also Bourne et al., 2014).

A systematic review of the literature on chemsex behaviours in MSM indicated that men tend to engage in chemsex because they believe that this will enhance their sexual encounters and increase the pleasurability of sex. Chemsex users tend to report better sexual experiences than when sober, given that some of the substances utilised reduce inhibitions and increase sexual pleasure (Maxwell et al., 2019). In their interview study of MSM in Malaysia, Lim et al. (2018) found that the desire to increase sexual pleasure and to engage in sexual exploration underpinned use of methamphetamine in sexualised settings.

In addition to noting the perceived pleasurability of chemsex in terms of sexual enhancement and prolongation, MSM have described a fear of rejection from potential sexual partners, which decreased when they engaged in chemsex. Moreover, it appeared that chemsex constituted a strategy for coping with societal rejection on the basis of sexual orientation (Lim et al., 2018). Engagement in chemsex can decrease the presence of negative affect associated with stressors, such as internalised homophobia and HIV stigma and, thus, protect feelings of self-esteem (Bourne et al., 2014). Some MSM who engage in chemsex do so in part because they wish to increase feelings of intimacy with partners but feel unable to do so in sober settings (Graf et al., 2018). James indicated how his low body image and self-esteem constituted a barrier to acquiring feelings of intimacy with his partner. Juan anticipated stigma from sexual partners, and perhaps thought of this as an obstacle to finding a sense of intimacy in potential sexual and/or romantic connections. The use of drugs can reduce these concerns via disinhibition.

The positive affect experienced in chemsex sessions can lead to a form of psychological dependence as some people may become immersed in this environment, which they find pleasurable and as meeting their sexual and social needs, and, thus, lose the ability to enjoy sex outside of it. On considering why MSM keep revisiting chemsex, despite the potential harms, the intense experience of both connection and sexual pleasure as powerful reinforcers must be recognised. Indeed, Bourne et al. (2014) have shown that chemsex users come to find 'sober' sex unsatisfactory, leading to an inability to engage in sex without the use of psychoactive drugs. Thus, chemsex can constitute a strategy for enhancing identity and wellbeing.

Psychological issues: what comes first – the adversity or the chemsex?

Reflective point

What are the main sources of psychological adversity among MSM?
Is chemsex the cause of, or the response to, psychological adversity?

The predisposing factors

There are indications in the literature that chemsex is associated with psychological adversity that existed before chemsex participation. In their online survey of 1648 MSM, Hibbert, Brett, Porcellato and Hope (2019) found that 41% of respondents reported recent sexualised drug use, and that the practice was associated with lower satisfaction with life but greater sexual satisfaction. It could be hypothesised that MSM who are dissatisfied with their lives are more likely to engage in chemsex, which they then perceive to provide greater sexual satisfaction. Moreover, the authors of that study found that low sexual self-efficacy was a significant predictor of engaging in chemsex, suggesting that decreasing self-control may lead to the practice.

The high prevalence of chemsex in MSM living with HIV has been noted earlier in this chapter. Pakianathan et al. (2018) found that MSM reporting chemsex behaviour were more likely to report recent HIV infection. This may mean that chemsex constitutes a behavioural response (possibly as a coping strategy) to the social psychological stressors associated with HIV infection. Indeed, Juan became immersed in the chemsex scene soon after his HIV diagnosis to attempt to escape the stressors associated with this psychologically adverse event in his life. In their study of HIV-positive gay men, Pufall et al. (2018) found that the practice was associated inter alia with diagnosed depression/anxiety. It appears that, for some MSM, chemsex may constitute a form of escapism in that it enables those facing social and psychological stressors, such as a recent HIV infection, to disconnect from their reality and to seek respite in a context in which these social psychological stressors cease to threaten identity. For instance, MSM may derive confidence about their physical appearance or sexual performance in this context (as highlighted in James's case) and those living with HIV report that HIV status is a non-issue, thereby ceasing to constitute a source of stigma or a basis for sexual rejection (as indicated in Juan's case).

When the party is over: the unwanted impact

In their interview study, Smith and Tasker (2018) found that, although chemsex can initially be construed as exciting and conducive to self-exploration, it can come to represent an isolating and distressing phenomenon in the people's lives over which they have little control. This reiterates the notion that it is challenging for self-efficacy. The negative effects of chemsex appear to be wide-ranging. In a study of 510 MSM in Dublin (Glynn et al., 2018), it was found that one in four MSM reported that chemsex was having an adverse impact on their lives and almost a third of respondents reported a desire for help or advice in relation to chemsex. Furthermore, Hegazi and colleagues (2017) found that 42% of the chemsex users who participated in their study perceived the practice to have had an adverse impact on their physical or mental health or their careers. There is a need to understand the identity principles that might be challenged as a result of engaging in chemsex. This should constitute the focus of future research.

Chemsex and identity threat: a complicated, bidirectional relationship

As much of the existing research is correlational, and therefore can only document associations, it is difficult to draw conclusions about what comes first – does chemsex cause MSM to experience identity threat or is it a response to identity threat?

In view of the evidence presented, it is likely that chemsex is both the cause and product of identity threat. There is a general (although not rigid) pattern of those who have a more significant history of psychological adversity being more likely to become involved in the practice, which is likely to be due to longstanding coping tendencies. The unwanted consequences of chemsex can then have a detrimental impact on psychological and emotional states, perhaps more so for those with a more considerable history of mental health issues. There is mounting evidence regarding the exposure to trauma for those who participate in chemsex, and this is likely to build on existing adverse experiences. This is perhaps particularly pertinent for people living with HIV as there are high levels of trauma in this population (Applebaum et al., 2015). Negative outcomes and harms such as experiencing or witnessing disturbing events, sexual assault or criminal activity outside of someone's normal moral compass can lead to feelings of shame, fear and a general sense of being out of control (Maxwell et al., 2019; Morris, 2019). These experiences will no doubt act as exacerbating and re-traumatising factors (see Chapter 6).

Attitudes towards chemsex vary among MSM. For James, chemsex is the cause of psychological distress and he feels compelled to engage in the practice due to pressure from his friends and partner, while for Juan it is clearly a strategy for coping with the stigma and rejection he faces on the basis of his positive serostatus. Some MSM view chemsex as harmless and engage in the practice transiently, while others clearly experience physical and psychological health problems as a result of it. In their qualitative interview study with 10 gay men who were experiencing difficulties with chemsex and wished to cease the practice, Van Hout, Crowley, O'Dea and Clarke (2019) found that chemsex constituted a maladaptive form of escapism for participants who, nonetheless, felt compulsively attached to the practice and, thus, unable to leave the chemsex scene. This gives credence to the complexity of the phenomenon. The remainder of the chapter focuses on potential pathways to supporting MSM struggling with chemsex.

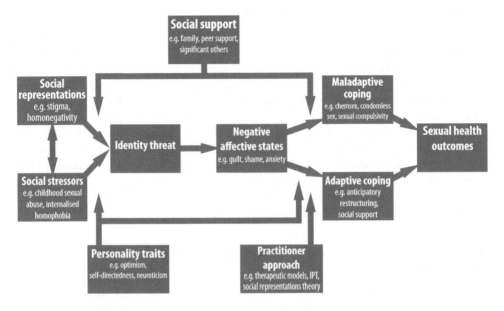

Figure 7.1 A framework for understanding self-identity, wellbeing and sexual health among MSM
(from Jaspal, 2018)

So how can we help promote wellbeing?

In this chapter, various social and psychological stressors and their potential impact for identity processes have been described. Effective coping is key to both psychological and physical wellbeing. Drawing on much of this empirical evidence, Jaspal (2018) has proposed a multi-level model that can enable practitioners to predict, and to intervene in order to mitigate, poor sexual health (and other health and mental health) outcomes associated with chemsex (see Figure 7.1).

Healthcare practitioners can use this model to help make sense of why some MSM participate in chemsex, and why some continue to do so even when engagement in it is causing considerable harm. The model is applied in light of what the evidence base tells us about the kind of issues and events that many MSM experience.

A vulnerable starting point

Unfortunately, human beings all experience what can be loosely described as 'adverse events'. These are essentially social representations, events and situations that can cause psychological stress. MSM have been, and continue to be, exposed to negative social representations of their sexual identity. On the one hand, this is as a result of their social-isation in heteronormative contexts, whereby heterosexuality is considered 'normal' – the implicit message being that homosexuality is 'abnormal' – thereby creating the conditions for a negative self-view. On the other hand, a more explicit negative message comes from the experience of overt homophobia (Jaspal, 2019). Some come to internal-ise the homophobia that they encounter (create an internal negative view of the self, based on the messages they have received), leading to self-stigma. In addition to these negative social representations of their identity, there is a higher prevalence of particular social stressors among gay men, such as childhood sexual abuse, homophobia and increased HIV risk. Some of these stressors are evident in the two case studies presented at the beginning of this chapter.

The complex relationship between harm and coping

Both these negative social representations and the adverse stressors have the potential (when adequate support was not available) to undermine the principles of self-esteem, continuity, self-efficacy and so on, leading to identity threat. When thinking about chemsex, for some MSM, engagement in itself may be construed as an adverse event because of the stigma associated with it. Chemsex may also give rise to other adverse/traumatic events and situations, which cause threats to identity. For instance, some chemsex users report difficulties in maintaining friendships, relationships and their employment, all of which can challenge their sense of continuity, self-efficacy and self-esteem (e.g. Bourne et al., 2014). However, not everyone exposed to negative social representations or social stressors will necessarily experience identity threat. The relationship between the adverse event and identity threat is likely to be mediated by personal history and personality traits, on the one hand, and by the availability of social support, on the other hand. For instance, an individual with high levels of neuroticism might be more prone to identity threat than an individual who has high levels of optimism. However, it is important to acknowledge that personality traits can shift depending on context. Moreover, MSM who possess a high-quality social support network are able to draw on that network in order to minimise the negative psychological consequences of the adverse event, thereby initiating effective coping before its onset.

Understanding distress responses

If the adverse event does threaten identity, the individual may experience negative psychological and emotional states, such as guilt, shame or anxiety. As a rough rule of thumb, negative psychological and emotional responses are likely to be accentuated if the adverse event challenges more than one principle. Indeed, as demonstrated in this chapter, an HIV diagnosis can pose 'hyper-threats' to identity because it simultaneously undermines various, if not all of, the identity principles which underpin how a person makes sense of and values themselves. Furthermore, people tend to favour some identity principles over others and this is related partly to what they value generally. An adverse event that threatens a favoured identity principle, understandably, may induce a more marked distress response. For instance, an individual who values conservation (such as tradition and conformity) may place greater importance on the continuity principle of identity than somebody who values openness to change (such as self-directedness and stimulation) who may, conversely, be more concerned about maintaining a sense of distinctiveness.

The impact of coping strategies

As a theory of identity threat and coping, identity process theory predicts that the threatened individual reacts to the threat by deploying coping strategies. Coping can be thought of as occurring at three distinct levels: intrapsychic, interpersonal and intergroup.

The ways of coping can also be meaningfully differentiated into adaptive and maladaptive strategies, based on the outcomes of each approach. Examples of adaptive coping include thinking about the situation differently and accessing social support that allows the person to feel understood and to make sense of what has happened. Examples of maladaptive coping can include denial, sexual compulsivity and indeed chemsex. MSM may engage in chemsex in order to cope with social and psychological stressors, such as rejection from sexual partners on the basis of HIV status, poor body image, low self-esteem and so on. Therefore, it is recognised that, although some coping responses can have unwanted outcomes, the initial intent is one of self-protection.

Reflective point

Some people can unintentionally use coping strategies that could be considered maladaptive in the longer term. How might you support someone to think about the impact of the strategies used and to explore alternative options?

What would be important about your approach, given that the person may be experiencing psychological issues, such as shame, low self-esteem, etc?

How can we help reduce the risk of harm?

One way to address problematic chemsex participation is to consider how clinicians may help service users think about different ways of coping. There are several factors that will influence coping and the (sometimes unconscious) choice of strategy, which include personality/personal history, the availability of social support and the healthcare practitioner:

- First, personality traits will predispose an individual to cope in particular ways. For instance, the individual who values the 'status quo' (conservation) may be less inclined to elect a coping strategy such as anticipatory restructuring (e.g. changing their view of a situation) due to their desire to maintain a sense of continuity between past, present and future. They may not wish to entertain the idea of change because they strive to hold onto the past. On the other hand, the individual with a personality profile that favours sensation-seeking and hedonism may react to threat by engaging in risk behaviours, such as chemsex.
- Second, the availability of social support is a significant determinant of coping strategy. Put simply, only those who actually possess a social support network can make use of it. The socially supported person is more likely to engage in potentially helpful strategies, such as discussing sensitive issues (which may include HIV diagnosis) and to make use of the support offered by others. However, support is a complex arena in itself, and the nature and quality of the support are likely to influence its helpfulness. A person who lacks a social support network does not have the option of making sense of their problems. Being unable to gather alternative perspectives, they will have only their own, which may be a negative framework if they have a history of difficult experiences (refer to Chapters 4 and 6). This can then exacerbate any psychological/emotional issues. MSM who face social and psychological adversity may then benefit from accessing social support to minimise the risk of selecting chemsex as a coping strategy. Neither James nor Juan appear to have

access to social support, which seems to have led to them to engage in chemsex to fill the gap relating to unmet needs.

- Third, practitioners working with MSM at risk of poor sexual health outcomes have the potential to help service users explore alternative coping strategies. Tenets of social psychological theory, such as identity process theory, can enable the practitioner to gauge their patients' awareness, understanding and potential behaviour in any given context. This can also allow the practitioner to work alongside service users to think about, and perhaps predict, patterns of behaviour, allowing them to identify and alter unhelpful patterns of coping. For instance, a newly diagnosed gay man who has not spoken about his sexual identity to others due to anticipated homophobia is also likely to conceal his HIV status from others, precluding access to social support. The practitioner may intervene by introducing other options regarding social support networks, for example, LGBT and/or HIV community support services. In short, the choice of coping strategy plays a fundamental role in sexual health outcomes among MSM facing identity threat.

Important aspects of a healthcare clinician's approach

The discussion above has considered in detail how belonging to one or several marginalised groups (e.g. MSM, HIV) can have an adverse impact on psychological and emotional wellbeing. As a result of this, MSM can engage in coping strategies that aim to redress the unmet needs that come with this experience. However, this can inadvertently lead to participation in risky activities, such as chemsex, which can lead to further distress and increase feelings of shame. Feelings of shame and low self-esteem may already exist for MSM who have experienced homophobia and have received negative messages relating to their sexuality, which are embedded in heteronormative, or indeed homophobic, societal attitudes. Therefore, the manner in which healthcare clinicians offer support is important if it is to benefit the service user and minimise further distress.

Perhaps most importantly, a non-judgemental approach is essential to avoid any exacerbation of shame that a person may already be experiencing. Some stories about chemsex can be shocking to healthcare practitioners, as it may be far from anything they have experienced or spoken of in their personal world. However, it is important for practitioners to manage their responses, as outright expressions of shock may imply negative judgement. For example, the service user may worry that the practitioner perceives them to be 'abnormal' or 'disgusting'. As well as emotional expression/non-verbal communication, the choice of language when exploring the person's experiences must be sensitive. One example might be that, although we have understood some coping strategies to be 'maladaptive' from a theoretical point of view, it would not be helpful to use this language when working with someone. It may insinuate that they are a 'maladaptive coper', which may (unintentionally) communicate a message that they are somehow inherently wrong or damaged, thus exacerbating shame. Healthcare workers will therefore need to practise with self-awareness in order to ensure that service users feel able to communicate openly, which is essential for effective healthcare intervention (refer to Chapters 2, 4, 5 and 6).

Delivering care to people participating in chemsex is complex, particularly as we are still learning about what makes an effective healthcare approach. However, in general, it will be helpful to avoid questions or statements that make assumptions or that may appear to come from a critical or blaming stance. Adopting a curious perspective to gather information and responses from the service user, while expressing understanding of their situation, is likely to be validating for the person. A validating experience is then more likely to lead to the development of a trusting healthcare relationship, through which high-quality support can be offered and alternative coping options explored. A collaborative approach with the service user is best placed to increase their sense of self-efficacy as it allows a sense of agency in the process.

Care delivery for chemsex users

Given the level of harms and the rise in chemsex-related deaths, there have been calls for it to become a public healthcare priority (McCall et al., 2015). As a relatively new area of health need, sexual health and addiction services are responding reactively as best they can, although neither, on its own, can be expected to be equipped to manage the complexity of the issue. Researchers in the field are advocating the need for integrated, person-centred and holistic multi/interdisciplinary team approaches, given the inter-related nature of sexual, psychological and substance use needs (e.g. Glynn et al., 2018; Pufall et al., 2018; Sewell et al., 2017). It seems clear that professionals with expertise that relate to these areas will be better positioned to support chemsex users if they work together, and alongside the person. This will help gain a full understanding of the often mutually exacerbating issues and how they relate to the person in their individual and social context. Establishing relationships between NHS and community services is likely to be essential as partnership working has the potential to meet even broader needs. Overall, there is a requirement for multidimensional approaches that involve mental health screening and support, substance use interventions, goal-focused approaches and conversations around prevention of adverse outcomes and harm minimisation. Additionally, community-led projects that include health promotion through creative outlets (e.g. films, theatre, online education projects) have the promise to address the complexities of chemsex on a wider scale (Stardust et al., 2018).

Conclusions

In this chapter, it is suggested that, for some MSM, chemsex may constitute an unhelpful strategy for coping with psychological adversity, even though intentions may be rooted in attempts to address unmet needs and self-protection. However, it is acknowledged that many MSM engage in chemsex transiently and are able to maintain a sense of self-efficacy, enabling them to disengage from the practice when they wish to do so. In the case studies outlined at the beginning of the chapter, James and Juan clearly view chemsex as a potential means of enhancing their identity and wellbeing, although they acknowledge the secondary challenges that chemsex can induce in their lives. The empirical research summarised in this chapter supports the hypothesis that chemsex may provide temporary respite from identity threat but that it is likely to result in secondary threats associated with disruption to other aspects of one's life. Moreover, chemsex can result in harm to mental and sexual health outcomes for MSM. It is suggested that practitioners can intervene to help explore alternative coping to chemsex participation among MSM at risk, and to reduce the risk of negative health outcomes in those who do engage in chemsex. Chemsex is a complex practice with physiological, social and indeed psychological dimensions. Not all of these dimensions have been empirically examined. Yet, they must be understood by clinicians and practitioners working with MSM who engage in chemsex. It is hoped that this chapter will stimulate further empirical research into the social psychology of chemsex and enhance both prevention and treatment efforts in this context.

Notes

1 It is acknowledged that a wide range of terms are used to describe men who have sex with men, such as 'gay', 'bisexual', 'queer' and others. In this chapter, the term 'men who have sex with men' is used.
2 Grindr is a geospatial social networking mobile application for MSM.
3 'Chems' are psychoactive substances that are used in sexualised settings.

Useful resources

Antidote @London: LGBT Drug and Alcohol Support: http://londonfriend.org.uk/get-support/drug sandalcohol/#.XTMFbcrRbmo
Chemsex First AIDS: A Community Booklet: www.davidstuart.org/Chemsex%20First%20Aid% 20action%20sheet.pdf
Chemsex Support at 56 Dean St: http://dean.st/chemsex-support/
Jaspal, R. (2018). *Enhancing Sexual Health, Self-Identity and Wellbeing among Men Who Have Sex With Men: A Guide for Practitioners*. London: Jessica Kingsley Publishers.
Understanding Chemsex, Terrence Higgins Trust: www.steveretsonproject.scot/media/1348/tht_chem sex_guide.pdf

References

Applebaum, A. J., Andres Bedoya, C., Hendriksen, E. S., Wilkinson, J. L., Safren, S. A., & O'Cleirigh, C. (2015). Future directions for interventions targeting PTSD in HIV-infected adults. *Journal of the Association of Nurses in AIDS Care*, 26, 127–138.

Barrett, P., O'Donnell, K., Fitzgerald, M., Schmidt, A. J., Hickson, F., Quinlan, M., Keogh, P., O'Connor, L., McCartney, D., & Igoe, D. (2019). Drug use among men who have sex with men in Ireland: Prevalence and associated factors from a national online survey. *International Journal of Drug Policy*, 64, 5–12.

Bourne, A., Reid, D., Hickson, F., Torres Rueda, S., & Weatherburn, P. (2014). *The Chemsex Study: Drug Use in Sexual Settings among Gay & Bisexual Men in Lambeth, Southwark & Lewisham*. London: Sigma Research, London School of Hygiene & Tropical Medicine. Available at www.sig maresearch.org.uk/chemsex Accessed 7 December 2016.

Bourne, A., Reid, D., Hickson, F., Torres-Rueda, S., & Weatherburn, P. (2015). Chemsex" and harm reduction need among gay men in South London. *International Journal of Drug Policy*, 26(12), 1171–1176.

Daramilas, C., & Jaspal, R. (2016). HIV diagnosis and identity processes among men who have sex with men (MSM) in London, Athens and New York. *Social Psychological Review*, 18(2), 6–16.

Dolling, D. I., Desai, M., McOwan, A., Gilson, R., Clarke, A., Fisher, M., Schembri, G., Sullivan, A. K., Mackie, N., Reeves, I., Portman, M., Saunders, J., Fox, J., Bayley, J., Brady, M., Bowman, C., Lacey, C. J., Taylor, S., White, D., Antonucci, S., Gafos, M., McCormack, S., Gill, O. N., Dunn, D. T., Nardone, A., & PROUD Study Group. (2016). An analysis of baseline data from the PROUD study: An open-label randomised trial of pre-exposure prophylaxis. *Trials*, 17, 163. doi:10.1186/s13063-016-1286-4.

Evers, Y. J., Van Liere, G. A. F. S., Hoebe, C. J. P. A., & Dukers-Muijrers, N. H. T. M. (2019). Chemsex among men who have sex with men living outside major cities and associations with sexually transmitted infections: A cross-sectional study in the Netherlands. *PLoS ONE*, 14(5), e0216732. doi:10.1371/journal.pone.0216732.

Frankis, J., Flowers, P., McDaid, L., & Bourne, A. (2018). Low levels of chemsex among men who have sex with men, but high levels of risk among men who engage in chemsex: Analysis of a cross-sectional online survey across four countries. *Sexual Health*, 15(2), 144–150.

Glynn, R. W., Byrne, N., O'Dea, S., Shanley, A., Codd, M., Keenan, E., Ward, M., Igoe, D., & Clarke, S. (2018). Chemsex, risk behaviours and sexually transmitted infections among men who have sex with men in Dublin, Ireland. *International Journal of Drug Policy*, 52, 9–15.

Graf, N., Dichtl, A., Deimel, D., Sander, D., & Stöver, H. (2018). Chemsex among men who have sex with men in Germany: Motives, consequences and the response of the support system. *Sexual Health*, 15(2), 151–156.

Hegazi, A., Lee, M. J., Whittaker, W., Green, S., Simms, R., Cutts, R., Nagington, M., Nathan, B., & Pakianathan, M. R. (2017). Chemsex and the city: Sexualised substance use in gay bisexual and other men who have sex with men attending sexual health clinics. *International Journal of STDs and AIDS*, 28(4), 362–366.

Hibbert, M. P., Brett, C. E., Porcellato, L. A., & Hope, V. D. (2019). Psychosocial and sexual characteristics associated with sexualised drug use and chemsex among men who have sex with men (MSM) in the UK. *Sexually Transmitted Infections*, 95(5), 342–350.

Jaspal, R. (2018). *Enhancing Sexual Health, Self-Identity and Wellbeing among Men Who Have Sex With Men: A Guide for Practitioners*. London: Jessica Kingsley Publishers.

Jaspal, R. (2019). *The Social Psychology of Gay Men*. London: Palgrave.

Jaspal, R., & Breakwell, G. M. (eds.) (2014). *Identity Process Theory: Identity, Social Action and Social Change*. Cambridge: Cambridge University Press.

Kenyon, C., Wouters, K., Platteau, T., Buyze, J., & Florence, E. (2018). Increases in condomless chemsex associated with HIV acquisition in MSM but not heterosexuals attending a HIV testing center in Antwerp, Belgium. *AIDS Research & Therapy*, 15, 14. doi: 10.1186/s12981-018-0201-3.

Kohli, M., Hickson, F., Free, C., Reid, D., & Weatherburn, P. (2019). Cross-sectional analysis of chemsex drug use and gonorrhoea diagnosis among men who have sex with men in the UK. *Sexual Health*, Online First. doi: 10.1071/SH18159.

Kwan, T. H., & Lee, S. S. (2019). Bridging awareness and acceptance of pre-exposure prophylaxis among men who have sex with men and the need for targeting chemsex and HIV testing: Cross-sectional survey. *JMIR Public Health Surveillance*, 5(3), e13083. doi: 10.2196/13083.

Latini, A., Dona, M. G., Alei, L., Colafigli, M., Frasca, M., Orsini, D., Giuliani, M., Morrone, A., Cristaudo, A., & Zaccarelli, M. (2019). Recreational drugs and STI diagnoses among patients attending an STI/HIV reference clinic in Rome, Italy. *Sexually Transmitted Infections*, Online First. doi:10.1136/sextrans-2019-054043.

Lawn, W., Aldridge, A., Xia, R., & Winstock, A. R. (2019). Substance-linked sex in heterosexual, homosexual, and bisexual men and women: An online, cross-sectional "Global drug survey". *Journal of Sexual Medicine*, 16(5), 721–732.

Lea, T., Hammoud, M., Bourne, A., Maher, L., Jin, F., Haire, B., Bath, N., Grierson, J., & Prestage, G. (2019). Attitudes and perceived social norms toward drug use among gay and bisexual men in Australia. *Substance Use & Misuse*, 54(6), 944–954.

Lim, S. H., Akbar, M., Wickersham, J. A., Kamarulzaman, A., & Altice, F. L. (2018). The management of methamphetamine use in sexual settings among men who have sex with men in Malaysia. *International Journal of Drug Policy*, 55, 256–262.

Macfarlane, A. (2016). Sex, drugs and self-control: Why chemsex is fast becoming a public health concern. *Journal of Family Planning and Reproductive Health Care*, 42, 291–294.

Maxwell, S., Shahmanesh, M., & Gafos, M. (2019). Chemsex behaviours among men who have sex with men: A systematic review of the literature. *International Journal of Drug Policy*, 63, 74–89.

McCall, H., Adams, N., Mason, D., & Willis, J. (2015). What is chemsex and why does it matter? *British Medical Journal*, 351, h5790. doi:10.1136/bmj.h579.

Morris, S. (2019). Yes, has no meaning if you can't say no: Consent and crime in the chemsex context. *Drugs and Alcohol Today*, 19, 23–28.

Pakianathan, M., Whittaker, W., Lee, M. J., Avery, J., Green, S., Nathan, B., & Hegazi, A. (2018). Chemsex and new HIV diagnosis in gay, bisexual and other men who have sex with men attending sexual health clinics. *HIV Medicine*, Online First. doi: 10.1111/hiv.12629.

Pollard, A., Nadarzynski, T., & Llewellyn, C. (2017). O13 'I was struggling to feel intimate, the drugs just helped. Chemsex and HIV-risk among men who have sex with men (MSM) in the UK: Syndemics of stigma, minority-stress, maladaptive coping and risk environments. *Sexually Transmitted Infections*, 93(A5), doi: 10.1136/sextrans-2017-053232.13.

Pufall, E. L., Kall, M., Shahmanesh, M., Nardone, A., Gilson, R., Delpech, V., Ward, H., & Positive Voices study group. (2018). Sexualized drug use ('chemsex') and high-risk sexual behaviours in HIV-positive men who have sex with men. *HIV Medicine*, 19(4), 261–270.

Roux, P., Fressard, L., Suzan-Monti, M., Chas, J., Sagaon-Teyssier, L., Capitant, C., Meyer, L., Tremblay, C., Rojas-Castro, D., Pialoux, G., Molina, J. M., & Spire, B. (2018). Is on-demand HIV Pre-exposure Prophylaxis a suitable tool for men who have sex with men who practice chemsex? Results from a substudy of the ANRS-IPERGAY trial. *Journal of Acquired Immune Deficiency Syndromes*, 79(2), e69–e75. doi: 10.1097/QAI.0000000000001781.

Sewell, J., Miltz, A., Lampe, F. C., Cambiano, V., Speakman, A., Phillips, A. N., Stuart, D., Gilson, R., Asboe, D., Nwokolo, N., Clarke, A., Collins, S., Hart, G., Elford, J., Rodger, A. J., & the Attitudes to and Understanding of Risk of Acquisition of HIV (AURAH) Study Group. (2017). Poly drug use, chemsex drug use, and associations with sexual risk behaviour in HIV-negative men who have sex with men attending sexual health clinics. *International Journal of Drug Policy*, 43, 33–43.

Smith, V., & Tasker, F. (2018). Gay men's chemsex survival stories. *Sexual Health*, 15(2), 116–122.

Stardust, Z., Kolstee, J., Joksic, S., Gray, J., & Hannan, S. (2018). A community-led harm-reduction to chemsex: Case study from Australia's largest gay city. *Sexual Health*, 15(2), 179–181.

Stevens, O., Moncrieff, M., & Gafos, M. (2019). Chemsex-related drug use and its association with health outcomes in men who have sex with men: A cross-sectional analysis of Antidote clinic service data. *Sexually Transmitted Infections*, Online First. doi:10.1136/sextrans-2019-054040.

Tan, R. K. J., Wong, C. M., Chen, M. I., Chan, Y. Y., Bin Ibrahim, M. A., Lim, O. Z., Chio, M. T., Wong, C. S., Chan, R. K. W., Chua, L. J., & Choong, B. C. H. (2018). Chemsex among gay, bisexual, and other men who have sex with men in Singapore and the challenges ahead: A qualitative study. *International Journal of Drug Policy*, 61, 31–37.

Van Hout, M. C., Crowley, D., O'Dea, S., & Clarke, S. (2019). Chasing the rainbow: Pleasure, sex-based sociality and consumerism in navigating and exiting the Irish chemsex scene. *Culture, Health & Sexuality*, 21(9), 1074–1086.

Weatherburn, P., Hickson, F., Reid, D., Torres-Rueda, S., & Bourne, A. (2016). Motivations and values associated with combining sex and illicit drugs ('chemsex') among gay men in South London: Findings from a qualitative study. *Sexually Transmitted Infections*, 93(3), 153–154.

8   The seemingly intractable problem of HIV-related stigma

Developing a framework to guide stigma interventions with young people living with HIV

Tomás Campbell

Chapter description

This chapter will address how stigma is created and will focus particular attention on the creation and maintenance of HIV-related stigma. The effects of HIV stigma in the lives of young people with HIV will be examined and the kinds of interventions that have addressed these issues will be explored. As a result of reading this chapter, you will be introduced to a framework that may help to address HIV-related stigma within clinic practice.

Introduction

The introduction of antiretroviral therapy (ART) in the mid-1990s has saved the lives of millions of children with HIV (Mellins et al., 2009). Due to the success of early identification of HIV and effective treatment with ART, most children and young people with HIV in the United Kingdom (UK) survive into adolescence and adulthood (Foster et al., 2009). There are about 1951 children and young people in the UK living with HIV, of whom approximately 65% are now over the age of 15 years (Collaborative HIV Paediatric Study: Summary data, 2016) and most are of African origin (Judd et al., 2007). In international terms, however, the majority (90%) of young people living with HIV reside in sub-Saharan Africa (WHO, 2014).

Young people living with HIV, both in the UK and worldwide, experience the ordinary challenges of adolescence but may be also exposed to HIV-related stigma that interferes with their ability to adjust to and cope with their diagnosis (Rao et al., 2007). HIV stigma is a multi-faceted construct that has complex and mostly negative effects on the lives of people living with the condition. They may face particular and multiple challenges and stressors, including medical concerns, increased prevalence of psychological and behavioural issues as well as the exposure to HIV-related stigma (Wilkins et al., 2007).

Despite these issues, young people in the UK who are HIV positive are an under-researched group with regard to the psychosocial impact of the condition (Foster et al., 2009) and especially with regard to the impact of stigma. Generally, being a member of a stigmatised group results in relatively poorer outcomes across a range of health and social factors compared with groups that are not stigmatised.

> **Reflection point**
>
> What was your experience of adolescence?
> Did you feel you always fitted in with your peers?
> What was it like to worry about "being normal"?
> Could you discuss your worries with anyone?
> Did you seek information about any of your worries from the adults around you?
> If not, what stopped you? If yes, did their responses help you?

The experience of stigma and discrimination, and the increased number of negative life events that result from these, represent threats to physical, social and psychological well-being. Such experiences harm psychological well-being of young people by reducing expectations of oneself and others, undermining learning in educational settings, or reducing access to adequate health care.

What is HIV-related stigma?

Most HIV-related stigma research and theory is based on Goffman's (1963) work, which described stigma as a type of "spoiled identity" which occurs when a person or group possess a particular attribute that is viewed by others in society as an "undesirable difference". In this conceptualisation, the undesirable difference "reduces the bearer from a whole and usual person to a tainted, discounted one". The mechanism for this process is a societal one by which the undesirable difference is identified and located in an individual or group.

Subsequent work on the creation and development of stigma has attempted to explain further the mechanisms by which the experience of stigma is created and how it affects the thoughts and behaviours of both those who enact stigmatising behaviours and attitudes and those who are affected by stigma (Link & Phelan, 2001).

In this model, stigma is created when four distinct but related components converge:

1. Differences amongst people are articulated and labelled as either good or bad.
2. Dominant cultural beliefs link labelled persons to undesirable characteristics (or negative stereotypes).
3. Labelled persons are placed in distinct categories that facilitate the separation of "us" from "them".
4. Labelled persons experience status loss and discrimination that leads to unequal outcomes (e.g. health, economic, social).

These factors are further dependent upon the existence of inequalities in social, economic and political power that enables these four components of stigma to unfold.

> **Reflection point**
>
> Think about how people with HIV are usually considered:
>
> • What are the differences attributed to them?

- What values are placed on those differences?
- How does the labelling of those differences change the behaviours of the people around them?

Why is HIV stigmatised?

From the very early days of the emergence of the condition, HIV was associated with considerable social and political stigma. HIV/AIDS was quickly associated with gay men, drug users and sex workers – groups of people already stigmatised in most societies. Susan Sontag (1991), writing about the metaphors associated with HIV and AIDS in Europe and North America, observed how HIV was linked with notions of morality, sin and punishment. This observation is seen in the names first given to HIV. In the early days of the emerging epidemic and before the virus was identified, the condition was first referred to as the "gay cancer" and later as Gay-Related Immune Deficiency (GRID).

Through the linking of the condition with a group of people who had a stigmatised identity and who engaged in stigmatised sexual practices (gay men initially, but subsequently intravenous drug users and sex workers), the diagnosis both intensified the existing stigma of groups of people who were HIV-positive, and the new condition itself gained the stigma of having been acquired through shameful sexual or drug-use practices. In this way, HIV was interpreted by many as a "gay plague", as punishment for the immorality of "gays" as well as the immoral behaviour of other marginalised groups.

In the 40 years since its emergence, HIV has affected all countries and continents and has spread beyond the original affected groups. Indeed, HIV is now concentrated in sub-Saharan African, where millions have died and many more millions currently live with HIV. Sub-Saharan Africa is also home to 90% of people living with HIV, amongst whom AIDS-related mortality is increasing (WHO, 2014). Most of these people identify as heterosexual but the impact of stigma remains as strong as ever. Indeed, as the late Nelson Mandela (2002) remarked:

> The stigma and discrimination inflicted on these children (with HIV) are atrocious and inexcusable. And likewise, it is inexcusable to subject any person infected or affected by HIV or AIDS to such abuse and rejection. We must therefore tackle the stigma and discrimination associated with HIV/AIDS with even greater urgency. We must show that we care for all those affected by this terrible condition and that we are doing something about it.

Stigma may be a layered experience

HIV-related stigma can also be considered as a layered experience (Swendeman et al., 2006). This idea refers to HIV being particularly prevalent in certain groups or associated with particular sexual behaviours (e.g. gay, transgendered or alcohol/drug-using behaviours) that are already stigmatised. In this way, HIV-related stigma also becomes attached to other "traits or behaviours that are undesirable" (Goffman, 1963) and may deepen the experience of stigma. The interaction of personal characteristics that may already have stigma attached to them (e.g. black ethnic origin, asylum seekers, gay men) and HIV provides a context in which the contribution and importance of any one factor becomes blurred and stigma is experienced at many levels.

The process of stigma generates disregard for the discounted person and others like them, and they come to be considered as unworthy of equal regard or equal worth. This may further result in social sanctions (discrimination) against those who possess that attribute. Discrimination can create a sense of powerlessness, in that it implies a lack of control over one's life, as an important part of one's experience has to be hidden and may be found out with potentially disastrous consequences. There may also be possible exclusion from valued social groups and activities (e.g. family events, school, the workplace, etc). Given the experience of devaluation, exclusion and lack of control caused by discrimination, the impact of stigma and the perception of discrimination have negative effects on well-being for the affected person. This includes an effect on the psychological status of the discounted person, as the experiences threaten any positive self-concept of the person with the undesirable attribute.

What are the mechanisms through which HIV-related stigma operate?

At an individual level, the feeling of being stigmatised becomes internalised. This process occurs when a person who is living with HIV endorses societally derived negative attitudes associated with the condition and accepts them as applicable to themselves. This process of devaluation occurs when people who are HIV positive believe that they now belong to a group of people whom others view negatively (Pantelic, 2015). Once these attitudes have been incorporated into the person's own beliefs, the result is an experience of "internalised expectations of rejection" (Link, 1987). This internalisation of a sense of rejection because of HIV-positive status can become characterised by feelings of shame, guilt and worthlessness (Lee et al., 2002). Additionally, as well as creating feelings such as shame, internalised stigma can also exacerbate existing emotions of this nature that have derived from previous adverse experiences (see Chapter 6).

The process of internalising HIV-related stigma may also be conceptualised as a psychosocial stressor that affects the discounted person in different ways. This complex process creates a sense of powerlessness over the person's life that reduces a sense of self-efficacy. This is the psychological notion of being able to set personal goals or aspirations and believe that one has the personal characteristics and capability to achieve these. It can also reduce expectations of self, others and quality and enjoyment of life. There may be an anticipation of negative treatment by others (typically by a dominant group member). Additionally, as there is an expectation of negative responses, the maintenance of positive self-regard becomes difficult. This can sometimes manifest in poor self-care behaviours, as is illustrated in the case study below.

Case study: Eva

Eva was born in London of Zambian parents and she was diagnosed with HIV when she was 2 years old. She acquired it vertically and is the only child (two other siblings) in her family with the condition. She commenced medication at diagnosis as her CD4 was 100 and her viral load was 230,000 copies. The anti-retroviral treatment was effective and her health improved. However, there were many other issues facing the family, including threat of deportation, insecure housing and her father's mental health was poor. HIV was not discussed in the family and Eva was not told about her status until she was 12 years old. This was a very difficult time for her. Subsequently, she did not thrive at school, took risks in sexual relationships and struggled to take her medication. She was sexually assaulted when she was 16. Her adherence to her medication was patchy and her CD4 dropped to 150 and her viral load rose to 150,000 copies.

She was referred to a psychologist at the age of 18. Eva told the psychologist that she was drinking a lot of alcohol to improve her mood, but she was also aware that when she drank in company, her judgement was impaired and she was less able to take care of herself – physically, emotionally and sexually. The focus of the intervention was to establish a safe and trusting environment, where the issues of the sexual assault, HIV secrecy and the adherence to medication could be explored in a sensitive way. Eva realised that her drinking was associated with trying to cope with feelings of anxiety about HIV. She also talked about her sense of being a different person when she drank, someone who was fun, optimistic and lively. This was different from how she usually felt about herself, which was a feeling of being tainted, unwanted and unlovable. With the psychologist she was able to explore how the secrecy about her HIV status had made her feel that there was something wrong with her and that HIV was somehow her fault. They were able to find ways in which Eva was able to discuss her feelings with her parents to let them know how the stigma relating to being HIV positive had affected her sense of self-esteem. Eva reduced her alcohol intake and was able to consider ways in which to better manage her feelings of anxiety.

In a meta-analysis of 110 studies that explored the relationship between perceived discrimination and psychological well-being, Pascoe and Smart Richman (2009) discussed the mechanisms through which these factors result in poorer health. First, increased stress leads to behaviours that avoid or minimise stress. This includes the avoidance of situations and issues that are perceived to cause stress, such as taking medication, being reminded of HIV and sharing of status. This avoidance can clearly have implications for healthcare engagement and therefore affect health outcomes. Second, stress increases engagement in unhealthy behaviours as a way of managing stress. Typical behaviours include poor adherence to medication, increased use of drugs, tobacco and alcohol, avoidance of scheduled medical appointments and reduced engagement in positive lifestyle factors, including poor diet and lack of exercise. See Chapters 3 and 6 for further discussion of the complexities and impacts of different coping strategies.

Young people living with HIV and stigma

HIV-related stigma negatively affects many aspects of the lives of young people living with HIV, including their mental health, self-acceptance, their ability to discuss their status with others and adherence to ART (Mavhu et al., 2013; Mburu et al., 2014; Rongkavilit et al., 2010). However, there has been little specific British literature on the impact of HIV-related stigma and young people in the UK. Most adults living with HIV have acquired it in adulthood via sex, transfusion or drug use. Young people who acquired HIV perinatally have lived with HIV all their lives. They may not always have known their diagnosis and little is known about the gradual realisation of the presence of the condition and, as the young person matures, the unfolding and often unwelcome recognition of the complexity of both the condition and societal attitudes toward HIV (Campbell et al., 2011).

Table 8.1 The effects of HIV-related stigma

Unwanted outcomes	Research studies
Depression and anxiety	Rongkavilit et al., 2010 Andrinopoulos et al., 2011 Clum et al., 2009
Poorer mental health	Boyes & Cluver, 2013 Logie & Gadalla, 2009
Decreased self-esteem	Varni et al., 2012 Tanney et al., 2012
Less engagement with safer sex practices	Cluver et al., 2013 Meade & Sikkema, 2005
Poorer adherence to ART	Sayles et al., 2009 Dlamini et al., 2009
Reduced attendance at medical appointments	Magnus et al., 2010 Aggleton et al., 2005
Increased substance misuse	Varni et al., 2013 Clum et al., 2009

As HIV-positive serostatus is often not evident, the management of social relationships and serostatus discussion to avoid stigma and discrimination has been suggested as an added source of stigma-induced stress amongst young people (Rao et al., 2007). Stigma affects the degree to which people living with HIV choose to share their status, given the potential negative social consequences of such discussions. Young people living with HIV are often apprehensive about sharing their HIV status with parents, friends and sexual partners for fear of a stigmatising reaction (Hightow-Weidman et al., 2013; Hogwood et al., 2013). The experience also may affect support-seeking and the likelihood of being offered social support.

Therefore, HIV-related stigma and its consequences (e.g. discrimination, prejudice, violence, etc.) have been identified as stressors that have negative consequences for young people with HIV (Miller & Kaiser, 2001). For adolescents and young adults living with HIV, stigma negatively influences their quality of life and adherence to care (Harper et al., 2013; Martinez et al., 2012; Steward et al., 2008) (see Table 8.1).

The experiences of stigma in a cohort of young people living with HIV and who use substances in three US cities was the focus of a questionnaire-based study (Swendeman et al., 2006) that distinguished between experiences of enacted stigma (actual experiences of stigma and discrimination) and perceived stigma (a fear or anticipation of stigma, and an internal sense of shame). These two dimensions were captured by questions that focused on: personalised stigma (i.e. social rejection); disclosure concerns; negative self-image (i.e. internalised shame); and concern with public attitudes about people with HIV. Eighty-nine per cent (89%) reported ever having experienced perceived stigma and 64% reported having ever experienced enacted stigma. The results also indicated that 31% of participants had had some experience of stigma within the previous three months. Males reported less perceived stigma than females and females tended to have higher levels of anxiety and depression. This study reflects the research conducted with adults and confirmed the association of stigma with altered mood, especially for females.

Reflection point

If you had HIV, with whom would you discuss it?
How would you decide with whom to discuss it?
What kinds of reactions would you expect from others?
Why would you want to discuss your status?
What would stop you discussing it with others?

HIV-related stigma: the impact of sociocultural context

The effects of stigma emerge in different ways in the lives of people with HIV in the UK. Experiences of discrimination are common, with some studies reporting that up to 50% of participants had experienced stigma as a result of their HIV status (Campbell et al., 2011; Weatherburn et al., 2003). Most of the evidence comes from UK research with adults. In an ethnically mixed sample of 1385 participants, nearly a third of respondents (29.9%) said they had been discriminated against because of their HIV status, with nearly half (49.6%) reporting that this involved their dentist or primary care physician (Elford et al., 2008). Evidence indicates that the experience of stigma is exacerbated for those who belong to already marginalised groups. The influence of structural inequality is highly pertinent within the area of HIV, as many people affected often belong to subcultures stigmatised in society based on factors such as ethnicity, sexuality, mental health and socioeconomic status (Watkins-Hayes, 2014). A qualitative study of gay men and heterosexual African people with HIV in England reported that prevalent social discourses of homophobia, racism and xenophobia underpin individuals' experiences of HIV-related stigma (Dodds, 2006). In addition to this, there are factors and issues within subcultures that can add to, or reinforce, stigma related to living with HIV.

The African and Afro-Caribbean communities in the UK tend to be religious and the role of religious belief and participation can be a double-edged sword with regard to coping with HIV. Religious belief can assist individuals to better cope by providing a sense of community, having a belief in a higher power and belief in redemption. However, a qualitative study focused on the experiences of HIV-positive adults of Caribbean origin noted high rates of perceived stigma in this population (Anderson et al., 2008). Participants reported high levels of HIV-stigmatising behaviour and attitudes in others and attributed this to a combination of fear of contamination, homophobia and ignorance of HIV that was reinforced by religious beliefs. The authors noted that religion serves a double role in Caribbean culture – both underpinning stigma and assisting in coping with HIV – a phenomenon also noted by other researchers (Chinouya & Keefe, 2005).

In relation to internalised stigma stemming from social discourses, it was found that this led to problematic influence on interpersonal relationships for black MSM, in that they were less likely to share their status with partners and family members (Overstreet et al., 2013). Within the gay community, it has been shown that perceived HIV-related stigma from HIV-negative men toward HIV-positive men had a detrimental impact on mental health. Issues identified were increased depression, avoidant coping and suicidal ideation (Courtenay-Quirk, Wolitski, Parsons, Gomez and the Seropositive Urban Men's Study Team, 2006). A review of HIV-related stigma within the gay community acknowledged that those living with HIV experienced discrimination in many forms, including ageism, judgements on physical appearance, rejection, violence and social exclusion through practices such as serosorting (choosing sexual partners based on HIV-positive or -negative status). Regarding the latter, although some studies report positive aspects of serosorting, others argue that it increases stigma and can actually lead to increased risk of HIV transmission, through lack of testing and/or sharing of status. Additionally, it was posited that the practice is closer to "seroguessing" as decisions are based on perceived, rather than actual, HIV status. The study reflected on increasing divides within gay communities relating to HIV status, which has implications for the mental health of MSM living with the condition (Smit et al., 2012).

With regard to the links between stigma and mental health, nearly 50% of the 1576 participants who responded to the 2015 UK Stigma Index survey reported that they had felt shame, guilt and self-blame with regard to their HIV status in the preceding year. Almost 20% had felt suicidal because of their HIV status (at some point) and suicidal feelings were more common in people who had been more recently diagnosed (Stigma Survey UK, 2015).

Campbell et al. (2016) explored experiences of HIV-related stigma in a group of UK-based young people. In a mixed gender sample, females reported more enacted stigma experiences than males (77% vs. 25%), e.g. more females than males reported losing friends because of their status. Females also reported more serious experiences of being hassled or threatened because of their status. Males reported feeling less stigmatised than females on measures of perceived stigma except with regard to shame, to which there was an equal percentage of response. Feeling socially rejected was the most common experience in males and females, followed by feeling shame about their HIV status. A third of both males and females reported feeling shame because of their status.

Interventions to address HIV-related stigma

There have been few interventions to address the impact of HIV-related stigma in the lives of young people with HIV. There are different reasons for this: the notion of HIV-related stigma has been hard to define, there is little concurrence in the literature about how to operationalise the term (Mahajan et al., 2008) and stigma prevention/intervention efforts are not a priority or remain unfunded (Piot, 2006). It has been also difficult to measure the extent and impact of stigma, both on individuals living with HIV and wider healthcare and societal structures. HIV-related stigma may operate at the level of the individual and also at organisational and societal levels, often affected by different cultural or national settings.

Much of the research to date has focused on adults' perceptions of stigma, the impact on mental health and the barriers thrown up by societal stigma to accessing HIV testing, health care and ART. Interventions in the UK have sought to change negative perceptions that the general public might hold about people with HIV through mass media campaigns, education about transmission and enactment of laws to prevent discrimination. However, little is known about the effectiveness of these interventions, although recent UK data suggest HIV stigma is stubbornly resistant to change. The National AIDS Trust 2014 Survey (National AIDS Trust, 2014) reported that when it comes to the impact of HIV, there are considerable knowledge gaps among the general public regarding HIV treatment, and, worryingly, significant growth in public misunderstandings and myths regarding how HIV is transmitted.

Although there has been some modest improvement in attitudes in recent years, and a majority may hold somewhat supportive attitudes to varying degrees, significant minorities do not do so, or do not do so clearly. The views of these minorities have the potential to make life difficult for people with HIV. Stigma is not only observed in wider society, but can also present itself in healthcare settings (see Chapter 1). For example, the 2015 Stigma Survey reported that people living with HIV reported high rates of stigma and discrimination when attending for dental care in the previous 12 months (Okala et al., 2018). Some people also worry about seeking employment due to fears about potential discrimination.

Managing HIV in the workplace

There is no obligation on employees to tell their employers about their HIV status except in certain professions (e.g. surgery or dentistry, where there is a risk of exposure to bodily fluids or blood).

The availability of ART means that most people who are HIV positive should not become too ill to work. However, if HIV does become symptomatic (i.e. the person starts experiencing related infections), it may be helpful to have a discussion about their situation as the person may require time off work due to illness or may require certain adjustments to be made to their job role, hours of work, etc., in order to allow them to continue working.

From an employer's perspective, the most important thing is to ensure that a person with HIV is not discriminated against in the workplace. People living with HIV are legally protected from discrimination in the workplace and during recruitment under the Equality Act 2010, which, for example, prohibits the use of pre-employment health questionnaires before the offer of a job has been made.

Interventions for young people

There is little published literature about effective anti-stigma interventions for young people. Kidd et al. (2003) developed an anti-stigma intervention for use in African countries, and while the interventions were not specifically targeted at young people, the toolkit aimed to support HIV trainers to confront HIV stigma, promote more care and support for people living with HIV and to defend their rights. However, given the range of negative psychosocial and medical outcomes that young people living with HIV may experience due to HIV-related stigma, it is important develop tailored interventions to equip them with the practical skills needed to address and cope with the negative effects that stigma can have. Interventions should aim to promote adjustment to HIV and effective self-care behaviours. Such interventions may be delivered when adolescents and young adults are newly diagnosed or have been told about their status (Campbell et al., 2016; Hosek et al., 2002). However, a longer-term approach may also be helpful (Campbell et al., 2010).

Harper et al. (2014) described a group-based intervention for adolescents and young adults newly diagnosed with HIV and its impact over time on four dimensions of HIV stigma:

- personalised stigma
- concerns about sharing status
- negative self-image
- concern with public attitudes about people with HIV.

In this intervention, HIV-related stigma was addressed in a holistic manner by providing HIV/AIDS-related information, facilitating the acquisition of coping skills and providing contact with other young people living with HIV in order to improve social support. This approach was underpinned by the notion that HIV-related stigma is manifested both through negative attitudes towards people with HIV but also by internalised negative feelings and beliefs about HIV held by young people living with HIV about themselves and others. The intervention aimed to build and promote resistance skills that would address the external and internal aspects of HIV-related stigma, working both at the individual/intrapersonal level as well as at the group/interpersonal level.

This was achieved by promoting individual-level coping skills and group-based social support focused on:

(a) decreasing negative feelings toward self and others living with HIV
(b) increasing planned and strategic HIV sharing with others and building supportive networks to reduce fears and feelings of rejection
(c) building skills to address HIV-related discrimination and other forms of stigma.

The evaluation of the intervention reported that both male and female participants experienced small overall reductions in HIV-related stigma in three areas: personalised stigma (experiences of rejection for having HIV or fears that others will reject them because of their HIV status), status sharing concerns (worries related to keeping their HIV status secret or controlling who knows their HIV status); and negative self-image (negative feelings toward self for having HIV). However, these effects were not maintained at the three-month follow-up for personalised stigma or concerns about sharing status, and were only minimally maintained for negative self-image. The intervention had no effect on concerns with public attitudes toward people with HIV.

Support for such interventions has been seen in research in the United States and South Africa within populations of youth and adults living with HIV. Results have demonstrated the negative effects of stigma on individuals who are newly diagnosed with HIV, such as it being associated with lower rates of retention in medical care (Fortenberry et al., 2012; Naar-King et al., 2007). Campbell and Griffiths (2016) described a model for delivering an anti-stigma group workshop for UK-based HIV-positive young people in which there were three components:

- First, an explanatory framework was developed to explain what stigma is, what the effects are and why are people stigmatised.
- Second, participants were invited to consider which groups of people have been historically stigmatised and the possible reasons why.
- Third, participants worked together to identify the domains of their lives in which they had personally experienced stigma and developed self-statements to counter the effects of stigma.

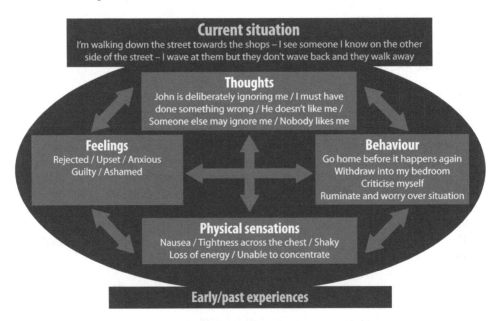

Figure 8.1 An example of the links amongst thoughts, emotions, physical sensations and behaviours

This intervention was based on two psychological models, one of which was cognitive-behavioural therapy (CBT) and narrative therapy. Strategies based on CBT were utilised to give participants an explanatory structure within which to understand what stigma is and the cognitive, emotional and behavioural responses to it. An example of this can be seen in Figure 8.1.

The CBT framework informed the development of strategies to new self-statements to counter the negative effects of stigma. By noticing the ways that thoughts, feelings, physical sensations and behaviours relate to each other, it is possible to begin to break negative patterns and cycles. Participants also took part in an exercise called "a letter from my future self". This technique derives from narrative therapy and encouraged participants to consider how they might use the tools they have learned in a practical way in the coming year. Participants were invited to consider their personal goals and elaborate the process by which these might be achieved and to congratulate themselves (in advance) for their success.

This intervention was evaluated by recording participants' responses to three questions about their experiences of the intervention (Campbell et al., 2011) and analysing the data into themes. Responses indicated that the young people expressed optimism for their ability to cope with stigma-related challenges and emphasised seeking help from family members and health professionals. They also emphasised the benefits of taking ART and of maintaining good self-esteem as counters to negative events. The results presented a picture in which the young people felt confident to face HIV-related challenges. However, as we knew these young people well and were knowledgeable about the ways in which they and their families coped with HIV, we considered that the responses were perhaps unrealistic about the effectiveness of their strategies. These results emphasised to us that developing effective responses to stigma was a long-term goal and required regular intervention.

Exploring the evidence base for addressing HIV-related stigma

There have been a number of systematic reviews to assess the evidence for the type and effectiveness of interventions to address HIV-related stigma. Brown et al. (2003) reviewed 22 studies that had focused on stigma reduction, most of which had focused on reducing stigmatising attitudes and behaviours in health providers and groups within the general population (e.g. school children) by changing individual-level fears, attitudes or behaviours. Brown et al. (ibid.) concluded that there were categories of intervention:

- first, the provision of information about HIV-related stigma
- second, skills-building (e.g. participatory learning sessions to discuss/reduce negative attitudes)
- third, the provision of counselling/support (e.g. support groups for people with HIV)
- lastly, contact with affected groups (e.g. interactions between people with HIV and their friends and colleagues).

The authors concluded that some stigma-reduction interventions appeared to work in the short term, but it was unclear about which components were most effective and what duration of intervention was most effective.

Subsequently, Sengupta et al. (2011) in a systematic review of later studies, examined 19 HIV stigma reduction interventions that measured HIV stigma pre- and post-intervention. The review found that information, skills-building, counselling and people with HIV testimonials seemed to reduce stigmatising attitudes amongst participants.

Stangl et al. (2013) in their systematic review discussed that stigma reduction efforts had improved in the intervening years, but that most efforts were still devoted to reducing misinformation and stigmatising attitudes amongst groups within the general population.

Most studies that are reported in the literature focus on reducing stigmatising attitudes in people who are themselves not HIV positive. While this is essential in reducing the social and psychological burden on people who live with HIV, there is a dearth of interventions to assist in addressing HIV-related stigma amongst people who are HIV positive.

Group-based interventions

There is now evidence that interventions that are solidly based within a theoretically driven framework can be useful in equipping young people living with HIV with the skills necessary to cope more effectively with HIV-related stigma. The most effective interventions seem to comprise structured individual sessions followed by multiple group-based intervention sessions. These interventions appear to offer young people the best opportunity to acquire better coping skills in a social context with other young people with HIV. Group-based approaches also facilitate participants to build social connections within the groups, and perhaps to create a supportive network of other youth.

Components of effective group-based interventions seem to share a number of features. First, the provision of information about the nature and function of stigma is important in order to provide an explanation of how these processes work. This enables young people to consider and understand how the process of stigma works and allows them to place their own experiences within an articulated and explicable framework. Second, it is important that there is a discussion about how the experience of stigma emerges in the lives of young people. As previously discussed, stigma may emerge in many different forms and may not immediately be experienced as the effect of stigma. Lastly, the intervention needs to contain ways of identifying personal emotional and cognitive responses to HIV stigma and ways in which the effects can be recognised and countered.

A cognitive-behavioural approach to managing negative thoughts and emotions can be useful. This is a psychological approach to identifying negative thoughts, feelings and beliefs about the self that underpin behaviours that are consonant with the underlying beliefs. Thus, if a person's underlying beliefs about themselves are negative, the thoughts and feelings they may have about themselves in given situations are also likely to be negative. Behaviours, especially in domains associated with the negative beliefs (medication, status sharing, healthcare), are also likely to be affected negatively thus reflecting the underlying stigmatised beliefs.

A CBT approach starts with the identification of negative beliefs about oneself and then proceeds to an exploration of how personal behaviours reflect these beliefs. This can be a very powerful process for young people with HIV who may have never encountered a systematic exploration of how they may feel about themselves and examine how their previously unspoken feelings are reflected in important self-care behaviours, particularly with regard to managing their HIV condition.

The next step is to explore how powerful and usually automatic beliefs can be reduced in their impact and intensity. This might take the form of finding alternatives to the emotional and behavioural responses to the experience of HIV stigma (e.g. not avoiding discussions of HIV, not assuming that others will react negatively to a sharing of HIV status, seeing adherence of medication as an act of self-care). Maintaining a hopeful and optimistic approach is important while emphasising that each person approaches these issues from a different perspective and each will have a different solution to the unique set of circumstances and challenges in their own lives. Asking young people with HIV to imagine themselves a year hence, having at that point addressed a personally important stigmatising experience, and writing a letter that outlines the steps undertaken to achieve this, can be a powerful and motivating strategy.

Finally, the process of exploring these issues in a supportive group context cannot be underestimated. Through the sharing of stories and experiences, young people can readjust their previously unarticulated expectations of themselves and others and forge new bonds of acceptance of themselves and others.

Reducing the negative effects of HIV stigma: what works?

Providing frameworks for understanding:

- helping young people to understand how stigma is formed and operates
- using cognitive behavioural therapy approach to understand relationships between thoughts, feelings, physical responses and coping behaviours
- giving information about the links between stigma and the effects on mood, behaviour and discussion about status with others and adherence to medication
- encouraging young people with HIV to meet each other, share experiences and form meaningful connections
- developing practical skills to cope with and address situations in which stigma occurs

Whilst it is always important to acknowledge and validate a person's experience of stigma and discrimination, learning to understand the processes of stigma, and discovering ways to address and respond assertively to experiences of it, can be extremely empowering for young people.

Working with an individual young person

Clinicians have a unique opportunity to address HIV-related stigma in practical ways in their clinical work. Clinicians often feel powerless to address the effects of stigma, as it is a reality for people living with HIV. Additionally, they may not understand the mechanisms by which stigma affects their patients and are not able to articulate ways in which patients can identify and address the impact of stigma in their lives. Clinicians may also misattribute behaviour and difficulties in coping with HIV to other factors, such as personality issues, poor adjustment to HIV status, complex family or relationship issues, immaturity, poor understanding of the condition or unwillingness to engage with healthcare when these issues might be better considered and understood within a framework of HIV-related stigma.

Within clinical settings, HIV stigma may be addressed by:

1. **Discussing the patient's experience of HIV**, paying particular to any difficulties with disclosure of status to family and friends, difficulties in adjusting to HIV status and changes to a sense of self-esteem.
2. **Explaining the nature of stigma** and what are the mechanisms and effects. It might be useful to explain how HIV became stigmatised in the early days of the condition and how that association between HIV and immoral or sanctioned behaviours are still prevalent.
3. **Discussing the patient's own views about HIV** would help to identify their own attitudes. Previously held attitudes towards people with HIV may be positive or negative (or a mixture of both) and may underpin and contribute towards their attitudes towards their own changed serostatus.
4. **It will be useful to broaden the discussion of stigma** to consider groups of people in society and in history who have also been stigmatised. This will help to identify the wider societal reasons underpinning the development of stigma, the mechanisms through which this was achieved and the effects on the groups concerned. It will also emphasise that the experience is common and may help to reduce the sense of being singled out for exceptional treatment, which is a consequence of stigma.
5. **Discussion about the impact of shame and guilt**. Past behaviours (especially those associated with having led to acquiring the condition) and desires (especially sexual ones) may now intensify the experience of stigma.
6. **Exploration of where the effects of stigma are emerging in one's life**: not discussing HIV status with others (particularly family members and sexual partners), poor or non-adherence to medication, poor self-care in other domains (alcohol, tobacco and drug use) and poor engagement with HIV healthcare professionals.

Learning points

- As HIV is a stigmatised condition, it is probably not possible for any individual **not** to be affected by stigma in some way.
- Stigma is associated with guilt and shame, especially when it comes to past and future sexual/romantic relationships.
- The experience of HIV stigma intersects with other sources of psychological distress.

Points for discussion with patients

- What is the function of stigma?
- Where does HIV stigma emerge in your life?
- How do you think of yourself as a person with HIV?
- What do you imagine others would think of you if they were aware of your status?
- Are you aware of any feelings of shame or guilt related to your status?
- Do you try to conceal your status from others?
- Are you worried about "being found out"?

Bringing the evidence together: points for clinicians

The current approach of stigma reduction programmes and interventions are mainly directed toward groups within the general population. They aim to reduce the negative attitudes and discriminatory behaviours that badly affect young people with HIV. However, this is not enough, and effective interventions require delivery in all contexts and environments in which young people access care, treatment and support. Such contexts range from the clinic-based environment to community-based organisations.

Clinicians assuming responsibility

The challenge for health professionals is to find effective ways in which to address these issues so that the impact of stigma does not become a major negative component in the ability of young people to cope with their status. Future interventions to reduce HIV-related stigma can benefit from existing evidence-based research, which emphasises that intervention efforts are achievable and can be successful. It is clear that such interventions require urgent implementation to best address the issues faced by millions of young people and particularly in countries and regions most affected by the condition. Health professionals are well placed to undertake these interventions as we have regular contact with young people, we have established helpful and trusting relationships with them and we are able to both track their developmental progress and anticipate future health care needs.

Clinicians cannot assume or rely upon that others will undertake these tasks and roles, as many young people will not be engaged with community-based organisations that may undertake such work, nor can we rely on the family structures within which they live to adequately equip them with the tools necessary to address these issues. This points to a need for comprehensive and ongoing educational programmes for clinicians on all aspects of HIV-related stigma. Such training might be difficult to establish and also may be a challenge to maintain due to lack of trained staff, budget considerations and clinical time pressures. However, as outlined in this chapter, the problem of stigma and its effects are complex and effective interventions require time and resources through which staff can properly consider the issues and explore the impact on their own clinical work and the young people with whom they work.

The most important component of an anti-stigma intervention is the confidence of the health professional to deliver it. Clinicians often feel powerless to address the worst aspects of HIV-related stigma because they may not have an explanatory framework within which they can speak confidently to young people about the nature, impact and effects of stigma. Clinicians may require further ongoing support in order to increase familiarity with important concepts and develop confidence in speaking about the issues with young people. It is vital that all staff who have clinical contact with young people have as comprehensive an understanding of the nature and effects of stigma as possible in order that they do not underestimate its effects on the health-related behaviours of young people. If staff are not fully aware of the impact of stigma, it might be too easy to attribute clinical problems (e.g. non-adherence, poor appointment attendance) to other factors (e.g. immaturity, carelessness, lack of consideration for themselves and/or clinic staff).

Consider family-based and systemic working

Families and caregivers of young people also may require information and training about the long-term effects of stigma on themselves (if they are HIV-positive care-givers) and on the young people they are caring for. The experiences of stigma need to be identified by health professionals within clinical consultations and effective interventions need to be offered to counter the negative impact of stigma. Many young people grow up in homes where there is at least one parent or caregiver who also has HIV. The experience of HIV-related stigma may also have adversely affected the ability of their caregivers to effectively parent them. This points to the need to introduce targeted interventions to parents and families who are affected by HIV in order to equip them with skills to effectively tackle the effects of stigma in their own lives and that of their children.

What is advantageous versus what is achievable?

Stigma reduction interventions can be delivered as a group intervention and there are many advantages to this: it can be a useful time-effective strategy for clinicians, participants have the opportunity to discuss their own experiences with others, and supportive ongoing relationships are key to reducing personal isolation and distress. However, group interventions can also be difficult to establish as young people may have concerns about being judged by others or have fears about discussing personal experiences. Therefore, individual interventions may be more achievable in the short term and have the advantage of being opportunistic in nature. However, clinic visits are often quick and many young people (because of the stigma associated with being in an HIV clinic) wish to get the appointment over with as quickly as possible. This may make it difficult for the clinician to introduce discussions about stigma and have enough time to explore the complexities of how HIV-related stigma might be operating in the life of the young person. Clinicians may have to plan in advance for such discussions and allow enough time for them. Discussions may need to occur on an ongoing and long-term basis as the lives of young people and their personal challenges change quickly during adolescence and young adulthood.

Be mindful of complex needs

There are groups of young people for whom additional consideration is required. Young women and young gay people living with HIV may need further support to reduce stigma than young men. Such support should focus increased time on helping participants to address discrimination and negative societal stereotypes for these groups especially related to issues of pregnancy, vertical transmission and gay sex.

Additionally, as young people are more vulnerable to poorer mental health, close monitoring of mental health status and early referral to supportive mental health services should be considered.

Summary

This chapter has explored the prevalence and impact of stigma for people living with HIV, and in particular for young people who are diagnosed with the condition. It has considered theoretical viewpoints in relation to how stigma is developed and functions and applied this to the experiences of the HIV population. Thought has been given to how the experience of stigma can have multiple layers and how those who belong to marginalised groups are potentially more intensely affected. The unwanted outcomes of HIV-related stigma were explored and reflections on the processes that lead to these outcomes were made. Consideration was then given to interventions for HIV, on a wider societal level, but more attentively to how healthcare professionals can begin to design interventions to support young people living with HIV to address the impact of HIV-related stigma. Different approaches and useful theoretical frameworks were discussed and evaluated in terms of their utility for young people. Finally, the evidence was drawn together to offer helpful recommendations for clinicians in terms of how they can best strive to support young people who are living with a condition that is so often stigmatised.

Resources

The diminished self: HIV and self-stigma:
www.aidsmap.com/The-diminished-self-HIV-and-self-stigma/page/2657859/
HIV stigma and discrimination:
www.avert.org/professionals/hiv-social-issues/stigma-discrimination
Reduction of HIV-related stigma and discrimination:
www.unaids.org/en/resources/documents/2014/ReductionofHIV-relatedstigmaanddiscrimination

References

Aggleton, P., Wood, K., Malcolm, A., & Parker, R. (2005). *HIV-related stigma discrimination and human rights violations: case studies of successful programmes*. Geneva: UNAIDS.

Anderson, M., Elam, G., Gerver, S., Solarin, I., Fenton, K., & Easterbrook, P. (2008). HIV/AIDS-related stigma and discrimination: accounts of HIV-positive Caribbean people in the United Kingdom. *Social Science & Medicine*, 67, 790–798.

Andrinopoulos, K., Clum, G., Murphy, D. A., Harper, G., Perez, L., Xu, J., & Adolescent Medicine Trials Network for HIV/AIDS Interventions. (2011). Health related quality of life and psychosocial correlates among HIV-infected adolescent and young adult women in the US. *AIDS Education and Prevention*, 23, 367–381.

Boyes, M., & Cluver, L. D. (2013). Relationships among HIV/AIDS orphanhood, stigma, and symptoms of anxiety and depression in South African youth: a longitudinal investigation using a path analysis framework. *Clinical Psychological Science*, 1, 323–330.

Brown, L., Macintyre, K., & Trujillo, L. (2003). Interventions to reduce HIV/AIDS stigma: what have we learned? *AIDS Education and Prevention*, 15, 49–69.

Campbell, T., Beer, H., Wilkins, R., Griffiths, J., Sherlock, E., & Merrett, A. (2010). I look forward. I feel insecure but I am OK with it. The experience of young HIV+ people attending transition preparation events: a qualitative investigation. *AIDS Care*, 22, 2, 263–269.

Campbell, T., & Griffiths, J. (2016). "I can still be happy, I can still get my life again": psychological interventions with children, young people and families living with HIV in the United Kingdom. In: P. Liamputtong (Ed.). *Children, young people and living with HIV/AIDS: A cross-cultural perspective* (pp. 399–420). Dordrecht: Springer.

Campbell, T., Griffiths, J., Wilkins, B., & Marinho, G. (2011). Hopes, dreams and ambitions: A qualitative investigation into the views and concerns of older HIV+ adolescents about their future challenges and support needs. *HIV Medicine*, 12, 22.

Campbell, T., Griffiths, J., & Wilkins, R. (2016). Young HIV positive people and experiences of HIV stigma in the UK: a pilot study. *HIV Nursing*, 16, 4, 123–127.

Chinouya, M., & Keefe, E. O. (2005). God will look after us: Africans, HIV and religion in Milton Keynes. *Diversity & Equality in Health and Care*.

Clum, G., Chung, S. E., & Ellen, J. M. & Adolescent Medicine Trials Network for HIV/AIDS Interventions. (2009). Mediators of HIV-related stigma and risk behavior in HIV infected young women. *AIDS Care*, 21, 1455–1462.

Cluver, L., Orkin, M., Boyes, M. E., Sherr, L., Makasi, D., & Nikelo, J. (2013). Pathways from parental AIDS to child psychological, educational and sexual risk: developing an empirically-based interactive theoretical model. *Social Science & Medicine (1982)*, 87, 185–193.

Collaborative HIV Paediatric Study (CHIPS). Summary data. (2016). Available at: http://www.chips cohort.ac.uk/patients/summary-data/ (accessed December 2016).

Courtney-Quirk, C., Wolitski, R. J., Parson, J. T., Gòmez, C. A., & The Seropositive Urban Men's Study Team. (2006). Is HIV/AIDS stigma dividing the gay community? Perceptions of HIV-positive men who have sex with men. *AIDS Education and Prevention*, 18, 56–67.

Dlamini, P. S., Wantland, D., Makoae, L. N., Chirwa, M., Kohi, T. W., Greeff, M., … Holzemer, W. L. (2009). HIV stigma and missed medications in HIV-positive people in five African countries. *AIDS Patient Care and STDs*, 23, 377–387.

Dodds, C. (2006). HIV-related stigma in England: experiences of gay men and heterosexual African migrants living with HIV. *Journal of Community & Applied Social Psychology*, 16, 472–480.

Elford, J., Ibrahim, F., Bukutu, C., & Anderson, J. (2008). HIV-related discrimination reported by people living with HIV in London, UK. *AIDS and Behavior*, 12, 2, 255–264.

Fortenberry, J. D., Martinez, J., Rudy, B. J., Monte, D., & Adolescent Trials Network for HIV/AIDS Interventions. (2012). Linkage to care for HIV-positive adolescents: a multisite study of the adolescent medicine trials units of the adolescent trials network. *Journal of Adolescent Health*, 51, 551–556.

Foster, C., Judd, A., Tookey, P., Tudor-Williams, G., Dunn, D., Shingadia, D., ... Lyall, H. (2009). Young people in the United Kingdom and Ireland with perinatally acquired HIV: the pediatric legacy for adult services. *AIDS Patient Care and STDs*, 23, 159–166.

Goffman, E. (1963). *Stigma. Notes on the management of spoiled identity.* New York: Simon and Shuster.

Harper, G. W., Fernandez, I. M., Bruce, D., Hosek, S. G., & Jacobs, R. J. & Adolescent Medicine Trials Network for HIV/AIDS Interventions. (2013). The role of multiple identities in adherence to medical appointments among gay/bisexual male adolescents living with HIV. *AIDS and Behavior*, 17, 213–223.

Harper, G. W., Lemos, D., & Hosek, S. G. (2014). Stigma reduction in adolescents and young adults newly diagnosed with HIV: findings from the project accept intervention. *AIDS Patient Care and STDs*, 28, 543–554.

Hightow-Weidman, L. B., Phillips, G., Outlaw, A. Y., Wohl, A. R., Fields, S., Hildalgo, J., & LeGrand, S. (2013). Patterns of HIV disclosure and condom use among HIV-infected young racial/ethnic minority men who have sex with men. *AIDS and Behavior*, 17, 1, 360–368.

Hogwood, J., Campbell, T., & Butler, S. (2013). I wish I could tell you but I can't: Adolescents with perinatally acquired HIV and their dilemmas around self-disclosure. *Clinical Child Psychology and Psychiatry*, 18, 44–60.

Hosek, S. G., Harper, G. W., & Domanico, R. (2005). Predictors of medication adherence among HIV-infected youth. *Psychology, Health & Medicine*, 10, 166–179.

Hosek, S. G., Harper, G. W., & Robinson, W. L. (2002). Identity development in adolescents living with HIV. *Journal of Adolescence*, 25, 355–364.

Judd, A., Doerholt, K., Tookey, P. A., Sharland, M., Riordan, A., Menson, E., ... Duong, T. (2007). Morbidity, mortality, and response to treatment by children in the United Kingdom and Ireland with perinatally acquired HIV infection during 1996–2006: planning for teenage and adult care. *Clinical Infectious Conditions*, 45, 918–924.

Kidd, R., Clay, S., & Chiiya, C. (2003). *Understanding and challenging HIV stigma: toolkit for action.* Washington, DC: International Center for Research on Women.

Lee, R. S., Kochman, A., & Sikkema, K. J. (2002). Internalized stigma among people living with HIV-AIDS. *AIDS and Behavior*, 6, 309–319.

Link, B. G. (1987). Understanding labeling effects in the area of mental disorders: an assessment of the effects of expectations of rejection. *American Sociological Review*, 52, 96–112.

Link, B. G., & Phelan, J. C. (2001). Conceptualizing stigma. *Annual Review of Sociology*, 27, 363–385.

Logie, C., & Gadalla, T. M. (2009). Meta-analysis of health and demographic correlates of stigma towards people living with HIV. *AIDS Care*, 21, 742–753.

Magnus, M., Jones, K., Phillips, G., Binson, D., Hightow-Weidman, L. B., Richards-Clarke, C., ... Cobbs, W. (2010). Characteristics associated with retention among African American and Latino adolescent HIV-positive men: results from the outreach, care, and prevention to engage HIV-seropositive young MSM of color special project of national significance initiative. *JAIDS Journal of Acquired Immune Deficiency Syndromes*, 53, 529–536.

Mahajan, A. P., Sayles, J. N., Patel, V. A., Remien, R. H., Ortiz, D., Szekeres, G., & Coates, T. J. (2008). Stigma in the HIV/AIDS epidemic: a review of the literature and recommendations for the way forward. *AIDS*, 22, S67–S79.

Mandela, N. (2002). Closing address at the 14th International AIDS conference, Barcelona, Spain, 12 July 2002.

Martinez, J., Harper, G., Carleton, R. A., Hosek, S., Bojan, K., Clum, G., & Ellen, J. & The Adolescent Medicine Trials Network, J. (2012). The impact of stigma on medication adherence among HIV-positive adolescent and young adult females and the moderating effects of coping and satisfaction with health care. *AIDS Patient Care and STDs*, 26, 108–115.

Mavhu, W., Berwick, J., Chirawu, P., Makamba, M., Copas, A., Dirawo, J., ... Mungofa, S. (2013). Enhancing psychosocial support for HIV positive adolescents in Harare, Zimbabwe. *PLoS One*, 8, e70254.

Mburu, G., Hodgson, I., Kalibala, S., Haamujompa, C., Cataldo, F., Lowenthal, E. D., & Ross, D. (2014). Adolescent HIV disclosure in Zambia: barriers, facilitators and outcomes. *Journal of the International AIDS Society*, 17.

Meade, C. S., & Sikkema, K. J. (2005). HIV risk behavior among adults with severe mental illness: a systematic review. *Clinical Psychology Review*, 25, 433–457.

Mellins, C. A., Elkington, K. S., Bauermeister, J. A., Brackis-Cott, E., Dolezal, C., McKay, M., ... Abrams, E. J. (2009). Sexual and drug use behavior in perinatally HIV-infected youth: mental health and family influences. *Journal of the American Academy of Child & Adolescent Psychiatry*, 48, 810–819.

Miller, C. T., & Kaiser, C. R. (2001). A theoretical perspective on coping with stigma. *Journal of Social Issues*, 57, 73–92.

Naar-King, S., Bradford, J., Coleman, S., Green-Jones, M., Cabral, H., & Tobias, C. (2007). Retention in care of persons newly diagnosed with HIV: outcomes of the Outreach Initiative. *AIDS Patient Care and STDs*, 21, S–40.

National AIDS Trust. (2014). *HIV public knowledge and attitudes*. London: National AIDS Trust.

Okala, S., Doughty, J., Watt, R. G., Santella, A. J., Conway, D. I., Crenna-Jennings, W., ... Benton, L. (2018). The People Living with HIV STIGMA Survey UK 2015: stigmatising experiences and dental care. *British Dental Journal*, 225, 143–150.

Overstreet, N. M., Earnshaw, V. A., Kalichman, S. C., & Quinn, D. M. (2013). Internalized stigma and HIV status disclosure among HIV-positive black men who have sex with men. *AIDS Care*, 25, 466–471.

Pantelic, M., Shenderovich, Y., Cluver, L., & Boyes, M. (2015). Predictors of internalised HIV-related stigma: a systematic review of studies in sub-Saharan Africa. *Health Psychology Review*, 9, 469–490.

Pascoe, E. A., & Smart Richman, L. (2009). Perceived discrimination and health: a meta-analytic review. *Psychological Bulletin*, 135, 531–554, doi:10.1037/a0016059.

Piot, T. (2006). AIDS: from crisis management to sustained strategic response. *The Lancet*, 368, 526–530.

Rao, D., Kekwaletswe, T. C., Hosek, S., Martinez, J., & Rodriguez, F. (2007). Stigma and social barriers to medication adherence with urban youth living with HIV. *AIDS Care*, 19, 28–33.

Rongkavilit, C., Wright, K., Chen, X., Naar-King, S., Chuenyam, T., & Phanuphak, P. (2010). HIV stigma, disclosure and psychosocial distress among Thai youth living with HIV. *International Journal of STD & AIDS*, 21, 126–132.

Sayles, J. N., Wong, M. D., Kinsler, J. J., Martins, D., & Cunningham, W. E. (2009). The association of stigma with self-reported access to medical care and antiretroviral therapy adherence in persons living with HIV/AIDS. *Journal of General Internal Medicine*, 24, 1101.

Sengupta, S., Banks, B., Jonas, D., Miles, M. S., & Smith, G. C. (2011). HIV interventions to reduce HIV/AIDS stigma: a systematic review. *AIDS and Behavior*, 15, 1075–1087.

Smit, P. J., Brady, M., Carter, M., Frenandes, R., Lamore, L., Meulbroek, M., & Thomson, M. (2012). HIV-related stigma within communities of gay men: a literature review. *AIDS Care*, 24, 405–412.

Sontag, S. (1991). *Illness as Metaphor and AIDS and its Metaphors*. London: Penguin Books.

Stangl, A. L., Lloyd, J. K., Brady, L. M., Holland, C. E., & Baral, S. (2013). A systematic review of interventions to reduce HIV-related stigma and discrimination from 2002 to 2013: how far have we come?. *Journal of the International AIDS Society*, 16.

Steward, W. T., Herek, G. M., Ramakrishna, J., Bharat, S., Chandy, S., Wrubel, J., & Ekstrand, M. L. (2008). HIV-related stigma: adapting a theoretical framework for use in India. *Social Science & Medicine*, 67, 1225–1235.

Stigma Survey UK. (2015). HIV in the UK: changes and challenges; actions and answers. The People Living with HIV Stigma Survey UK 2015 National Findings. Available at: www.stigmain dexuk.org/reports/2016/NationalReport.pdf (accessed May 2017).

Swendeman, D., Rotheram-Borus, M. J., Comulada, S., Weiss, R., & Ramos, M. E. (2006). Predictors of HIV-related stigma among young people living with HIV. *Health Psychology*, 25, 501.

Tanney, M. R., Naar-King, S., & MacDonnel, K. & Adolescent Trials Network for HIV/AIDS Interventions 004 Protocol Team. (2012). Depression and stigma in high-risk youth living with HIV: a multi-site study. *Journal of Pediatric Health Care*, 26, 300–305.

Varni, S. E., Miller, C. T., McCuin, T., & Solomon, S. (2012). Disengagement and engagement coping with HIV/AIDS stigma and psychological well-being of people with HIV/AIDS. *Journal of Social and Clinical Psychology*, 31, 123–150.

Watkins-Hayes, C. (2014). Intersectionality and the sociology of HIV/AIDS. Past, present, and future research directions. *The Annual Review of Sociology*, 40, 431–457.

Weatherburn, P., Ssanyu Sseruma, W., Hickson, F., McLean, S., & Reid, D. (2003). Project NASAH: an investigation into the HIV treatment information and other needs o African people with HIV resident in England.

WHO. (2014). *Health for the world's adolescents*. Geneva: World Health Organization.

Wilkins, R., Campbell, T., & Beer, H. (2007). Preparing HIV-positive young people for the challenges of adult life: a group work approach. *AIDS & Hepatitis Digest*, 119, 1–4.

9 Multidisciplinary management of neuropathic pain in HIV care

Sarah Blackshaw, Hoo Kee Tsang and Catherine Heaton

Chapter description

This chapter will look at some of the difficulties that people living with HIV have with chronic pain, particularly neuropathic pain (which is pain as a result of problems with the nerves in the body). We will discuss some of the reasons that people develop neuropathic pain, and look at why an approach that combines medication, physiotherapy and psychological techniques is most effective.

HIV is now considered to be a chronic disease with a life expectancy closer to that of the general population (Gueler et al., 2017; Teeraananchai et al., 2017). As life span increases, the management of co-morbid conditions with the aim of maintaining quality of life becomes equally important. Pain is a common symptom in people with HIV, and research has considered the prevalence of pain in people with HIV, with one study reporting it to be over 90% (Wandeler, Johnson, & Egger, 2016).

During the 1990s a number of studies highlighted the under-recognition and under-treatment of pain in people with HIV (Bernard et al., 1999; Breitbart et al., 1996). Under-treatment more often affects women and non-white populations (Sambamoorthi et al., 2000; Tsao, Stein, & Dobalian, 2010). People with HIV and pain suffer a higher incidence of sleep disturbance, severe fatigue, anxiety and depression, substance misuse, overall work impairment and activity impairment than those without pain. This has been linked to significant clinical and economic costs (Mann et al., 2016; Miaskowski et al., 2011; Wilson et al., 2016).

Reflective point

Think about the last time you had pain – from an illness, or injury perhaps.
What if that pain did not go away over time?
How do you think you would feel?
How do you think you would behave?
What do you think you would do?
How might other people respond to you?

Understanding neuropathic pain

Many pain syndromes have been described in people with HIV, including abdominal pain, headaches, throat pain, peripheral neuropathy, arthralgia, back pain and herpes zoster (Perry et al., 2013). HIV may also be associated with a higher incidence of fibromyalgia, with cohort studies identifying an incidence of 11–14% compared with 0.2–6.6% in the general population (Dotan et al., 2016; Marques et al., 2016). However, the most common complaint that people living with HIV present to pain clinic with is neuropathic pain, which is "Pain caused by a lesion or disease of the somatosensory nervous system" (IASP, 1994).

What causes neuropathic pain?

There are two main causes of neuropathic pain in people living with HIV – as a consequence of taking some of the older medications available to manage HIV such as Stavudine, or as a secondary issue to the HIV itself. The medical community is not sure what causes this secondary issue, which is known as "distal sensory peripheral neuropathy", but there are a number of theories, including that the virus itself can cause problems with the nerves.

In 2010 the World Health Organization started a programme to phase out the use of Stavudine. At the end of 2011 its use had reduced significantly in Europe but continued to rise globally due to the increased uptake of treatment. The 2016 World Health Organization guideline continues to recommend the discontinuation of Stavudine in first-line treatment (WHO, 2013, 2016). It is important to remember that even though these medications are not used in the UK, there are still many countries, particularly in Africa, where these medications are still used a lot. This means that, unfortunately, neuropathic pain as a consequence of taking medication is unlikely to be completely eradicated in the near future.

How do people present with neuropathic pain?

Distal sensory peripheral neuropathy and drug-induced peripheral neuropathy can be difficult to tell apart just from speaking to the person about their symptoms. The short amount of time between the onset of symptoms and the start of antiretroviral medication may be the only feature that helps to identify a drug-induced neuropathy.

People commonly present with symmetrically altered sensation such as numbness, pins and needles, and a burning sensation affecting the toes and soles of the feet. Patients may describe their symptoms as: aching, painful and numb; burning; more severe in the soles of the feet; and worse at night. Symptoms can gradually progress up the legs to the knees. Late-stage symptoms can develop in the hands. Pain associated with the condition can range from mild to debilitating, with varying impact on activities of daily living (De la Monte et al., 1988; Verma, 2001).

> I've always had a little bit of pain, but it seemed to get worse over time. It's in the soles of my feet and it feels like I'm walking over hot coals. Sometimes my feet go numb, and that makes me really frightened.
>
> When the pain started I found it really difficult to walk. Standing for any amount of time makes my feet burn, and then the burning spreads up my legs. I try not to walk around much, as that makes the pain worse.

How to assess someone with neuropathic pain

If someone comes to see you complaining of pain, there are a number of different ways this can be assessed. Within a pain clinic, the person is usually seen by a pain consultant first (doctors who are usually trained as anaesthetists). Sometimes, it may be a physiotherapist who the patient sees first, or a clinical nurse specialist. A full medical and medication history is taken, which asks questions such as:

- How long have you had the pain, and how long have you had HIV?
- What medication have you been taking to manage the HIV? Have you been taking anything to manage the pain?
- Does the pain stop you from doing anything (such as walking for long periods of time, lying down, doing things that you like to do such as hobbies)?
- How is your mood at the moment? Do you feel worried about the pain?

Reflective point

It is always important to remember that people may be sensitive about discussing their HIV diagnosis for a variety of reasons.
What might some of those reasons be?
Can being cautious in discussing HIV inadvertently reinforce feelings of stigma in some people?

In addition to this, a full clinical examination is often done, where a person is asked to walk so the clinician can see whether they are favouring one leg over the other. Altered gait may have an impact later on, in terms of pain developing in other areas as various muscles compensate for their increased use. Objective examination of a patient with neuropathic pain should focus on the location of pain and identifying any neurological abnormalities; in particular, detecting abnormal responses to sensory stimulus.

One common feature of neuropathic pain is **allodynia**, which is defined as pain due to stimulus that does not normally provoke pain. Three types of neuropathic allodynia are reported based on the initiating stimulus: mechanical (touch), thermal (warm/cold) and movement. **Hyperalgesia** can also be present, which is defined as painful sensation of abnormal severity following a noxious stimulus. There are several simple tests for detecting abnormal responses and, where possible, the symptomatic site should be compared with a non-painful (control) site – so, touching the leg where the pain is felt, and then checking how it compares with the patient's other leg. Allodynia is best assessed by lightly brushing a piece of cotton wool over the symptomatic area. If pain is elicited in contrast to the control site, allodynia is present. Hyperalgesia and **hypoalgesia** are assessed by examining pinprick thresholds (PPT). A raised PPT (patient cannot feel sharpness at the site of symptoms) suggests hypoalgesia, a lowered PPT (patient feels exaggerated pain compared with control site) indicates hyperalgesia. To test thermal sensations, the responses to cold water/ hot water within plastic containers can be compared at the site of symptoms and the control site.

Screening tools

Pain is essentially a subjective experience described with patient-specific symptoms. Consequently, standardised screening tools for neuropathic pain, such as the neuropathic pain questionnaire (Krause & Backonja, 2003), Leeds Assessment of Neuropathic Symptoms and Signs (Bennett, 2004) and DN4 (Bouhassira et al., 2005), have been developed to classify neuropathic pain on the basis of patient-reported verbal descriptors of pain qualities. Most of these questionnaires comprise questions about burning pain, paraesthesias, pain attacks, mechanical and thermal hypersensitivity, and numbness. The clinical strength of the screening tools is that they can be used to identify potential patients with neuropathic pain, particularly by non-specialists. Their ease of use for both clinicians and patients makes these screening tools attractive because they provide immediate information to guide further assessment/management. However, these screening tools do not identify about 10–20% of patients with clinician-diagnosed neuropathic pain (Cruccu & Truini, 2009). In summary, there is good evidence that screening tools can offer guidance for further diagnostic evaluation, although they should not replace clinical judgement.

> The doctor listened to what I had to say about my pain, and about how my daughter has to help me when I need any shopping. She gave me a questionnaire to complete about my pain. She also touched my foot with cotton wool, which was horrible – it really hurt. I told her that I don't even touch my foot myself unless I really have to.

Reflective point

If someone came to you with pain in their feet, what would you do?

How would you assess them?

When would you consider referral to a specialist pain clinic (think about whether you feel competent to treat the level of pain the person is experiencing, whether you feel able to explain chronic versus acute pain to the person, and whether there might be any other options in a pain clinic that are not available to you in your service)?

Case study

Myra is a 56-year-old woman who presents at your HIV clinic. She has had HIV for 30 years and has always felt that she manages it well, but two years ago she started to notice a burning sensation in her feet when she stood for a long period of time. This gradually progressed and now she struggles to walk more than 50m without severe burning pain in both her feet. She has also noticed pins and needles in her feet, and sometimes feels that her left foot will go completely numb.

Myra works as an accounts administrator in a busy office, but has struggled to attend work consistently over the last two years due to her pain and is currently on extended sick leave. She spends most of her day sitting with her legs elevated to try to control her pain. At first, her friends from work would visit her on weekends, but Myra tearfully notes that they no longer come to see her and feels that they have forgotten about her. She lives with her husband and has two grown-up children who live close by, but as she spends most of her time indoors she often does not want to spend time with them as she feels they would find her boring now. The pain has also impacted on her intimate relationship with her husband, as Myra often finds that she is too tired and in too much pain to have sex. Myra says she feels quite desperate as she talks with you, and that her life is completely hopeless at the moment.

How is Myra's pain condition affecting her functioning? How is it affecting her emotionally? Considering that her pain is chronic, what would you do to try to help her? (You may wish to revisit these questions at the end of the chapter, to see if your answers have changed.)

Medical management of HIV-associated pain

First, it is always important to make sure that the person's HIV is being treated with the best medication and in the most helpful way. If possible, discontinue any drugs that may be increasing the pain. Once new antiretroviral therapy is established, the focus of treatment is symptomatic pain management, as the pain is unlikely to go away completely over time.

> The doctor told me that the pain in my foot is chronic, which he said means it won't go away. I didn't realise that before, and I got upset when he told me. I thought doctors could cure things like pain. Now I know that I have to learn to live with it, but it's really hard to do that.

There are no medications licensed for the treatment of HIV sensory neuropathy. Evidence for medication is extrapolated from studies of neuropathic pain where the participants did not have HIV. The National Institute for Clinical Excellence (NICE) updated its guidance for the management of neuropathic pain in 2013. A systematic review of the pharmacological treatments for HIV sensory neuropathy in 2010 identified randomised control trial evidence of analgesic efficacy superior to placebo for smoked cannabis, recombinant human nerve growth factor (rhNGF), and high dose (8%) topical capsaicin (Phillips et al., 2010). Cannabis is not a legal therapeutic option in the UK, although it may be in other countries around the world, and there are (at the time of writing) no plans to develop recombinant human nerve growth factor for clinical use in HIV sensory neuropathy.

There are randomised control trials on other treatments such as amitriptyline 100mg/day, gabapentin 2.4g/day, pregabalin 1200mg/day, lamotrigine 600mg/day, Acetyl L carnitine 1g/day, mexilitine 600mg/day, prosaptide 16mg/day, topical capsaicin 0.075%, and peptide-T 6mg/day. None appeared more effective than placebo (Phillips et al., 2010).

Opioids (drugs such as tramadol, codeine and morphine) have been recommended as part of the World Health Organization's analgesic ladder. How effective opioids are in the management of HIV sensory neuropathy has not been assessed. Opioids can also interact with antiretroviral therapy, which can cause other difficult side effects such as changes in the plasma levels of both types of medications. There are studies highlighting an association between HIV and an increased incidence of substance and medication misuse, and so it is recommended that long-term opioid therapy should include universal opioid precautions such as clearly documented risk assessments, consent, agreed treatment goals, therapeutic boundaries, and ongoing assessments (Krashin, Merrill, & Trescot, 2012; Önen et al., 2012). Living with chronic pain is very distressing, and as medication can sometimes work well for a short period of time, it is tempting to keep increasing the dosage, which is not always helpful as the side effects can be severe and include drowsiness, constipation, nausea and sometimes increased pain.

In the treatment of refractory distal sensory peripheral neuropathy, spinal cord stimulation is an option. This is a procedure whereby a small device is implanted into the back and applies electrical signals to the spinal cord. The device can be controlled by remote control. It is an invasive procedure as it involves an operation, and the evidence is limited and supported by case reports only (Knezevic et al., 2015).

Goals of medical management of neuropathic pain

The goal for treatment is to improve function and maintain quality of life. Reduction in pain may not always be possible, and it is very important not to promise patients this as an outcome. Evidence supports an interdisciplinary clinical approach to chronic pain management. Chronic pain remains a frequent symptom reviewed by HIV palliative care clinics (Perry et al., 2013). A 2015 longitudinal study following the pattern of peripheral neuropathy in antiretroviral naïve patients before the initiation of modern antiretroviral therapy found that the prevalence of peripheral neuropathy at seven years was 31%, and the prevalence of symptomatic peripheral neuropathy was 5% (Lee et al., 2015). Although targeted assessment continues to identify peripheral neuropathy in patients prescribed modern antiretrovirals, most of these patients do not have symptoms. One cohort study also identified that the prevalence of pain reduced with time (Mphahlele, Kamerman, & Mitchell, 2015). As insight into HIV sensory neuropathy improves, new targets for effective therapy may develop, but it will always be important to work in an interdisciplinary manner. It can be particularly helpful for pain clinics and HIV specialists to work together in managing chronic pain in people with HIV – this may mean being aware of the medications that someone is on, and the possible interactions between them, or liaising with the pain clinic to discuss what approach is being taken to manage pain, in order to best support the patient.

> I went to the pain clinic because I didn't know how to manage the pain in my feet any more. Paracetamol from the shop wasn't helping. They talked to me and told me that the pain probably won't go away, and they gave me some gabapentin and some amitriptyline, which helps me sleep but doesn't really take the pain away.
>
> When the doctor told me that the pain might not go away, I cried, but I'm happy she was honest with me. It means I can try to get on with my life.

The use of physiotherapy in managing neuropathic pain

Treatment

The goal of managing HIV-related peripheral neuropathy, like other chronic illnesses, is to control symptoms and prevent disability rather than cure disease. Thus, the objectives of chronic disease interventions include managing physical symptoms, improving independence and increasing quality of life. Physiotherapy is therefore important to help people to strengthen muscles that may not have been used for a while due to fear of pain and to help people to learn how to adapt to their pain.

A systematic review explored the effects of aerobic and progressive resistive exercise among adults living with HIV (O'Brien et al., 2008), and the results indicated that performing continuous aerobic or interval aerobic exercise, or a combination of continuous aerobic and progressive resistive exercise, for at least five weeks, is safe and may be beneficial for adults living with HIV who are medically stable. Exercise is associated with improvements in selected outcomes of cardiovascular fitness, weight and body composition (arm and thigh girth), and quality of life. The majority of results from individual studies demonstrated improvements in strength and psychological outcomes. It is therefore important to encourage people to exercise, even with neuropathic pain.

Physical exercise

The exercise programme should be modified according to an individual's physical function, health status, exercise response and stated goals. The use of both neuromuscular strength and cardiovascular health has become an important part of most recommended exercise regimes.

The key aims of physical activity programmes are usually to:

- Overcome the effects of physical deconditioning, as people may not have used their muscles for a while due to worries about the pain.
- Challenge and reduce fears of engaging in physical activity, and explain to people that they are not damaging themselves if they move, even though it hurts to do so.
- Reduce physical impairment and capitalise on recoverable function.
- Provide a safe and graded approach to re-engagement in physical activity, as doing too much too soon will lead to increased pain and anxiety.
- Help patients accept responsibility for increasing their functional capacity, as one physiotherapy session a fortnight is not going to provide helpful gains. It is up to the person to work on their goals in between sessions.
- Promote a positive view of physical activity.
- Introduce physically challenging, functional activities to rehabilitation.

Goal-setting and pacing

Engaging in activity may exacerbate pain immediately or after the activity has finished. Although it is explained to people that they need to remain active despite the pain, it is essential that they do not push themselves so far that they need to limit their activity due to the pain the next day. Conversely, some people avoid activity to such an extent that they do not progress and do not achieve improvement. This is usually because they fear that they are damaging themselves, as we are often taught that pain means danger. This is true of acute pain (the pain that signals a broken leg or sprained wrist) but is not accurate when managing chronic pain. Pain-related fear, particularly when accompanied by pain catastrophising (worrying about the worst possible outcome related to the pain) can lead to further avoidance and make the pain worse.

Reflective point

Have you ever been to the gym, or done more activity than you normally would during a day?
How did you feel the next day?
How did you manage this? Did this stop you from ever exercising again?
Did you recognise this as a sign you had overdone it the day before?

Chronic pain sufferers often report levels of activity that fluctuate dramatically over time. Patients often report they frequently persist at activities until they are prevented from carrying on by the pain. This leads them to rest until the pain subsides. Over time the periods of activity become shorter and those of rest lengthen. Achievements become smaller and disability increases, as the individual becomes physically deconditioned, characterised by reduced strength and aerobic capacity.

Note: "recovery" in this context does not mean the pain will be taken away completely.

Reflective point

Considering the fear avoidance model in Figure 9.1, how do you think other people would relate to a person with neuropathic pain who struggled to attend events and do activities due to their pain?
What do you think might happen to social relationships over time?
What might happen to romantic relationships over time?

However, whilst being mindful of concerns such as stigma which may be barriers to increasing activity, it is important to remember that people living with HIV may also struggle to access activities due to fear of stigma, or other psychosocial difficulties.

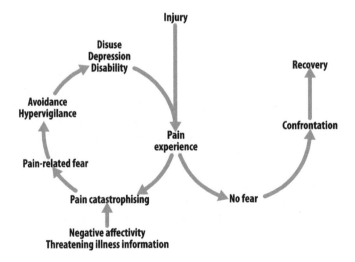

Figure 9.1 The fear avoidance model (adapted from Vlaeyen & Linton, 2012)

Being aware of the rationale for increasing activity, and that they are not going to damage themselves by being more active, can often help to support the person in returning to valued activities. The purpose of pacing and goal-setting is to regulate daily activities and to structure an increase in activity through a gradual pacing-up. Activity is paced up by timing activity or by the introduction of quotas of exercise interspersed by periods of rest or change in activity (Gill & Brown, 2009). Pacing is often difficult for people as they are not used to doing it, and sometimes have beliefs around whether they "should" be doing it, comparing themselves with how they used to be. We will discuss this further under "psychological management".

Functional goal-setting is fundamental to the rehabilitation programme. Goals should be meaningful to the patient and therefore set by the patient. Goals should be SMART: Specific; Measurable; Achievable; Rewarding; Timely.

Case example of goal-setting/pacing

Mr A has a diagnosis of HIV. He reports a recent onset of intermittent severe bilateral foot pain which is very variable with good and bad days. He also reports constant numbness when walking barefoot. He tries to capitalise on the good days by performing many of the tasks he is unable to do on the days when his pain limits his activity. This leads to an increase in his pain, to which he responds by restricting his activity until the pain subsides.

Mr A came up with his SMART goal as:

Specific: walk 20 minutes three times a week on flat ground.
Measureable: can measure distance covered to monitor progress.
Achievable: takes into consideration current activity levels.
Rewarding: takes him to the shop, so he is able to go and buy what he wants.
Timely: to be achieved in three months.

Calculating a baseline for Mr A involved taking a measurement of how far he could comfortably walk on three consecutive days. The average of these was then calculated and this was used as a baseline for Mr A, which was 10 minutes.

Mr A was started on a graded walking programme starting with 10 minutes' walking every other day for one week. This was increased by 1 minute every week until he was up to 20 minutes. This slow, steady approach to building up activity levels allows his body to adapt to the activity.

Little literature exists on HIV-associated neuropathy rehabilitation interventions other than exercise; however, desensitisation techniques are commonly used in clinical practice to reduce the sensitivity of the nerves. Desensitisation consists of lightly rubbing different textures (e.g. cotton wool, silk, towelling, etc.) over the area that is sensitive. The length of time that the exercise is done depends on your individual tolerance, and generally speaking, the more variety, the more likely a positive outcome. Gait re-education, balance training and use of orthotics are all further physiotherapeutic interventions that are clinically used for patients with neuropathic pain.

The use of psychological therapies in managing neuropathic pain

It is recognised by the International Association for the Study of Pain that pain is "an unpleasant sensory and emotional experience" (International Association for the Study of Pain. Pain, IASP Pain Terminology, 1994). All pain has an emotional component, meaning that the experience of pain can increase the incidence of difficulties such as anxiety and depression (Bair et al., 2003; McWilliams, Cox, & Enns, 2003). Chronic pain also increases risk of suicidal behaviour and self-harm, with risk of death by suicide being at least doubled in people with chronic pain (Tang & Crane, 2006).

Being in constant pain is understandably difficult to manage psychologically, as it changes the ways in which people relate to the world. After having a diagnosis such as HIV, which also changes your life in a number of ways, getting neuropathic pain can feel like a double blow:

> When they told me there was no cure for my pain, that they couldn't take it away, I felt really low. First I get HIV, and now this happens to me. The pain is a constant reminder of my HIV that I can't distract myself from. I was starting to come to terms with the HIV, but the pain made me feel like my life was over.

It is understandable to want to avoid pain – that is something we all try to do. But with chronic pain, that is not possible, and attempts to avoid pain and distress tend to increase these feelings in the long run. For example, staying at home rather than going out with friends because you are worried the pain will increase leads to refusing more and more invitations, until you go out very rarely in an attempt to control the pain. The problem is that the pain is still there, and it often does not change the more you rest.

> I stopped going out years ago. When the psychologist asked me if that has helped me manage the pain, I had to laugh. If I was managing the pain, I wouldn't be seeing her in the pain clinic!

There are a number of challenges to working with people with chronic pain and HIV. These include the fact that many people are reluctant to see a psychologist for an issue that they feel is completely physical, and that they may feel that the referring clinician thinks that their pain is not "real" or that "it's all in my head". It is important to reassure people that this is not the case before referring them to psychology. Additionally, people with chronic pain often come to see a psychologist following a number of medical interventions and may feel that psychology is their "last chance". The reasons for referral should therefore be discussed clearly with the person with pain before referring them and any worries should be addressed.

In relation to HIV, people often prefer to be seen within HIV specialist services due to fears around confidentiality. Unfortunately, HIV services cannot be specialist in every area of physical and mental health, and over the last few years there has been more recognition of the fact that people with HIV need to access other services within the healthcare system. Services may need to think carefully about how to respect a person's concerns around confidentiality whilst providing timely access to appropriate pain management – this may involve explaining to the person with HIV that pain medications can interact with HIV medications, and exploring their reasons for not wanting others to know about their diagnosis.

> When I found out they'd referred me to a psychologist, I thought, "they just think you're crazy. They think you're making it up." The first time I was referred, I never went to the appointment.
>
> I was really angry with the psychologist when I first saw him – I thought that he would say that the pain wasn't real, because that's what everyone seems to think. But he didn't say that at all. We talked about stress, and how that can make pain worse, and we're going to look at ways of coping with the pain.

Whilst there is no treatment for chronic pain that will completely resolve symptoms, psychological management strategies based on effecting behavioural change have been successful in helping people to manage their symptoms and continue to engage in activities that they find enjoyable and valuable. There are a number of different methods by which this is achieved, but the ones with the largest amount of evidence are cognitive-behavioural therapies, including acceptance and commitment therapy and compassion-focused therapy.

Cognitive-behavioural therapy

Cognitive behavioural therapy (CBT) in pain management aims to help people develop useful strategies for managing their pain and re-engage with activities they have previously avoided. Behaviour such as avoiding activity that is believed to increase pain levels leads to narrowing behavioural repertoires, which over time increases feelings of low mood and hopelessness, and increases anxiety when activity has to be engaged in. It is important to be clear that people's thought processes are not "wrong" or "bad" – rather, they are unworkable in the moment and lead to decreased function over time. This then has a knock-on effect on relationships and mood.

> The therapist talked about how being frightened of pain was normal, but that it wasn't working for me. We talked about ways to cope, including relaxing and breathing, and we also talked about my thoughts about pain – I often thought that if I went out and had to go home because of a flare-up, my friends would all laugh at me, but that wasn't the case. We came up with a plan that would let me practise doing things differently, and I started to go out again for a few minutes every day. Now I can go out for up to an hour, and I'm less worried about the future because I know how to cope with the pain.

Research suggests that cognitive behavioural ways of working are effective in helping people to manage chronic pain (relative to a waiting list control) and that CBT can produce significant changes in how people perceive their pain, how they cope, and how much activity they engage in (Morley, Eccleston, & Williams, 1999).

When working with people with HIV who also have pain, non-psychologist clinicians can be aware of how someone thinks about both of these issues – worries about the pain indicating damage or their HIV diagnosis meaning that they are a bad person – which can be useful to think about sensitively with the person once a relationship has been established. It is important not to use this information to seem "more clever" than the person with pain/HIV or to tell them that they are thinking about their situation "wrongly" – their thoughts are valid, but may not be helpful in the moment and may lead to difficult patterns of behaviour.

Acceptance and commitment therapy

Rather than challenging thoughts, which can be difficult for some people to do, acceptance and commitment therapy (ACT; pronounced as the word "act" and not as separate letters) encourages people to acknowledge and accept their difficult thoughts and emotions. ACT argues that pushing these thoughts away, rationalising or debating with them, or trying to get rid of them is ineffective in both control of thought processes and increase in behaviours that are important and useful. Instead, people are encouraged to take those thoughts and feelings with them whilst engaging in valued activities that may cause anxiety. The evidence base for ACT suggests that it is effective in enabling people with chronic pain to re-engage with previously avoided activities, in the service of doing something that is meaningful to them. This can be particularly useful in physical health contexts, as pain and HIV are both chronic conditions that cannot be taken away or "fixed".

> We talked about all the things that I had tried before, and that they weren't getting rid of the pain. It seemed like the more I tried to get rid of it, the worse the pain got. So we talked about ways to accept the pain – not like it, but accept that it is there and it isn't going away – and I started to see people again and go out more. The pain is still there, but I can do things again, so I'm happier.

The available research on ACT suggests that it is useful to people with chronic pain, and that the processes that it targets (acceptance, mindfulness, action in pursuit of valued living) do indeed correlate with improvements in psychological wellbeing (low mood and anxiety) and in disability, independent of changes to chronic pain (McCracken & Gutiérrez-Martínez, 2011). Again, it is important not to promise people that the pain will change, but they can still enjoy life in spite of the pain.

Compassion-focused therapy

People with chronic pain, and people with HIV, tend to have high levels of shame and self-criticism, which responds well to a compassion-focused approach (Bennett et al., 2016; Gilbert, 2009; Werner, Isaksen, & Malterud, 2004). This may be due to the stigma of living with a diagnosis such as HIV, or due to the fact that decreasing levels of activity when someone has pain can leave them vulnerable to feeling as though they are "failing" in some way (refer to Chapter 8). People are therefore taught strategies to treat themselves more gently, and to forgive themselves when it is difficult for them to complete activities due to pain. Asking for help can also be hard for people with chronic pain, so compassion is discussed in the context of the most compassionate thing not necessarily being the easiest.

> When the therapist talked about me being nicer to myself, I laughed. I didn't see how that would help. But we did some exercises, and I can see that I've always been so hard on myself, for no reason really. I try to be a bit kinder, to think about

what I need rather than beating myself up. It even helps with the pain a bit, because I can ask people to help me now rather than having to do it all myself, and I know that they care and really will help me when I need them to.

Pain management programmes

The "gold standard" of care for people with chronic pain is attendance at a pain management programme (PMP). These programmes are over 36 hours of group-based treatment for pain, including input from a variety of specialisms such as psychology, medicine, physiotherapy, occupational therapy, pharmacy technicians and expert patients.

For people with HIV, attending a group-based programme may be a daunting prospect. Many people are concerned about telling others that they have HIV, or that their status will be shared with the group without their consent. It is important to take time to discuss these concerns, to help people with HIV make a decision about whether a PMP is suitable for them and to prevent dropout, which may make people with chronic pain feel worse (as it is "another failed treatment").

> When they told me about the group, I didn't want to do it. I couldn't imagine sitting in a room full of people who might ask me why I had pain. She (the therapist) said I didn't have to do it if I didn't want to, and I've decided to work with her on my own for a little while, to work my way up to a group. I don't want to miss out, but I'm not ready to do it yet.
>
> The group was fantastic – lots of really useful information, and I didn't have to talk about my status, which made it less scary.

Reflection point

Think about a patient that you have seen previously with HIV-related pain.
Which of the different interventions above could you have offered them?
Do you feel that these interventions would be better on their own, or in combination with others?

Summary

Neuropathic pain can be a debilitating complication of living with HIV. People with neuropathic pain commonly present with burning, numbness or pins and needles in their feet, which can progress up their legs. There is no cure for neuropathic pain; instead, management of the pain focuses on a biopsychosocial approach. This involves a combination of appropriate medication, physiotherapy and psychological therapies (particularly cognitive-behavioural therapies) to help people to return to activities that are important to them and enhance their quality of life, in spite of their ongoing pain condition. Difficulties such as fear of telling people about HIV status, stigma and adjusting to managing another chronic health condition on top of HIV can make management of chronic pain more complicated. For this reason, interdisciplinary working can be a particularly helpful approach to managing both pain and HIV.

Resources

The British Pain Society website is full of useful information and resources about chronic pain: https://www.britishpainsociety.org/

Overcoming Chronic Pain – Frances Cole, Helen Macdonald, Catherine Carus and Hazel Howden-Leach. This book uses CBT to explore how to manage pain, as well as having practical information about sleep-related difficulties and pacing.

The Pain Toolkit is a self-help resource for managing chronic pain: https://www.paintoolkit.org/

Coping Successfully with Pain – Neville Shone. This book is written by a person with chronic pain and has many practical tips on how to manage pain.

References

Bair, M.J., Robinson, R.L., Katon, W., & Kroenke, K. (2003). Depression and pain comorbidity: A literature review. *Archives of Internal Medicine, 163(20)*, pp. 2433–2445.

Bennett, D.S., Traub, K., Mace, L., Juarascio, A., & O'Hayer, C.V. (2016). Shame among people living with HIV: A literature review. *AIDS Care, 28(1)*, pp. 87–91.

Bennett, M. (2001). The LANSS pain scale: The Leeds Assessment of Neuropathic Symptoms and Signs. *Pain, 92(1-2)*, pp. 147–157.

Bernard, N., Spira, R., Ybanez, S., Chêne, G., Morlat, P., Lacoste, D., Loury-Larivière, I., Nouts, C., Burucoa, B., Lebras, M., & Beylot, J. (1999). Prevalence and underestimation of pain in HIV-infected patients by physicians: A cross-sectional study in a day care hospital. *AIDS, 4; 13(2)*, pp. 293–295.

Bouhassira, D., Attal, N., Alchaar, H., Boureau, F., Brochet, B., Bruxelle, J., Cunin, G., Fermanian, J., Ginies, P., Grun-Overdyking, A., Jafari-Schluep, H., Lantéri-Minet, M., Laurent, B., Mick, G., Serrie, A., Valade, D., & Vicaut, E. (2005). Comparison of pain syndromes associated with nervous or somatic lesions and development of a new neuropathic pain diagnostic questionnaire (DN4). *Pain, 114(1-2)*, pp. 29–36.

Breitbart, W., Rosenfeld, B.D., Passik, S.D., McDonald, M.V., Thaler, H., & Portenoy, R.K. (1996). The under-treatment of pain in ambulatory AIDS patients. *Pain, 65(2-3)*, pp. 243–249.

Cruccu, G., & Truini, A. (2009). Tools for assessing neuropathic pain. *PLoS Medicine, 6(4)*: e1000045. doi:10.1371/journal.pmed.1000045.

De la Monte, S.M., Gabuzda, D.H., Ho, D.D., Brown, R.H., Jr., Hedley-Whyte, E.T., Schooley, R.T., Hirsch, M.S., & Bhan, A.K. (1988). Peripheral neuropathy in the acquired immunodeficiency syndrome. *Annals of Neurology, 23(5)*, pp. 485–492.

Dotan, I., Riesenberg, K., Toledano, R., Schlaeffer, F., Smolyakov, A., Saidel-Odes, L., Wechsberg, O., Ablin, J.N., Novack, V., & Buskila, D. (2016). Prevalence and characteristics of fibromyalgia among HIV-positive patients in southern Israel. *Clinical and Experimental Rheumatology, 34(2 S96)*, pp. 34–39.

Gilbert, P. (2009). Introducing compassion-focused therapy. *Advances in Psychiatric Treatment, 15 (3)*, pp. 99–208.

Gill, J., & Brown, C. (2009). A structured review of the evidence for pacing as a chronic pain intervention. *European Journal of Pain, 13*. pp. 214–216.

Gueler, A., Moser, A., Calmy, A., Günthard, H.F., Bernasconi, E., Furrer, H., Fux, C.A., Battegay, M., Cavassini, M., Vernazza, P., Zwahlen, M., & Egger, M. (2017). Life expectancy in

HIV-positive persons in Switzerland: Matched comparison with general population. Swiss HIV Cohort Study, Swiss National Cohort. *AIDS 28*; *31(3)*, pp. 427–436.

International Association for the Study of Pain. Pain, IASP Pain Terminology. (1994). Accessed at https://www.iasp-pain.org

Knezevic, N.N., Candido, K.D., Rana, S., & Knezevic, I. (2015). The use of spinal cord neuro-modulation in the management of HIV-related polyneuropathy. *Pain Physician*, *18(4)*, pp. 643–650.

Krashin, D.L., Merrill, J.O., & Trescot, A.M. (2012). Opioids in the management of HIV-related pain. *Pain Physician*, *15(3 Suppl)*, pp. ES157–68.

Krause, S.J., & Backonja, M.M. (2003). Development of a neuropathic pain questionnaire. *Clinical Journal of Pain*, *19(5)*, pp. 306–314.

Lee, A.J., Bosch, R.J., Evans, S.R., Wu, K., Harrison, T., Grant, P., & Clifford, D.B. (2015). Patterns of peripheral neuropathy in ART-naïve patients initiating modern ART regimen. *Journal of Neurovirology*, *21(2)*, pp. 210–218.

Mann, R., Sadosky, A., Schaefer, C., Baik, R., Parsons, B., Nieshoff, E., Stacey, B.R., Tuchman, M., & Nalamachu, S. (2016). Burden of HIV-related neuropathic pain in the United States. *Journal of the International Association of Providers of AIDS Care*, *15(2)*, pp. 114–125.

Marques, A.P., Santo, A.S., Berssaneti, A.A., Matsutani, L.A., & Yuan, S.L. (2016). Prevalence of fibromyalgia: Literature review update. *Brazilian Journal of Rheumatology*, *S0482-5004(16)*, pp. 30174–30177.

McCracken, L.M., & Gutiérrez-Martínez, O. (2011). Processes of change in psychological flexibility in an interdisciplinary group-based treatment for chronic pain based on acceptance and commit-ment therapy. *Behaviour Research and Therapy*, *49*. pp. 267–274.

McWilliams, L.A., Cox, B.J., & Enns, M.W. (2003). Mood and anxiety disorders associated with chronic pain: An examination in a nationally representative sample. *Pain*, *1–2(106)*, pp. 127–133.

Miaskowski, C., Penko, J.M., Guzman, D., Mattson, J.E., Bangsberg, D.R., & Kushel, M.B. (2011). Occurrence and characteristics of chronic pain in a community-based cohort of indigent adults living with HIV infection. *Jounal of Pain*, *12(9)*, pp. 1004–1016.

Morley, S., Eccleston, C., & Williams, A. (1999). Systematic review and meta-analysis of random-ized controlled trials of cognitive behaviour therapy and behaviour therapy for chronic pain in adults, excluding headache. *Pain (80)*, pp. 1–13.

Mphahlele, N.R., Kamerman, P.R., & Mitchell, D. (2015). Progression of pain in ambulatory HIV-positive South Africans. *Pain Management in Nursing*, *16(1)*, pp. 1–8.

O'Brien, K, Tynan, A.M., Nixon, S., & Glazier, R.H. (2008). Effects of progressive resistive exercise in adults living with HIV/AIDS: Systematic review and meta-analysis of randomized trials. *AIDS Care*, *20(6)*, pp. 631–653.

Önen, N.F., Barrette, E.P., Shacham, E., Taniguchi, T., Donovan, M., & Overton, E.T. (2012). A review of opioid prescribing practices and associations with repeat opioid prescriptions in a contemporary outpatient HIV clinic. *Pain Practice*, *12(6)*, pp. 440–448.

Perry, B.A., Westfall, A.O., Molony, E., Tucker, R., Ritchie, C., Saag, M.S., Mugavero, M.J., & Merlin, J.S. (2013). Characteristics of an ambulatory palliative care clinic for HIV-infected patients. *Journal of Palliative Medicine*, *16(8)*, pp. 934–937.

Phillips, T.J., Cherry, C.L., Cox, S., Marshall, S.J., & Rice, A.S. (2010). Pharmacological treatment of painful HIV-associated sensory neuropathy: A systematic review and meta-analysis of random-ised controlled trials. *PLoS One 28*; *5(12)*, p. 14433.

Sambamoorthi, U., Walkup, J., McSpiritt, E., Warner, L., Castle, N., & Crystal, S. (2000). Racial differences in end-of-life care for patients with AIDS. *AIDS Public Policy Journal*, *15(3–4)*, pp. 136–148.

Tang, N.K.Y., & Crane, C. (2006). Suicidality in chronic pain: A review of the prevalence, risk factors and psychological links. *Psychological Medicine (36)*, pp. 575–586.

Teeraananchai, S., Chaivooth, S., Kerr, S.J., Bhakeecheep, S., Avihingsanon, A., Teeraratkul, A., Sirinirund, P., Law, M.G., & Ruxrungtham, K. (2017). Life expectancy after initiation of combination antiretroviral therapy in Thailand. *Antiviral Therapies 10.3851/IMP3121*.

Tsao, J.C., Stein, J.A., & Dobalian, A. (2010). Sex differences in pain and misuse of prescription analgesics among persons with HIV. *Pain Medicine*, *11*(*6*), pp. 815–824.

Verma, A. (2001). Epidemiology and clinical features of HIV-1 associated neuropathies. *Journal of the Peripheral Nervous System*, *6*(*1*), pp. 8–13.

Vlaeyen, J.W.S., & Linton, S.J. (2012). Fear-avoidance model of chronic musculoskeletal pain: 12 years on. *Pain* (*153*), pp. 1144–1147.

Wandeler, G., Johnson, L.F., & Egger, M. (2016). Trends in life expectancy of HIV-positive adults on antiretroviral therapy across the globe: Comparisons with general population. *Current Opinion in HIV and AIDS*, *11*(*5*), pp. 492–500.

Werner, A., Isaksen, L.W., & Malterud, K. (2004). I am not the kind of woman who complains of everything': Illness stories on self and shame in women with chronic pain. *Social Science and Medicine*, *59*(*5*), pp. 1035–1045.

WHO. (2013). Consolidated guidelines on the use of antiretroviral drugs for treating and preventing HIV infection. *Recommendations for a Public Health Approach*.

WHO. (2016). Consolidated guidelines on the use of antiretroviral drugs for treating and preventing HIV infection. Recommendations for a public health approach – Second edition.

Wilson, N.L., Azuero, A., Vance, D.E., Richman, J.S., Moneyham, L.D., Raper, J.L., Heath, S.L., & Kempf, M.C. (2016). Identifying symptom patterns in people living with HIV disease. *Journal of the Association of Nurses in AIDS Care*, *27*(*2*), pp. 121–132.

10 The psychological impact of ageing with HIV

Shaun Watson and Alexander Margetts

Chapter description

When considering what 'ageing' means for people living with HIV, the age of 50 is increasingly used to record and analyse statistical information and is considered an age where people living with HIV are most at risk of developing HIV-related co-morbidities, such as cardiovascular disease. Older people are the fastest growing group of people living with HIV, with their care needs being explored within the scientific community in order to ensure safe, effective care. What is becoming increasingly more apparent is that within HIV care, interdisciplinary working is becoming critical to the sharing of knowledge and expertise when treating older people living with HIV. Within this chapter we will explore the concept of ageing further, highlighting its multiple meanings for different people and highlight how ageing affects the quality of life for people ageing with HIV.

Introduction: defining ageing and old age

All things age. Yet despite being universal, human ageing (and even more so 'old age') proves difficult to define. Once born, our age is initially measured socially in days (e.g. she's six days old). Days become weeks (he's three weeks old). Weeks become months (they're eight months old next week). And then months become years. As an adult, then, our age is typically measured in how many years old we are (chronological age), although sometimes this is rounded to the decade it falls in (e.g. someone might describe themselves as 68 years old or 'in my sixties'). Ageing is this process of becoming older. However, it has bleakly been described as 'a collection of changes that render human beings progressively more likely to die' or a 'progressive functional decline, or a gradual deterioration of physiological function with age, including a decrease in fecundity'. The language used in these definitions do not engender a positive experience, which could help explain why many people struggle with the notion that they are ageing.

Thinking points

- How old are you?
- Do you feel 'young' or 'old' for your age?

- How would you define young, middle-aged and old?
- What do you see as the positive and negative aspects of ageing?
- Which list is longer? Where have these different views and stereotypes come from?

Ageing represents the accumulation of physical, psychological and social changes, and age is a social construct that has been given positive and negative attributes: 'you're only as old as you feel'; 'you have a young outlook'; 'you're mature beyond your years', 'older and wiser'. We are influenced by society, images, social media and experience, with some cultures particularly valuing or disparaging older people. People are told they 'don't look their age' or to 'act their age', yet defining how we 'should' look and act is complex and individual. We describe age chronologically so that it can be treated as a precise and accurate marker to define our life by. This includes milestones such as age-specific events and 'significant birthdays', from pre-school health checks and vaccinations, school attendance, teenage years, adulthood, and also legal rights such as the ability to consent to sex, vote, get married and drink alcohol. Such legal markers vary across (and sometimes within) countries. There are consequently many different theories of ageing: biological, psychological and social (e.g. Bengtson & Settersten, 2016 for a comprehensive review).

What we think and feel about 'old age' (and thus implicitly 'young age') is individual too; some fear it, some embrace it. Crucially there is no clear definition of what 'old age' is: to some teenagers, 30 years old seems 'ancient'; to someone in their thirties reaching retirement might define old age, whilst someone in their nineties might wistfully reflect on their younger self when they were in their seventies.

Within HIV services, older age is usually categorised as beginning at 50 years, with Public Health England (PHE) and the British HIV Association (BHIVA) defining older age as 50 years onwards. Older age is associated with a complexity of physical, emotional, and societal changes and adaptations (Schäfer et al., 2010), with individuals of the same chronological age differing dramatically from each other in respect to their health status (Rockwood et al., 2000).

Thinking points

- Do you agree with PHE's categorising of what is considered to be old age for people living with HIV?
- How might this age marker affect someone approaching 50 years old living with HIV?

Psychological impact of ageing with HIV

The focus of this chapter will be the psychological impact of ageing with HIV and the following areas: emotional wellbeing, cognition, personality and isolation. Each will be briefly explored with regard to how they affect the wider population initially, and then the impact for people ageing with HIV. In order to do this it is necessary first to consider the unique history of HIV, and how ageing has been situated within this over the past decades.

The history of ageing with HIV

In the mid to late 1980s, for people living with HIV (and those who care for them), unless they were diagnosed in older age, ageing sadly was not an issue that required focus. With a poor prognosis and almost certain death within three to five years of an 'AIDS' diagnosis, many understandably cashed in pensions early and depleted their savings, sold property, gave up work, and tried to focus on living in the moment and enjoying the last few years they were told they had left. Men and women died despite their youth, with those left behind often struggling with premature and multiple bereavements. It became clear that a few people did survive despite little knowledge and no medication, often termed 'long-term non or slow progressors', or 'elite controllers'; however, these were very much the exception to the rule.

Fortunately, with the discovery, introduction and refinement of antiretroviral therapy (ART), living to older age is now both achievable and expected should the person be able to access and willing to take medication. Whilst initially people living with HIV would 'only' gain a couple of extra decades compared with no treatment, this has improved to near-normal life expectancy today (Trickey et al., 2017). Older age is therefore now something that needs to be addressed, discussed and planned for, both by people living with HIV and those who provide services for them.

Accelerated versus accentuated ageing

In the United Kingdom, approximately a third of people with HIV are now aged 50 and over. This has been steadily increasing, with projections estimating that in 2030 some 73% of people living with HIV will be 50 or over (Smit et al., 2015), up from 28% in 2010. It is therefore of ever-increasing importance that we understand the needs of those ageing with HIV, as whilst HIV can be well controlled with ART, the long-term effects of living with HIV and ART are still being discovered (High et al., 2012).

For example, one current area of exploration is whether HIV either accelerates and/or accentuates ageing (e.g. Sabin & Reiss, 2017). Accelerated ageing would occur if there is an ongoing issue for people living with HIV of age-associated co-morbidities occurring earlier than for those not living with HIV (i.e. 'normal ageing occurring sooner than expected'). Accentuated ageing refers to a one-off increase in the risk of age-associated co-morbidities after acquiring HIV, but any subsequent risks remain the same as for those who are not living with HIV (i.e. a greater burden of age-related damage). These can of course occur in combination, or may be different for different co-morbidities.

The role of inflammation has been shown to have a premature ageing effect (Mitnitski, Mogilner, & Rockwood, 2001; Pathai et al., 2013) and ageing with HIV and the long-term use of ART can increase a person's risk of several co-morbidities, with possible side effects including liver toxicity, cardiac and renal problems, osteoporosis, pancreatitis, lipodystrophy and peripheral neuropathy (Balderson et al., 2013; Grulich et al., 2007).

Biographic age versus chronological

A challenge to the 'over 50' definition of older age is the finding that 'biographic' age is as important, if not sometimes more so, than chronological. This refers to the age at time of diagnosis, and crucially if this was before or after the introduction of antiretroviral medications. For example Robinson (2011) found differences in experience of ageing between 'long-term survivors' and older men who have sex with men (MSM) diagnosed with HIV later in life. The former had issues regarding interruption of an imagined life trajectory, confusion about surviving beyond expectation at diagnosis, and lost camaraderie of a community politicised in the early era of the epidemic. The latter were less connected to the struggles of the earlier years, more concerned about sharing HIV status, thinking about a life possibly foreshortened, and the physical and emotional burden of starting treatment. Owen and Catalan (2012) found similar accounts, and explored narratives that could be either 'regressive' or 'progressive', and influenced by lived experience of HIV on personal health, emotional proximity to AIDS-related bereavements and the narrative interpretation of the history of the epidemic (Table 10.1). These narratives could either be stable or fluctuate, and although the research was MSM focused, many themes could also apply to heterosexual men and women.

Other aspects may be gender-specific and relate more to chronological age. For example, in a study of older women living with HIV, six themes were drawn out: sexual pleasure changes due to age, sexual freedom as women age, the role of relationships in sexual pleasure, changes in sexual ability and sexual health needs, sexual risk behaviours, and ageist assumptions about older women's sexuality (Taylor et al., 2016). Related to this, the menopause and coping with its associated symptoms can be a challenge for women (Lamont, 2012). The effect of menopause in women with HIV upon their physical, sexual and psychological health needs to be addressed, with currently limited understanding and literature upon this area of care (Loufty et al., 2013; Sherr et al., 2016).

Voyage into the unknown

Solomon et al. (2014) highlighted the issues raised by a group of people who are considered to be the first generation of people living with HIV who are ageing. The main

Table 10.1 HIV+ older MSM narratives (summarised from Owen & Catalan, 2012)

Regressive	*Progressive*
Biographical disruption	Continued storylines
Movement away from valued life objectives	Movement towards valued life objectives
More likely to be diagnosed pre-ART	More likely to be diagnosed post-ART
Felt stuck or trapped by past experience of HIV	Orientation to present not past, HIV a chronic condition
'Premature ageing' from multiple bereavements	Social and support networks not organised around HIV
Interrupted careers, dependency on benefits, hardship	Working lives not interrupted, fewer benefits
Ambivalence, fear and anxiety about ageing with HIV	Fewer anxieties about prospect of ageing with HIV

concerns that were raised were not knowing if what they were experiencing was HIV-related or part of the normal ageing process. This was also emphasised by their perceptions that healthcare providers were unprepared in their knowledge and skills around how they would age.

The Terrence Higgins Trust further explored the concerns of 246 men and women living with HIV aged over 50 in their *Uncharted Territory* report (THT, 2017). They highlighted:

- *50+ is not one category*: those employed identified different needs from those retired who were within the same age range.
- *Employment*: concerns regarding increase in the retirement age, competitive job market, and ability to work with multiple long-term conditions.
- *Finances and the benefit systems*: poverty twice the rate as the general population, 58% of respondents living below poverty threshold, 84% concerned about their financial future.
- *Social care system*: 81% concerned about who will care for them and how they will manage their lives, 25% felt they had no one to support them, concerns about discrimination and stigma in residential or nursing homes.
- *Healthcare management*: three times as many long-term conditions as the general population, concerns about polypharmacy and multiple appointments by different specialists, need for co-ordinated long-term condition management with support to self-manage, 79% concerned re: effects of long-term ART, 84% re: HIV care management and 80% re: uncertainty of long-term HIV.
- *GPs*: playing an increasing role in the care of people living with HIV, however a fifth stated their GP had never discussed ageing with HIV.
- *Isolation*: 82% experienced moderate to high levels of loneliness, 76% fearing a future of loneliness. A third stated that they felt socially isolated as they were ageing.
- *Women*: older women demonstrated lower levels of wellbeing, felt less financially stable and showed more concern about long-term effects of HIV and ART and caring for their family compared with their male counterparts.

Thus, we have moved from an era of palliative care to liaising and consulting with older age charities and gerontology services, discussing the management of long-term health and advising our clients about living healthy lifestyles that will maintain cardiac, respiratory, hepatic and bone health. It is an amazing turnaround and something that we should celebrate. However, as healthcare professionals working within HIV, we must continue to change our outlook, knowledge base, skills and the way we work. Equally as important is that we must recognise the legacy that past expectations and trauma may have had on our current clients (see Chapters 4 and 6).

Thinking points

- How might the history of HIV healthcare and when they were diagnosed affect someone's ageing process with HIV now?
- Does HIV accelerate or accentuate ageing?
- What uncertainties are there for people ageing with HIV? How would you feel if these applied to you?

Emotional wellbeing

Emotional health is a complex concept, and can be thought to consist of and be influenced by internal psychological processes, bodily state and sociocultural context (see Chapter 3).

Social, cultural and economic issues may affect our feelings of wellbeing and create some level of uncertainty. As we age we may get greater resolution, or drift, in such issues, leading to better or worse mental health. For example, there could be more experiences of loss and trauma, which might be associated with lower mood for one person. Conversely for another the same experiences might lead to more acceptance of loss, and post-traumatic growth from adversity, which might then connect to contentment and improved mood.

In older people generally, rates of depression are estimated at a fifth of people in the community, and for anxiety 1 in 20 people (NAT, 2017). It's important to hold in mind that the people living with HIV will share the same/similar issues and concerns that are related to growing older within the general population. However, there may also be significant differences as discussed elsewhere in this book, or accentuation of issues. Various studies have looked into the effects of HIV and ageing (Vance, Farr, & Struzick, 2008; Ghidei et al., 2013; Solomon et al., 2014), with anxiety and depression estimated at between 5% and 10% prevalence, although some studies show up to 48% (Rabkin, 2008). The role of depression has been linked to multiple issues, including poor cognitive and physical function (Vance & Struzick, 2007), health-induced stress and anxiety (Enriquez, Lackey, & Witt, 2008) and social isolation and loneliness (McDowell & Serovich, 2007).

For example, HIV can intersect with any of these aspects: poverty from changes in social support and benefits; physical health from the direct impact of HIV and/or its treatments; relationships and reduced social support (either from experienced or feared rejection due to HIV status, or loss of those who were also HIV+); discrimination due to HIV status in addition to age-related stigma; reduction in participation in meaningful activities due to closure of HIV services due to funding cuts and fear of engaging in 'mainstream' services due to feared or actualised stigma experiences (see Chapter 8).

Thinking points

- Who assesses emotional wellbeing in the interdisciplinary team?
- How can team members work together to ensure needs are met and understood?

Cognition

Cognition is used here to refer to the mental action or process of acquiring knowledge and understanding, through thought, experiences and the body's senses. For some people as they reach older age, their cognitive abilities start to deteriorate, either naturally and gently ('normal ageing') or significantly and abnormally (e.g. strokes, dementia). This is covered in more depth in Chapter 11, including the impact that HIV can have within this process and the role for the interdisciplinary team. However, in general, normal age-related changes are as shown in Table 10.2.

Table 10.2 Normal versus unusual age-related changes in cognitive functioning

Domain	Normal	Unusual
Memory	May forget parts of an experience	Forgets entire experience
Later free recall	Often remember later something temporarily forgotten	Does not remember at all
Recognition	Benefit from reminder cues	No recognition effect
Directions	Usually able to follow written or spoken directions	Not able to follow directions
Reminders	Usually able to use notes as reminders	Notes not effective as reminders
Self-care	Usually able to care for themselves	Unable to care for themselves
Cognitive efficiency	Slow loss, may accelerate in fifth decade onwards	Rapid loss
Processing speed	Some reduction/limitations in amount of information	Near complete loss or major slowing

However, it is important to note that cognitive decline does not occur for everyone, and neither is it necessarily rapid or progressive when it does. Indeed, many people still have the capability to develop and better utilise their cognitive capacity. Whilst a popular saying is 'you can't teach an old dog new tricks', research on stereotypes associated with ageing demonstrated that it is the stereotypes that impact upon beliefs about learning ability, not a lack of actual ability. These beliefs may then become self-fulfilling prophecies, leading to poorer performance in older adults (Levy, 2003) and becoming ingrained in a person's self-perception, affecting cognition and wellbeing. It may be that focusing upon affirming aspects of older age (e.g. wisdom, maturity, increased self-esteem and confidence) and promoting a positive yet realist image can have a beneficial influence on function and wellbeing, rather than the negatives such as potential declines in cognition and performance.

Therefore, when working with older people living with HIV, we should be mindful of the potential for cognitive difficulties and make necessary adaptations when they occur, but equally we should not patronise nor assume that older people will not be able to cope by virtue of their age alone.

Thinking points

- Who assesses cognition in the interdisciplinary team?
- How might different team members need to adjust their work if cognitive impairment was present in the person living with HIV?

Personality

Our personality is what makes us individuals with character traits, attitudes, habits and emotions. We show our personality from the way we conduct and carry ourselves, for example the way we dress (jewellery, make-up, tattoos, clothing) or display our likes and dislikes. Personality also predicts life events such as relationships, employment, health, wealth and happiness and is shaped by early experiences that create templates of expectation about the world, which influences interactions with it (see Chapter 6).

Common (and usually negative and pejorative) stereotypes of older adults played out in the media and social discourses include 'grumpy old men/women', 'cougars', 'dirty old men', loving grandparents, and 'dotty', 'dithering' or 'dementing' with so-called 'senior moments' (i.e. cognitive errors or mistakes). As well as being potentially offensive, these of course make many assumptions: that people weren't 'grumpy young people' first; that being sexual in old age should be taboo; that people have had children and grandchildren; that we all lose cognitive faculties as we age.

In general, it is assumed that in old age our personality changes, usually towards the 'grumpy' negative side. However, some may feel more at ease in old age; with the stress of work and family upbringing over, they may feel more free and relaxed. However, the influence of the individual's social environment on personality traits can be also very significant as well as life events and history. There has been much research into the changes in personality. Some have been attributed to life events such as retirement, becoming grandparents, grief and loss following the death of relatives and friends. There is some evidence that people experience changes to their agreeableness, conscientiousness and emotional regulation, with falling levels of neuroticism, openness and extraversion (Srivastava et al., 2003); these may be provoked by social marginalisation and the exclusion of older people. Of course we are capable of believing differently dependent on the context, so perhaps it is not so specific to age?

Importantly, our personality can be influenced by significant life events, both in childhood and adulthood. This does not mean that it will remain fixed in this state, but may lead to inclinations or habits to think and behave in certain ways which become our 'default' unless otherwise challenged. For many people living with HIV, the diagnosis, treatment and response of others to it can be significant life events. It is therefore vital to understand a person's experience of HIV and the wider history of HIV.

Thinking points

How is ageing portrayed in the media? What positive and negative examples are you aware of? How might the images and language used affect older people's self-esteem? How have you experienced your personality changing with age? What aspects have stayed relatively similar, and what facets have changed over the years? What might have caused these changes?

Consider a person living with HIV across their lifespan and how the following might change as they age: education, work, social life, finances, housing, sex, exercise, substance use, diet, health, medication, etc.

How might these factors impact on their wellbeing as they age? Who in the interdisciplinary team would assess and assist with each of these?

Isolation

Isolation and loneliness have been highlighted in many studies and reports (Age UK, 2010; Luo et al., 2012; Tzouvara et al., 2015). Within the UK, isolation is a huge issue which has led to a 'Minister of Loneliness' to tackle isolation and loneliness across all ages. Isolation can be defined as separation from social or familial contact, community involvement or access to services, whilst loneliness can be described as an individual's personal subjective sense of lacking these things, to the extent that they are wanted or needed (Age UK, 2010). Social relationships are important to wellbeing and central to the maintenance of health (Steptoe et al., 2013). Loneliness is debilitating and can lead to poor health, and isolation and loneliness have been shown to impair quality of life and wellbeing and together can affect mortality (Holt-Lunstad, Smith, & Layton, 2010). However, it is important to note that people who choose to be socially isolated might not feel lonely, and people who feel lonely might not be socially isolated.

Loss of peers and partners is a direct way that people can become more isolated as they age. However, some studies have demonstrated that the transition to living alone after decades of cohabiting may not have a negative effect upon the psychological or physical health of an individual (Stone, Evandrou, & Falkingham, 2013). Conversely, physical illness, severe hearing and sight loss, depression, language barriers and cognitive decline can create barriers to communication and interaction that can lead people to feel isolated even when in their usual group settings or relationships.

Furthermore, these might limit the ability to use more modern communication technologies. Shifts in the way we communicate have also impacted on people's perceptions of how connected they feel to other people and what format of interactions are expected. Texts, social media, video calling, and geolocation apps (e.g. Tinder, Grindr) may increase or decrease a person's sense of connectedness and community depending on how accessible they are for the person and their previous experience (or lack thereof) of using this medium.

For people living with HIV, isolation may include feeling separate from others due to one's differing HIV status, or from a loss of peer support. This may be due to either bereavement, changes in personal circumstances (e.g. not being able to travel), a new living environment (e.g. residential care, moving closer to family) or the closure of previously used resources (e.g. many social HIV drop-in centres have closed and gay bars and clubs have shut down or moved due to 'gentrification'). All of these lead to a reduction in face-to-face peer contact opportunities.

Thinking points

- If someone is isolated, how might this impact their HIV care?
- How might the interdisciplinary team respond to this? Who might take the lead? Who might provide overarching support?

Stigma

The role that stigma plays in HIV and ageing is complex. As discussed in Chapter 8, stigma can be something that an individual feels or experiences which leads to social isolation (Hawthorne, 2006), and can be feared or actualised. This has been linked to poor health outcomes, including an increased cardiovascular risk (Grant, Hamer, &

Steptoe, 2009), particularly in women (Hackett et al., 2012), decreased quality of life, increased hospitalisation and use of services, functional decline and death (Perissinotto, Cenzer, & Covinsky, 2012). The combined effects of HIV-related stigma, depression and isolation adversely affect HIV treatment adherence (Ware, Wyatt, & Tugenberg, 2006) and limit the use of social support due to fear of rejection (Berger, Ferrans, & Lashley, 2001; Grov et al., 2010).

People ageing with HIV have a 'double stigma' to potentially contend with: that for being HIV+, and that for ageing and being older (ageism). For many, there may also be further layers of stigma attached to being a member of an already socially marginalised group(s) (e.g. LGBTQ+ vs. homonegativity, transphobia or heteronormativity; immigrant status vs. nationalism; (dis)abled vs. ableism; female vs. patriarchal societies; BAME vs. institutionalised racism; lower social economic status vs. classism, etc.). Such stigma can occur within groups also, for example the emphasis (and reward) that a lot of gay culture places on being young (Robinson, 2011), with older gay men three times more likely to be single than heterosexual men (Taylor, 2012). This can lead to older gay men with HIV feeling that they are becoming disconnected from their friends, family and society, and they report feeling separated, alone, isolated and rejected by their community and peers (Power et al., 2010).

Thinking points

- What stigmas are you aware of against older people, people living with HIV, and people from marginalised communities?
- How can different members of the interdisciplinary team actively challenge such stigma?

If older people living with HIV are seen as less worthy than younger or negative peers due to aforementioned stereotypes, this may affect 'social competence' (the ability to process social interactions constructively to secure physical, emotional and intimate needs: Baltes & Baltes, 1990). This in turn could lead to a vicious cycle of social withdrawal (especially observed in older adults with HIV: Nichols, Speer, Watson et al., 2002), leaving stigma unchallenged and the person living with HIV marginalised.

Even those who may have successfully navigated HIV-related stigma to date may be presented with new fears and anxieties regarding discrimination (e.g. fear of having to 'go back into the closet'), as well as practical issues (e.g. divesting responsibility for HIV medication management for the first time). Thus services such as older-age residential and domiciliary care that are not currently culturally competent in working with people living with HIV must learn and adapt to meet their needs (NAT, 2015). If healthcare workers approach older people with adequate knowledge and an open, non-judgemental mind, the future generations of people ageing with HIV will be able to receive care that meets their needs (Stuart-Hamilton, 2000).

Case study: Timon, 81-year-old bisexual man living with HIV

Timon has lived alone (apart from lodgers) in a large town house. He acquired HIV in 2014. He has no close family and is supported by a community HIV specialist nurse, and attends a local HIV drop-in for lunch twice a week. Over the past six months he has become frail and forgetful, has fallen at home twice and had his bedroom moved from the second floor to the living room. He has erratic adherence and consequently has had several hospital admissions. On his last admission it was decided that he could no longer go home, and a nursing home was found. After two weeks he called the community HIV specialist nurse to say that he wasn't happy as the staff weren't supportive. He was feeling shame and embarrassment about his HIV status as he felt 'singled out' and was feeling anxious about talking not only about HIV but also expressing himself as a bisexual man (e.g. having a male calendar in his room) and said his friends who visited felt some hostility. On discussion with the staff they felt they had good knowledge of HIV and stated that Timon had his own crockery and cutlery and that staff used universal precautions when bathing and during personal care. Timon felt isolated in his room and wanted to go out to the social area, but staff were reluctant due to his HIV status 'for his own good'.

What do you think the key issues are for:

Timon?
The care home staff?
The HIV care team?

What can be done to help Timon?
What proactive measures could be implemented to avoid the scenario Timon faced?

Successful ageing with HIV

Early on, eight factors were described as being part of ageing successfully with HIV: the impact of HIV on length of life, biological health, cognitive efficiency, mental health, social competence, productivity, personal control, and life satisfaction (Baltes & Baltes, 1990). This has been updated by Catalan et al. (2017), who found that better quality of life for people over 50 years and living with HIV was strongly associated with: being male, being in a relationship, being in paid employment, having a higher level of income and not being on benefits. Also relevant, although to a lesser degree, were: being a man who had sex with men, having a higher level of education and being diagnosed after 40 years old. The most consistent findings were not being on benefits and being partnered. Whilst some factors cannot be changed, others might be more amenable to intervention (both individual and social/systemic). For example, Catalan et al. (2017), as part of the 'HIV and Later Life Project', explored mental health and wellbeing themes. Poorer psychological wellbeing was associated with: anticipatory ageing, the unknown, 'good days and bad days', anxiety and emerging stigma. However, wellbeing themes were also identified, structured around: peers and volunteering, empowerment, positive thinking, a 'game' narrative, living in the moment and spirituality, and acceptance. This echoes qualitative research by Emlet et al. (2010), who identified seven themes of resilience and strengths:

- *Self-acceptance*: feeling comfortable with oneself and who you are at the later stage of life.
- *Optimism*: a positive outlook on ageing with HIV, feeling upbeat about life and hopeful about continued wellbeing (albeit a conscious effort at times).
- *Will to live*: surviving and living well is possible with access to treatment, research and understanding.
- *Generativity*: wanting to give back to community and society with wisdom that comes from age and experience.
- *Self-management*: self-care, personal responsibility and self-control.
- *Relational living*: acceptance from formal and informal support systems including family, partners, friends, peers, societies and support groups.
- *Independence*: being self-supporting, self-reliant, looking to oneself as a resource, managing one's own care.

What are the different factors behind successful ageing with HIV, and who in the interdisciplinary team could help foster these?

Case Study: Mabel, 54-year-old woman living with HIV

Mabel is a nurse and mother of three grown-up children, the last one leaving home a couple of months ago. Mabel was diagnosed with HIV in 1993 after moving to the UK. She recently started the menopause, experiencing symptoms that included hot flushes, difficulty sleeping, low libido, vaginal dryness, and low mood. Mabel isn't sure how to distinguish between her menopausal symptoms and symptoms of HIV, or side effects of medication. This has her feeling a bit anxious. Despite her symptoms, which include hot flushes, night sweats and mood changes that affected her daily life, Mabel has said she does not want to go on hormone replacement therapy due to the medication she was already taking for HIV. She is separated from the father of her children, but does not feel able to meet new people, despite wanting a relationship. Mabel said she has recently reduced how often she attends her local church from weekly to monthly, although continues to find her faith and spirituality incredibly important. She was offered the opportunity of a promotion at work, but declined it, saying she did not think she would be good enough at it. Mabel has scored highly on the questionnaires in the clinic that screen for low mood and depression, but insists that 'everything is fine' and that she 'does not want to bother anyone and waste their time'.

What do you think the key issues are for:

- Mabel?
- The HIV care team?

What can be done to help Mabel?
What proactive measures could be implemented to avoid the scenario Mabel faces?

Individualised care

Health and social care workers must recognise the clinical, functional and individual implications of ageing, to help them to develop appropriate models of care, care pathways and care plans. Each person ageing with HIV is unique and will likewise require individualised care, with differing contributions from different members of the interdisciplinary team at different stages. Successful ageing with HIV is achievable, with an emphasis upon social engagement, resilience and optimism essential in the training of professionals, to promote wellbeing as people living with HIV age (Moore et al., 2013). As such, the below prompts may be useful for formulating their holistic care plan:

- *Diversity:* how might gender, sexuality, ethnicity, class, (dis)ability, spirituality, etc., affect the needs and resilience of the person growing older with HIV? What cultural and societal expectations do they and others have of ageing, and how does HIV intersect with these? What positions of disempowerment or privilege might they have, and how might these be similar to or different from those providing their care and support?
- *Communication*: within HIV services we may manage and support the same person for many years, but do we need to change the way we communicate with them as they age? Would offering a variety of communication tools, as well as knowing how best the person receives information, help within consultations? Consider encouraging clients to write down key points. Would offering longer appointments help for fuller assessment and the opportunity for full expression of concerns? Or perhaps more frequent but shorter appointments due to fatigue and concentration issues?
- *Monitoring risk*: how can we adapt services to incorporate NICE Guidance (2010) which suggests ensuring staff in contact with older people can identify those most at risk of a decline in their independence and mental wellbeing. This includes being aware that certain life events or circumstances are more likely to increase the risk of decline. For example:

  o older people whose partner has died in the past two years
  o are carers
  o live alone and have little opportunity to socialise
  o have recently separated or divorced
  o have recently retired (particularly if involuntary)
  o were unemployed in later life
  o have a low income
  o have recently experienced or developed a health problem (whether or not it led to admission to hospital)
  o have had to give up driving
  o have an age-related disability
  o are aged 80 or older.

- *Specialist clinics*: due to the complex nature of physical and psychosocial ageing with HIV, some HIV clinics have introduced 'over-50s' clinics providing 'one-stop' appointments with standardised assessments of issues known to particularly affect those over 50. Clinics such as these may be opportunities for an interdisciplinary approach. Do we need to start to consider what pathways services have to best support people ageing with HIV?

- *Social connectedness*: as people age, how do they view their roles within social relationships: who are their friends, family, and who supports them? Do they ever feel isolated or lonely? If so, what have they done to rectify this? With a reduction in HIV support services, finding onward referral resources may be difficult, but there may be online resources (e.g. Terrence Higgins Trust's 'MyHIV' and Positively UK's peer support programme). Alternatively, local mainstream services outside of HIV care (e.g. Age UK groups, walking or local community centre activities, gay men/women's groups, BME, church/faith support, etc.) can be accessed and may benefit from 'upskilling' of their HIV knowledge by consultation or training by HIV services.
- *Later-life care*: in order to support and ensure safe effective care as people living with HIV age, what is our role going to be in educating residential and nursing homes? How can we allay fears around HIV transmission or drug interactions with ART?

Does the current model of care need to be altered in order to ensure that people who are ageing with HIV are resilient and can make the changes that they need? And are people ageing with HIV aware of issues regarding death, wills, advance decisions/directives, pensions, etc.? These are topics which used to be routinely discussed when we were in the grip of an epidemic, but since we may have become uncomfortable raising such conversations – due to their connection with mortality and our wish to de-stigmatise – and emphasising how much HIV care and outlook has improved.

Conclusion

We are at the beginning of a new wave of effectively developing the care for older people with HIV, and how we respond now should shape and address any issues with future care. Ageing generally is often associated with negative attributes and stereotypes. For those living with HIV, not only are there these to contend with, but also the additional impact that HIV can have, both on known ageing wellbeing factors and others unique to HIV (some of which have yet to be discovered). Biographic age can be as important as chronological age, and both should be considered by the interdisciplinary team to optimise the holistic physical and psychological care of those growing older with HIV.

References

Age UK. (2010) *Loneliness and isolation: Evidence review*. Age UK, London. Available at: www. ageuk.org.uk/documents/en-gb/for-professionals/evidence_review_loneliness_and_isolation.pdf? dtrk=true (Accessed April 2017).

Balderson, B. H., Grothaus, L., Harrison, R. G., McCoy, K., Mahoney, C., & Catz, S. (2013). Chronic illness burden and quality of life in an aging HIV population. *AIDS Care*, 25, 4, 451–458.

Baltes, P. B., & Baltes, M. M. (1990). Psychological perspectives on successful aging: The model of selective optimization with compensation. In P. B. Baltes and M. M. Baltes (Eds.), *Successful aging: Perspectives from the behavioral sciences* (pp. 1–34). Cambridge: Cambridge University Press.

Bengtson, V. L., & Settersten, R. J. R. (2016). *Handbook of theories of ageing*. London: Springer Publishing Company..

Berger, B. E., Ferrans, C. E., & Lashley, F. R. (2001). Measuring stigma in people with HIV: Psycho-metric assessment of the HIV stigma scale. *Research in Nursing and Health*, 24, 518–529.

Catalan, J., Tuffery, V., Ridge, D., & Rosenfield, D. (2017). What influences quality of life in older people living with HIV? *AIDS Research and Therapy*, 14, 1, 22.

Emlet, C. A., Fredriksen-Goldsen, K. I., & Kim, H. J. (2013). Risk and protective factors associated with health-related quality of life among older gay and bisexual men living with HIV disease. *The Gerontologist*, 53, 6, 963–972.

Enriquez, M., Lackey, N., & Witt, J. (2008). Health concerns of mature women living with HIV in Midwestern United States. *Journal of the Association of Nurses in AIDS Care*, 19, 1, 27–46.

Ghidei, L., Simone, M. J., Salow, M. J., Zimmerman, K. M., Paquin, A. M., Skarf, L. M., McDonnel, J. L., & Rudolph, J. L. (2013). Aging, antiretrovirals, and adherence: A meta-analysis of adherence among older HIV-infected individuals. *Drugs & Aging*, 30, 10, 809–819.

Grant, N., Hamer, M., & Steptoe, A. (2009). Social isolation and stress-related cardiovascular, lipid, and cortisol responses. *Annals of Behavioral Medicine*, 37, 1, 29–37.

Grov, C., Golub, S. A., Parsons, J. T., Brennan, M., & Karpiak, S. E. (2010). Loneliness and HIV-related stigma explain depression among older HIV-positive adults. *AIDS Care*, 22, 630–639.

Grulich, A. E., van Leeuwen, M. T., Falster, M. O., & Vajdic, C. M. (2007). Incidence of cancers in people with HIV/AIDS compared with immunosuppressed transplant recipients: A meta-analysis. *Lancet*, 370, 9581, 59–67.

Hackett, R. A., Hamer, M., Endrighi, R., Brydon, L., & Steptoe, A. (2012). Loneliness and stress-related inflammatory and neuroendocrine responses in older men and women. *Psychoneur-oendocrinology*, 37, 1801–1809.

Hawthorne, G. (2006). Measuring social isolation in older adults: Development and initial validation of the friendship scale. *Social Indicators Research*, 77, 521–548.

High, K. P., Brennan-Ing, M., Clifford, D. B., Cohen, M. H., Currier, J., Deeks, S. G., … Justice, A. C. (2012). HIV and aging: State of knowledge and areas of critical need for research. A report to the NIH Office of AIDS Research by the HIV and Aging Working Group. *Journal of Acquired Immune Deficiency Syndromes (1999)*, 60(Suppl 1), S1–S18.

Holt-Lunstad, J, Smith, T. B., & Layton, J. B. (2010). Social relationships and mortality risk: A meta-analytic review. *PLoS Medicine*, 7, 7, e1000316.

Lamont, J. (2012). Female sexual health consensus clinical guidelines. *Journal of Obstetrics and Gynaecology Canada*, 34, 8, 769–775.

Levy, B. R. (2003). Mind matters: Cognitive and physical effects of aging self-stereotypes. *The Journals of Gerontology Series B: Psychological Sciences and Social Sciences*, 58, 4, P203–P211.

Loufty, M. R., Sherr, L., Sonnenberg-Schwan, U., Johnson, M., & D'Arminio, A. (2013). Caring for women living with HIV: Gaps in the evidence. *Journal of the International AIDS Society*, 16, 18509.

Luo, Y., Hawkley, L. C., Waite, L. J., & Cacioppo, J. T. (2012). Loneliness, health, and mortality in old age: A national longitudinal study. *Social Science & Medicine*, 74, 6, 907–914.

McDowell, T.L., & Serovich, J. M. (2007). The effect of perceived and actual social support on the mental health of HIV-positive persons. *AIDS Care*, 19, 10, 1223–1229.

Mitnitski, A. B., Mogilner, A. J., & Rockwood, K. (2001). Accumulation of deficits as a proxy measure of aging. *The Scientific World Journal*, 1, 323–336.

Moore, R. C., Moore, D. J., Thompson, W., Vahia, I. V., Grant, I., & Jeste, D. V. (2013). A case-controlled study of successful aging in older adults with HIV. *The Journal of Clinical Psychiatry*, 74, 5, e417.

National AIDS Trust. (2017a) Trans* people and HIV: How policy work improves HIV prevention, treatment and care for trans* people in the UK. Available at: www.nat.org.uk/sites/default/files/pub lications/NAT%20Trans%20Evidence%20Review%20V3%20Digital.pdf (Accessed April 2017).

National AIDS Trust. (2017b) Why we need HIV support services: A review of the evidence. Available at: www.nat.org.uk/publication/why-we-need-hiv-support-services-review-evidence (Accessed April 2017).

National Institute for Health and Clinical Excellence (NICE). (2010) *Older People: Independence and mental wellbeing* [Online]. Available at: www.nice.org.uk/guidance/ng32 (Accessed 5 April 2017).

Nichols, JE, Speer, D. C., Watson, B. J., Speer, D., Vergon, T., & Meah, J. (2002). *Aging with HIV: Psychological, social, and health issues*. San Diego, CA: Academic Press.

Nussbaum, P. (2003). *Brain health and wellness*. Tarentum, PA: Word Association Publishers.

Owen, G., & Catalan, J. (2012). We never expected this to happen: Narratives of ageing with HIV among gay men living with HIV in London UK. *Culture, Health and Sexuality*, 14, 1, 59–72.

Pathai, S., Bajillan, H., Landay, A. L., & High, K. P. (2013). Is HIV a model of accelerated or accentuated ageing? *The Journals of Gerontology Series A Biological Sciences and Medical Sciences* 2014 July, 69, 7, 833–842.

Perissinotto, C. M., Cenzer, I. S., & Covinsky, K. E. (2012). Loneliness in older persons: A predictor of functional decline and death. *Archives of Internal Medicine*, 172, 1078–1084.

Power, L., Bell, M., & Freemantle, I. (2010) A national study of ageing and HIV (50 plus). Terrence Higgins Trust. www.jrf.org.uk/sites/default/files/jrf/migrated/files/living-with-HIV-full.pdf (Accessed April 2017).

Rabkin, J.G. (2008). HIV and depression: 2008 review and update. *Current HIV/AIDS Reports*, 5, 4, 163–171.

Robinson, P. (2011). The influence of ageism on relations be- tween old and young gay men. In Y. Smaal and G. Willett (Eds.), *Out here: Gay and lesbian perspectives VI* (pp. 188–200). Clayton, Australia: Monash University Publishing.

Rockwood, K., Hogan, D. B., & MacKnight, C. (2000). Conceptualization and instrumentation of frailty. *Drugs Aging*, 17, 295–302.

Sabin, C. A., & Reiss, P. (2017). Epidemiology of ageing with HIV: What can we learn from cohorts? *AIDS*, 31, S121–S128.

Schäfer, I., von Leitner, E. C., Schön, G., Koller, D., Hansen, H., Kolonko, T., Kaduszkiewicz, H., Wegscheider, K., Glaeske, G., & van den Bussche, H. (2010). Multimorbidity patterns in the elderly: A new approach of disease clustering identifies complex interrelations between chronic conditions. *PLoS One*, 5, 12, 15941.

Sherr, L., Molloy, A., Macedo, A., Croome, N., & Johnson, M. A. (2016). Ageing and menopause considerations for women with HIV in the UK. *Journal of Virus Eradication*, 2, 4, 215.

Smit, M., Brinkman, K., Geerling, S., Smitt, C., & Thyagarajan, K. (2015). Future challenges for clinical care of an ageing population infected with HIV, a modelling study. *The Lancet Infectious Diseases*, 15, 7, 810–818.

Solomon, P., O'Brien, K., Wilkins, S., & Gervais, N. (2014). Aging with HIV and disability: The role of uncertainty. *AIDS Care*, 26, 2, 240–245. DOI: 10.1080/09540121.2013.811209

Srivastava, S., John, O. P., Gosling, S. D., & Potter, J. (2003). Development of personality in early and middle adulthood: Set like plaster or persistent change? *Journal of Personality and Social Psychology*, 84, 50, 1041–1053.

Steptoe, A., Shankar, A., Demakakos, P., & Wardle, J. (2013). Social isolation, loneliness, and all-cause mortality in older men and women. *Proceedings of the National Academy of Sciences*, 110, 15, 5797–5801.

Stone, J., Evandrou, M., & Falkingham, J. (2013). The transition to living alone and psychological distress in later life. *Age and Ageing*, 42, 3, 366–372.

Stuart-Hamilton, I. (2000). *The psychology of ageing*. London & Philadelphia, PA: Jessica Kingsley Publishers.

Taylor, J. (2012) Working with older lesbian, gay and bisexual people: A guide for care and support services. Stonewall, London. Available at: https://www.basw.co.uk/system/files/resources/basw_61548-9_0.pdf (Accessed April 2017).

Taylor, T. N., Munoz-Plaza, C. E., Goparaju, L., Martinez, O., Holman, S., Minkoff, H. L., & Levine, A. M. (2016). "The pleasure is better as I've gotten older": Sexual health, sexuality, and sexual risk behaviors among older women living with HIV. *Archives of sexual behavior*, 1–14.

Trickey, A, May, M. T., Vehreschild, J. J., Obel, N., & Gill, M. J. (2017). Survival of HIV positive patients starting antiretroviral therapy between 1996-2013 a collaborative analysis of cohort studies. *The Lancet HIV*, 4, 8, e349–e356.

Terrence Higgins Trust (2017) Uncharted Territory: A report into the first generation growing older with HIV. Available at: www.tht.org.uk/%7E/media/Files/Publications/Policy/uncharted_territory_final_low-res.pdf (Accessed April 2017).

Tzouvara, V., Papadopoulos, C., & Randhawa, G. (2015). A narrative review of the theoretical foundations of loneliness. *British Journal of Community Nursing*, 20, 7, 329–334.

Vance, D.E., Farr, K. F., & Struzick, T. (2008). Assessing the clinical value of cognitive appraisal in adults aging with HIV. *Journal of Gerontological Nursing*, 34, 1, 36–41.

Vance, D.E., & Struzick, T.C. (2007). Addressing risk factors of cognitive impairment in adults aging with HIV. *Journal of Gerontological Social Work*, 49, 4, 51–77. DOI: 10.1300/J083v49n04_04

Ware, N. C., Wyatt, M. A., & Tugenberg, T. (2006). Social relationships, stigma and adherence to antiretroviral therapy for HIV/AIDS. *AIDS Care*, 18, 8, 904–910.

11 Neurocognitive issues for adults in HIV care

Tomás Campbell and Alexander Margetts

Chapter description

If not treated, HIV can have profound effects on the brain and brain function. In this chapter we define neurocognitive impairment caused by HIV and review the evidence base for this. After considering the controversy regarding aetiology and prevalence rates, we discuss how it might be screened for and assessed in a clinical setting, with suggestions for management and neurorehabilitation.

HIV and HIV-associated neurocognitive disorder (HAND)

The term HIV-associated neurocognitive disorder (HAND) has been used to describe a spectrum of neurocognitive dysfunction associated with HIV infection (e.g. Clifford, 2017), which can be either chronic, or more rarely, acute.

Chronic

HIV can enter the central nervous system (CNS) during early stages of infection, and persistent CNS HIV infection and inflammation probably contribute to the development of HAND. HIV is both a neurotropic and immunotropic virus, meaning that it can cause progressive destruction to the immune system by the targeted destruction of CD4 lymphocytes causing neuropathological changes particularly within the basal ganglia and the white matter (Simioni et al., 2010).

HIV-associated neurological conditions may be directly caused by HIV, or indirectly through immune depletion and subsequent vulnerability to infection. There is also evidence that the inflammatory process may persist despite effective medical control of HIV (Simioni et al., 2010). Chronic activation of essential and specialised brain cells (microglia) has been suggested to be a major contributing factor for HAND (Vera et al., 2016). The brain can subsequently serve as a 'sanctuary site' or 'reservoir' for ongoing HIV replication, even when systemic viral suppression has been achieved.

As HAND can remain a problem for patients treated with antiretroviral therapy (ART), its effects on survival, quality of life and everyday functioning make it an important and unresolved issue.

Acute

Alternatively (or in addition), there may be a one-off acute, HIV-related neurological incident that causes damage. One form of this would be HIV-related encephalitis (HIVE: e.g. Cherner et al., 2002), in which there is a sudden onset inflammation of the brain. Another form could be Immune Reconstitution Inflammatory Syndrome (IRIS: e.g. Gray et al., 2005), in which the immune system begins to recover from a previously ill state (usually after initiation of ART in those who were treatment naive, or switching from a failing treatment) but then responds to a previously acquired opportunistic infection with an overwhelming inflammatory response, making symptoms worse.

In both cases immediate symptoms could include: fever, headache, confusion, and/or seizures. Therefore it may be misattributed or assigned as delirium or could be co-morbid with another infection, especially common in an ageing population (Britton & Russell, 2004) (refer to Chapter 10).

Some recent interesting research has also indicated approximately half of people may experience milder neurological issues at the time of diagnosis (Hellmuth et al., 2016); however, for the vast majority these issues subside, and causality from HIV (as opposed to other risk factors such as anxiety and drug use) has yet to be established.

Defining HAND

In 2007, a new and revised classification was proposed for HIV-related CNS impairment that included milder forms of neurocognitive disturbance and are now referred to as the 'Frascati criteria'. HAND has been divided into three categories (Anitinori et al., 2007) that reflect increasing severity and related impact on everyday functioning, ranging from asymptomatic, mild and dementia (Figure 11.1). This is determined by how many different cognitive skillsets (domains) are affected, to what level of severity compared with the general population (standard deviation, SD, from age and education appropriate norms), and the impact on daily functioning. Relating to HIV is a process of exclusion of other possible causes (such as delirium and/or other dementia). Furthermore, when HIV-attributable, this definition does not in itself differentiate between a chronic cause (i.e. long-term HIV) or an acute cause (e.g. HIVE, IRIS response).

Antiretroviral medication

For those diagnosed and able to access treatment, ART has transformed the condition from being one in which declining health led to certain death to a manageable long-term condition, with an expectation of good health and associated quality of life and a lifespan similar to the non-HIV population (Antiretroviral Therapy Cohort Collaboration, 2017).

Research findings for ART and HAND are mixed (e.g. Nightingale et al., 2014). Effective ART (depending on its ability to penetrate the blood–brain barrier and enter the CNS) may stop, slow or even reverse the symptoms of HIV cognitive impairment. However, some types of HIV medication have themselves been implicated in cognitive impairment via neurotoxicity.

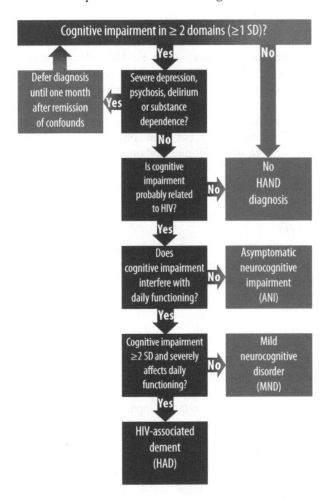

Figure 11.1 HAND definition and diagnosis (adapted from Woods et al., 2009)

Prevalence of HAND

Understandably researchers, healthcare professionals and people living with HIV want to know the prevalence, risk factors and likelihood of acquiring HAND. However, such data is somewhat controversial and difficult to obtain or estimate, because there are different definitions of HAND, and different populations of people living with HIV may have characteristics that make them more or less vulnerable to HAND and/or cognitive impairment in general. In addition, the availability of ART (alongside early detection of infection and rapid commencement of treatment) has led to dramatic improvements in medical morbidity and life expectancy, and this has also been reflected in improvements in neurological outcomes with a significant drop in the rate of HIV-associated dementia (Robertson et al., 2007).

Prior to the introduction of ART, prevalence estimates of HAND were approximately 16% (McArthur et al., 1993). More recent reviews estimate that neurocognitive impairment affects between 10% (Simioni et al., 2010) and 50% of individuals living with HIV (Heaton et al., 2010). These discrepancies may be attributable to differences in normative data sets and to how HIV-related neurocognitive impairment was defined in different studies.

While the prevalence of HAND may never accurately be known (and is liable to change as HIV management and treatment develops), it is clear that a significant minority of people living with HIV do experience HAND, and so research has focused on trying to understand who is at risk and what the impact is, neurologically, neuropsychologically and functionally.

Risk factors

The presence of risk factors will not necessarily equate to the development of HAND, and someone without risk factors may still experience HAND. However, they can be useful for clinicians and people living with HIV in estimating the likelihood of acquiring HAND, and crucially for changeable factors, potentially reducing this. A summary of possible risk factors is shown in Figure 11.2.

The variety of different risk factors requires a full interdisciplinary approach, and will vary for each client based on their personal history dictated by their culture, environment, age and wider health.

As previously discussed, accessing and adhering to ART is crucial in this; however, in and of itself it does not prevent HAND. There are risk factors for those stable on HIV medication. Yuen et al. (2017) in the CHARTER study examined risk factors for people living with HIV with undetectable viral load. They found that impaired kidney function, living with HIV for more than 15 years, educational status of less than 12 years, and protein levels in cerebrospinal fluid being mildly elevated or above, were found to raise

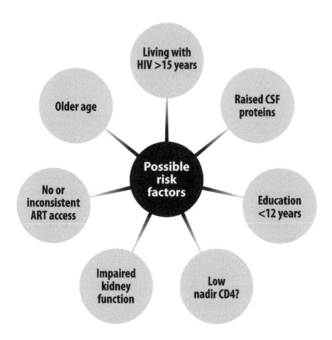

Figure 11.2 Possible risk factors for HAND

risk from background 2% rate (with none of these factors) to 95% (with all four of these factors) of cognitive impairment.

This is unsurprising as poor kidney function can relate to wider cardiovascular risk issues and increased risk of recurrent stroke and small brain infarctions, having lived longer with HIV means that someone may have been without effective treatment for longer, and reduced education levels may equate to reduced cognitive reserve (in which any cognitive functioning reduction will have a proportionally greater impact given a lower premorbid state).

Low nadir (lowest recorded) CD4 predicted neurocognitive difficulties in both eras, whereas degree of current immunosuppression, estimated duration of infection, and viral suppression in CSF (on treatment) were related to impairment only pre-ART. However, findings are not always consistent. For example, Winston et al. (2017) discussed risk factors to neurocognitive functioning in ART treatment naive participants. Results indicated that factors significantly and independently associated with poorer overall cognitive performance included: older age, fewer years of education, black ethnicity, lower height and lower plasma HIV RNA. Factors that were *not* associated with poorer cognitive functioning included current or nadir CD4 cell count, blood pressure or smoking status.

Learning task

Your client asks how they can avoid getting 'HIV dementia' – how might you respond?

- What would you tell them about the types and prevalence of HAND?
- How does ART affect this?
- What risk factors would you want to explore with them?
- Who would be responsible for assessing these?
- Who might help the client with any behavioural change indicated?

Reflection point

- What might it be like to be worried about your cognitive function?
- What issues might concern you?

HAND and neurological change

Neurological change refers to the physical changes to the brain. Neuroimaging and neuropsychological studies suggest that frontostriatal circuits (connections between the frontal lobes and basal ganglia) are affected initially, and there is a reduction in white matter volumes (the brain's connective tissue made from axons, which communicates information between the grey matter).

If the disease progresses, this may create structural abnormalities and impairment. Fortunately, this is unusual in a context where the disease may be effectively managed by early identification and prompt commencement of ART. However, it is important to note that there is an inconsistent pattern of impairments (Heaton et al., 2004), and so reliance on neuroimaging alone for a diagnosis of HAND will not suffice. Neurocognitive and functional change must also be assessed.

HAND and neurocognitive change

Neurocognitive change refers to changes in a person's ability to perform specific cognitive tasks. This has been noted since the beginning of the epidemic (Anitinori et al., 2007). These difficulties can range from subtle impairments in individuals with medically asymptomatic HIV infection, to profoundly disabling HIV-associated dementia (Underwood et al., 2017).

Cognitive difficulties identified have included motor skills impairment (our ability to move and use our body), cognitive speed issues (how quickly we can understand and process information), memory difficulties (particularly short-term memory) and executive functioning difficulties (e.g. planning, reasoning, decision-making, prioritising, emotional control).

The pattern of difficulties has changed since the introduction of ART. Impairment in motor skills, cognitive speed and verbal fluency were more commonly reported pre-ART, indicating sub-cortical involvement. These issues are similar to those found in Parkinson's disease, for which sometimes a differential diagnosis might be needed. However, even within Parkinson's disease alone there can be variation with cognitive symptoms (Kehagia, Barker, & Robbins, 2010).

In the ART era, memory, information processing, learning and executive function impairments are more commonly observed (Heaton et al., 2011). This pattern of difficulty is probably more cortical in origin, and more broadly similar to that observed in degenerative disorders such as Alzheimer's disease, providing a challenge for diagnosing HAND in people living with HIV in their older years (Turner et al., 2016).

HAND and functional change

Functional change refers to the day-to-day impact upon a person's life and activities. As cognitive difficulties may be subtle, they may be difficult to clinically assess; however, they may have an important impact on the lives of people living with HIV. For example, difficulties with prospective memory (the ability to 'remember to remember') may have an impact on workplace functioning as well as problems with medication adherence (Woods et al., 2011). Slower information processing, attention difficulties and executive functioning issues (e.g. impulsiveness, lack of motivation, emotional lability) may present difficulties with regard to both immediate and daily activities (such as driving or occupational functioning) or in the longer term, such as making important decisions about HIV management (e.g. whether or not to switch ART) or financial decision-making. Such difficulties may be underestimated or misunderstood by people living with HIV and clinicians, and therefore may not be properly assessed. Difficulties may be also wrongly attributed to disorganised lifestyles, stress or the emotional impact of HIV. Therefore, it is essential that the whole interdisciplinary team is aware of what HAND is, as it may present in a variety of forms and affect care in different ways (e.g. Figure 11.3).

Conversely, people living with HIV may *over*-estimate the existence of HAND by assuming functional change is related to this (or become overly sensitive to normal change/fluctuations). Laverick et al. (2017) found in the CIPHER study that approximately one in five people reported cognitive decline, but that co-morbid conditions of depression and/or anxiety, and social circumstances such as being unemployed and/or experiencing difficulties in affording basic needs, should be assessed and addressed before making the conclusion that the underlying problem is HAND (e.g. Figure 11.4).

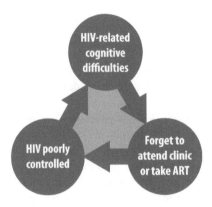

Figure 11.3 Example of a vicious cycle of cognitive difficulties and HIV care: A

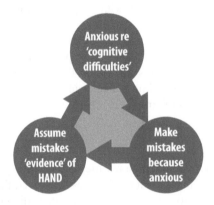

Figure 11.4 Example of a vicious cycle of cognitive difficulties and HIV care: B

Mood disorders (anxiety and/or depression) are common in people living with HIV due to issues such as stigma and inequalities (Chapters 6 and 8). As such there are specific standards for the provision of psychological support for people living with HIV (BHIVA, 2018; BPS, BHIVA & Medfash, 2011).

The symptoms of depression can range from mild to severe and can affect memory, motivation and self-care (Rodkjaer et al., 2016). Such symptoms may be co-morbid with HAND and indeed may be more distressing for the people living with HIV. The management of mood may become the focus for both the clinician and the people living with HIV, thus disguising the presence of HIV-related cognitive difficulties. It can be difficult to distinguish between mood versus HAND issues, particularly in a busy clinic environment where appointments are time limited.

Client factors are also important as people living with HIV may fear that HIV has affected their brain and cognitive functioning and they may deliberately under-report, hide or dismiss symptoms due to this anxiety (e.g. a concern it may affect their ability to drive, work or care for others). Given the significant impact that HAND can have, and that it may be over- or under-reported, clear and unbiased assessment methods are required, which will now be discussed.

Learning task

1   In what ways can HAND affect a client neurologically?
2   In what ways can HAND affect a client neuropsychologically?
3   In what ways can HAND affect a client functionally?
4   Why might HAND be over- or under-reported?

Reflection point

•   What might it be like to live with cognitive difficulties?
•   Think about what aspects of your life could be affected.

Neuropsychological assessment

The assessment of HAND can be complex, and will require joint working and information-sharing within the interdisciplinary team. Confounding issues such as clients having English as a second language (when assessments are in English), varying insight, a lack of culturally appropriate norms or tests, pre-existing physical and sensory disabilities, drug/alcohol use, and/or the presence of a mood disorder can further complicate matters. In any assessment the client's effort ('doing one's best') must be considered and can be influenced by factors such as anxiety, low mood, pain, fatigue and, in rare cases, 'secondary gain' (perceived benefits from a sick role, such as care, avoidance of duties or financial compensation).

The neuropsychological assessment process can comprise:

1.   presentation/screening
2.   clinical history
3.   neurocognitive assessment
4.   functional assessment.

Not everyone will necessarily need to progress from one section to the next. A neuropsychological assessment is differentiated from a neurological assessment, which will be more focused on medical form and function (e.g. assessment of sensory neuron and motor responses and, when appropriate, further medical investigation such as lumbar puncture and neuroimaging).

1.   Presentation/screening

Most clients will themselves be directly reporting their concerns. However, in some cases, it might be a partner, close friend or family member, or one of their healthcare team. The degree of insight and cooperation with assessment is important as it might affect the validity of tests (if someone does not view themselves as having a problem they may not engage with tests properly, which could negatively affect the results) or their response if difficulties are found.

Screening questions

National guidelines recommend annual screening for cognitive impairment (BPS et al., 2011). This does not mean every person living with HIV needs a complete neurocognitive assessment each year. Rather, it is not enough to assume clients will spontaneously self-report difficulties. Therefore cognitive function and health should be asked about on an annual basis by clinicians providing HIV care. This is covered in more depth in the annual health review standard (NHIVNA, 2017).

Simioni et al. (2010) suggest asking three questions regarding cognitive function:

1. Do you experience frequent memory loss (e.g. you forget the occurrence of special events, even the more recent ones, appointments, etc.)?
2. Do you feel that you are slower when reasoning, planning activities or solving problems?
3. Do you have difficulties paying attention (e.g. to a conversation, a book or a movie)?

For each the client can answer: (a) never, (b) hardly ever, (c) yes, definitely. In their research they found that 84% of those who answered one or more of the above with 'definitely' had cognitive impairment. However, so did 64% of those who did not answer any with 'definitely', and so one should not rely upon screening questions alone.

2.   Clinical history

If concerns exist about cognitive function, the next stage would be to gather clinical history specific to this. This may be from a variety of sources and require an interdisciplinary approach, covering:

*   *Presenting difficulties*: once the client has described their issues, it is important to check for further clarification and symptoms they may not have considered.
*   *HIV health*: in general, the poorer the HIV health has been/is, the more likely that there might be cognitive impairment.
*   *Wider health history*: other possible health-related causes (physical and mental health) should be considered.
*   *Premorbid ability*: it is important to try and ascertain at what level someone would be expected to perform before they noticed they had any difficulties, as this will affect interpretation of the results. For example, a score of 'average' in verbal skills for a university lecturer in languages might be an under-achievement, whilst the same score for someone who was not able to access education growing up could be a major accomplishment.
*   *Demographics*: this will help with selecting appropriate norms so people are compared against others of their age and background.

3.   Neurocognitive assessment

Assessment of cognitive functioning is considered within the context of domains (areas) of cognition. Neuropsychological domains commonly affected by HAND include attention and mental flexibility, psychomotor speed, working memory, memory retrieval, episodic memory, verbal fluency and executive functioning (Winston et al., 2017). A neurocognitive assessment can range from short screening tools to comprehensive test batteries.

Table 11.1 Neurocognitive screening tests

Generalist	HIV-focused
Montreal Cognitive Assessment (Nasreddine et al., 2005) Mini Mental State (Folstein, Folstein, & McHugh, 1975) Addenbrooke's Cognitive Examination (Hsieh et al., 2013)	HIV Dementia Scale (Power et al., 1995) International HIV Dementia Scale (Sacktor et al., 2005)

Screening tests

Many short/brief screening neurocognitive tests and batteries exist. Some are generalist and some, in theory, are 'HIV specific' (see Table 11.1).

Advantages compared with full neurocognitive assessments are that they are much quicker, cheaper and can be administered by a variety of different healthcare professionals (if appropriate training and supervision is provided).

However, as with any screening test, compromises are made with regards to sensitivity and specificity. They may miss more subtle cognitive changes (being focused upon dementia-level symptoms), some have limited norms and many were developed to research a subcortical profile only. Therefore, currently no one screening tool can be recommended (Joska et al., 2016; Skinner et al., 2009; Zipursky et al., 2013).

Full neurocognitive assessment

A full neurocognitive assessment is indicated when there is a reported history of significant concerns, corroboration of such difficulties (either by interview report, screening tests or direct observation), and exclusion or stabilisation of other modifiable confounding factors such as alcohol, drug use and/or mood difficulties. Clients may benefit by having neurocognitive issues confirmed and appropriate management strategies can then be enacted by the interdisciplinary team. Conversely, if no cognitive issues are identified, this may be reassuring for the client that there has been no significant decline and/or any cognitive changes are attributable to causes other than HIV.

This will require supervision or direct involvement by a suitably trained and qualified healthcare professional, such as a clinical psychologist or clinical neuropsychologist. There are a variety of different neuropsychological assessment tests available, assessing different cognitive domains. There is no gold-standard test or tests, rather the selection of tests used will depend on different factors, such as the client's reported difficulties, how thorough the assessment is, available norms, experience of the assessor, if retesting is planned and what tests are available locally.

Computerised testing

Historically neurocognitive tests have been 'pencil and paper' tests. However, as technology progresses, there is a move to computerised and online testing options, several of which have been used with people living with HIV (e.g. Cogstate, Maruff et al., 2009;

CANTAB, Sahakian et al., 1995). Advantages include reduced tester burden, wider access, greater standardisation in administration of tests and more accurate data collection (e.g. timing of delivery/responses). Disadvantages include their dependence on a certain level of computer literacy and competence, needing access to computers/tablets (and thus power points), a potential loss of behavioural data (if clients complete the tests unobserved) and less ability to respond clinically (e.g. if a client becomes unwell, is distressed or confused, etc.).

Repeat assessments

Sometimes clients will have already completed a neuropsychological assessment, either in their current service or a prior/different one. This provides an opportunity for comparison between previous and current results to help monitor for change (if any).

Practice effects are important factors to consider; if the same or similar tests are used, clients can benefit from their experience of previous assessment and so perform better on the second assessment. The longer the time difference, the more this will be mitigated. In addition, some memory tests (e.g. BMIPB; Coughlan, Oddy, & Crawford, 2007) have 'alternative' forms with different information to reduce the impact of previous presentations of verbal or visual information.

Finally, sometimes the same tests will not be available and so analogous tests assessing the same domains will need to be used.

4.   Functional assessment

As the diagnosis of HAND often rests on determining the impact upon everyday functioning, it is important to consider the issues involved in assessing functional impairment. This might be assessed by different members of the interdisciplinary team and in different ways.

Currently, there are no widely agreed-upon clinical measures of everyday functioning (Morgan & Heaton, 2009). Performance-based assessments of everyday functioning are sometimes used in research settings, but the lack of normative data coupled with lengthy administration protocols makes it unlikely that such an approach could be widely used clinically.

More commonly, assessments of everyday functioning rely on self-report questionnaires such as Lawton and Brody's (1969) modified Activities of Daily Living scale (Heaton et al., 2004) and the Patient's Assessment of Own Functioning (PAOFI; Chelune, Heaton, & Lehnam, 1986). Collateral reports by significant others and caregivers may be helpful, particularly in cases of significant cognitive impairment and poor insight.

Underwood et al. (2017) reported that associations between cognitive impairment and client-reported outcome measures are weak. Self-reported functional abilities can be confounded by the presence of factors such as mood disorders (e.g. over-reporting due to depressive or anxiety symptoms) or socioeconomic issues (e.g. under-reporting to retain parental, legal and work responsibilities), which must be carefully considered in assessing self-report validity.

> **Learning task**
>
> - What are the different stages of a neuropsychological assessment?
> - Who in the interdisciplinary team might contribute to the assessment?
> - What clinical history is required?
> - When might a full neurocognitive assessment be indicated, and when would it not?
>
> **Reflective point**
>
> - What might it be like to undergo the neuropsychological process? How would you feel at the different stages?

Differential diagnosis

If the assessment process indicates that someone has cognitive impairment, it is important not to assume that it is necessarily because of HIV. There are many other things that can also cause cognitive impairment, either for a short time or permanently, that need to be considered and ruled out by the assessing clinician (usually a clinical psychologist).

> **Reflective task**
>
> - Is your cognitive performance always the same?
> - What factors have you noticed affect your cognitive ability?
>
> **Learning task**
>
> - What different factors can you identify that might cause permanent cognitive impairment? Write these down and compare them with our list (Table 11.2).

Ageing

Following initial brain development and maturity (e.g. Somerville, 2016) it is not technically the 'age' of the brain that matters, but its health and what it has experienced in that time (risk factors usually accumulating with age). Many tests have norms adjusted for age, and so the general effects of this should be able to be discounted.

As people living with HIV with ART have a normal life expectancy and live into older age (or acquire HIV at an older age), the risk of other dementias and cerebral vascular accidents increases (e.g. Turner et al., 2016). Many physical, neurological and psychological health conditions associated with older age can cause cognitive impairment, and so a diagnosis of HAND is a diagnosis of exclusion. Thus 'pure' cases are rare, with most people having multiple risk factors.

Table 11.2 Possible causes of neurocognitive impairment other than HAND

Drug use	Vascular dementia	Psychosis
Alcohol	CO poisoning	Depression
Cholesterol	Multiple sclerosis	Fatigue
Pain	Liver problems	Smoking
Alzheimer's	Medication	Stroke
Parkinson's	Toxins exposure	Motor neurone disease
ADHD	Sleep apnoea	Vitamin deficiencies
Syphilis	Encephalitis	Concussion
Hepatitis	Lack of effort	Head injury
Cardiac problems	Delirium	Epilepsy
Hypoxia	Anxiety	Intellectual disability

Discussing the results

Once the assessment has been carried out, the results need to be shared with the client and their interdisciplinary team.

Reflective task

- If you had a cognitive impairment, how would you like to be told?
- Who would you like to tell you?
- What questions might you have?

We should not assume that telling someone they have cognitive impairment is 'bad news'. For example, some clients are relieved that difficulties have been found because this means that they are not 'making it up'. Conversely, if someone is convinced they have cognitive issues but the results indicate that they do not, they might question the validity or sensitivity of the tests, or be worried that they have 'wasted your time'.

For some clients, confirmation of cognitive difficulties can be an upsetting process; it can be emotionally difficult to learn that HIV has had an impact on cognitive functioning, and clients may have been struggling for some time as they may have minimised or underestimated their difficulties. A sensitive but straightforward approach is required when providing verbal feedback. The client may need time to adjust to the information and discuss their priorities with regards to intervention. The written report should list the outcomes of the assessment, key domains of difficulty and rehabilitation strategies to support and preserve current functioning.

When cognitive impairment has been detected, clients often have three common and understandable questions:

i) What caused it?
ii) Will it get worse?
iii) What can I do to make it better?

A good assessment will have prepared clients in advance for how easy/possible it will be to answer these questions.

i)   What caused it?

Being able to answer this will depend on the clinical history, how many different risk factors there are, and how clear the cognitive profile is. Sometimes causation might be clear, other times differential diagnosis or co-morbidity exists. Neurology assessments and neuroimaging might be required in this process.

ii)   Will it get worse?

Unless the test is a repeat test, it is not normally possible to say definitively if the cognitive profile is stable. The clinical history may give some clues (e.g. if the issues suddenly started and have not changed for several years). Sometimes cognitive impairment can improve (for example if medications have been changed or it was attributed to mental health difficulties or substance use which has since improved). Encouragingly, recent research indicates that in cases of impairment, most cognitive profiles appear to remain stable over time rather than deteriorate (e.g. 77% stable, 13% deteriorate, 10% improved; Sacktor et al., 2016).

iii)   What can I do to make it better?

When clients ask this, they often initially think about medication and/or 'brain training' exercises rather than the broader role of neurorehabilitation.

Neurorehabilitation

Neurorehabilitation is the process of recovering from, and/or minimising the impact of, neurological damage and the resulting cognitive and functional impairment. Most clients will not have access to ongoing specialist neurorehabilitation advice and support. Instead it will usually be managed by the current interdisciplinary HIV care team, who can work together to address either in-house or by signposting to relevant support services.

General principals

Neurorehabilitation approaches require a high degree of motivation and commitment by clients. Success also depends upon the client being surrounded by a supportive network of health and rehabilitation professionals, and ideally positive social support.

Current neuropsychological approaches to rehabilitation emphasise a 'compensatory' rather than a 'restorative' approach. Thus, the aims of rehabilitation are to help the client adapt and adjust to the difficulty they experience, and learn new strategies to cope, drawing on their strengths and any areas of preserved cognitive functioning (compensation). This is different from aiming to recover all neurocognitive functioning to a pre-morbid level (restoration), which usually is what clients initially hope for. For example, if someone had poor verbal memory difficulties but good visual memory, they might be encouraged to draw or imagine what they want to remember, rather than repeated verbal rehearsal.

The client needs to understand their cognitive deficit(s) in as much depth as possible and identify what specific problems it causes in their daily lives. This will help to identify the practical and real-life issues that require attention. Goals for rehabilitation and the identified strategies will need to be achievable and personally meaningful for clients.

Most clients will be unable to retain the amount and complexity of the information discussed. Therefore, verbal sessions should be supported with written information, including: the nature of their difficulties, rehabilitation strategies, where to access information (such as online or support groups) and reinforcing that the most effective way of preserving current abilities and preventing deterioration is adherence to ART to maintain an undetectable viral load and healthy CD4 count.

It can also be helpful if the client is accompanied by a supportive relative or friend who can assist and encourage the client to clarify information and ask questions. However, some clients will not have talked about their HIV diagnosis with others, and so may not wish to explain their impaired neurocognitive functioning or ask for support, for fear this will lead to them needing to explain the cause of their impairment as HIV.

Rehabilitation interventions

Clients whose neuropsychological needs are in more than one domain, or who are more impaired, may need onward referral to community-based neurorehabilitation teams, which may provide individual or group input. For those with singular or milder impairment, intervention may be provided by the interdisciplinary team.

There is little research currently on the most effective rehabilitation interventions for people with HAND, and the evidence base for such interventions comes mainly from the traumatic brain injury literature.

The goals for rehabilitation need to be functional, relevant and meaningful for the client. The choice of particular strategies should be the client's and they should be encouraged to test a range to find which suits them best. Rehabilitation strategies should be based on three key approaches: metacognitive strategy instruction, distraction minimisation and verbal self-instruction, all within the context of a client's mood and systems (e.g. work, family, friends).

Metacognitive strategy instruction

Metacognitive strategy instruction refers to a broad range of problem-solving rehabilitation approaches. Learning to break tasks into smaller components is important, alongside reviewing progress in the task and problem-solving and generating solutions to any issues that arise (Levine et al., 2000; Rath, Hennessy, & Diller, 2003).

For those with memory and recall problems, external memory aids (e.g. diaries, calendars, notebooks, smartphones, tablets, etc.) are used, in which important information (e.g. appointments, shopping lists, reminders) is recorded. It is important to ensure the client knows how to use the tools, as learning new skills may be impaired.

Distraction minimisation

The minimisation of distractions to the client's attention is important. Attention is a complex mechanism involving several cognitive components (e.g. attentional vigilance and the ability to react to stimuli).

Clients should be aware of the distracting effects of different stimuli and aim to reduce these and create a quiet environment as far as is possible (e.g. turning off background radio and/or TV, reducing social media alerts on smartphones, avoiding open-plan working environments) in order to remain focused on a task.

Verbal self-instruction

Verbal self-instruction refers to encouraging the client to verbalise (either out loud or sub-vocally) the steps needed to achieve a task and why (Turkstra & Flora, 2002). This encourages a focus on the task and may help with problem-solving.

The use of 'wh' questions (what, when, where, who) can provide a framework for clients to address situations in which they may have difficulties (Marshall et al., 2004).

Group-based neurocognitive rehabilitation

Group-based approaches to cognitive rehabilitation for people living with HIV have been described (e.g. McCarthy, Marnoch, & Campbell, 2016). A group approach has the advantage of facilitating supportive relationships, reducing the impact of stigma (particularly important for people living with HIV) and utilising scarce clinical resources in the most effective way (e.g. Table 11.3), assuming local potential participant numbers are substantial enough.

Reducing other risk factors

Clinicians and clients should be aware that there are many potential causes and effects of cognitive difficulties. The interaction amongst these factors may make it difficult to attribute cognitive loss to just one factor (e.g. the impact of HIV), but also allows for mitigation of others.

Whilst not the direct intervention that some clients might envisage, reduction of other neurocognitive risk factors is an important change that clients can make, to either reduce co-morbid effects or avert future impact (which may now be greater due to a reduced cognitive reserve). Thus, thorough assessment of mental health, social health, substance use (alcohol, smoking and recreational), blood pressure, diet, weight and exercise are important components of holistic, interprofessional care.

Table 11.3 Example of neurorehabilitation group programme (adapted from McCarthy, Marnoch, & Campbell, 2016)

Session	Content
1: Introduction to Cognition	What is cognition? Areas reported affected by clients with HAND: sharing of individual experiences (optional): sharing of goals (optional)
2: Attention and Mood	Psycho-education; Mood; CBT model; CBT formulation
3: Memory Psycho-education	Psycho-education; Types of memory; Memory processes
4: Memory Strategies	Internal; External; Sharing strategies; Practising strategies
5: Executive Function	Planning; Organising; Problem-solving; Multiple demands on cognition; Strategies for planning and organisation
6: Integration, Practice and Evaluation	Review

Learning task

- Should clients aim to restore, or compensate for, their neurocognitive impairment?
- What are metacognitive instruction, distraction minimisation and verbal self-instruction? How might they each help clients?
- How might a neurorehabilitation group help clients?
- What other lifestyle factors could a client consider improving?

Reflective point

- What support would you want and need if you had cognitive difficulties?

Utilising the learning

Case study 1: 'LH': Black-African, 58-year-old African woman

- Referred by HIV consultant. Diagnosed with HIV 15 years ago.
- Diagnosed with epilepsy seven years previously.
- Concerns regarding ongoing memory loss and confusion reported over past several years.
- Primary school level education: English her second language.
- Good adherence to both ART and epilepsy meds.
- CD4 was 650 at time of referral and viral load was undetectable.
- Nadir VL and CD4 were 240 and 400 respectively.
- Attended for clinical interview appointment at wrong time (12.30pm not 2pm), wrong date (25th not 22nd), and wrong month (September not August).

Differential diagnosis

- HAND? Tumour? Epilepsy related?

Assessment

- Mood scales normal. Performed well on neurocognitive domains including attention (trail-making test), psychomotor speed (digit symbol substitution), semantic ability (verbal fluency test) and executive functioning.
- Performed poorly on tests of working memory (backwards digit span) and delayed memory (story recall).

Outcome

- Mild to moderate working and delayed memory impairment (epilepsy-related accelerated forgetting) due to the neurocognitive impact of epilepsy.

Rehabilitation

- Education with regard to the assessment results and the practical implications on her life. Practical strategies to assist with memory including the use of memory aids (calendars, reminders, diary) and instructions about problem-solving.

Case study 2: 'KN': White-French, 39 years old, identifies as non-binary gender

- Referred by HIV physician. Self-reported concern over attention and cognitive function. English second language, but fluent.
- MSc level education.
- HIV diagnosis 2009: VL and CD4 nadir 20,000 and 350 respectively.
- Not currently on treatment (CD4 in 500s, VL 15,000) as stopped taking ART in context of one-year crystal methamphetamine addiction. Now 'only' sporadic use.
- Behaviourally very anxious. Has been unemployed for past year, recently returned to work and struggling.

Differential diagnosis

- HAND? Mood disorder? Drug-related impairment?

Assessment

- Mood scales indicated very high anxiety levels and moderate depression. Performance on attention test (trail-making test) a little impaired. Psychomotor speed (digit symbol substitution), semantic ability (verbal fluency test), executive functioning immediate and delayed recall within normal range.

Outcome

- Mood issues and consequences of intermittent drug use most likely cause of cognitive concerns. Advice given about the impact of mood on attention and recall, as well as drug use.

Rehabilitation

- Referral to services for intervention to address mood and drug use.

Case study 3: 'RM': White-British male, 64 years old

- Referred by neurologist: reported decline over past decade in concentration and short-term memory. Recently changed HIV medication regime.
- Long-term HIV (diagnosed 1986). Nadir CD4 90, current 400–500, undetectable viral load. Hepatitis B encephalitis 1975. Previous Hepatitis C. Mood currently good, managed depression throughout life. Self-reports that he is dyslexic. Drives.
- Two previous neuropsychological assessments in 1994 and 2010 found intellectual ability above average, lower scores in visual than verbal memory, no other major issues, and no significant change over time once age accounted for.

Differential diagnosis

- Mood problem? HAND? Early dementia?

Assessment

- No overall change in cognitive profile, improvements in some domains, deterioration in others, majority stable.

Outcome

- Results fed back to client that no overall change, however they remain concerned and highlight recent examples of impact on life (leaving taps on and flooding kitchen, pan left on stove). Discussion re: safety to drive.

Rehabilitation

- Group neurorehabilitation support.

Summary

Although rare for those able to access effective HIV treatment, HAND remains an understandable concern for both clients and clinicians. It can be either acute or chronic in presentation, and differ in level of severity. Alongside HIV, there are other neurocognitive risk factors which may be considered as a differential diagnosis, or be co-morbid. With these different factors, an ageing population and ever-evolving ART regimes, there is no singular 'HIV cognitive profile'.

Instead, a comprehensive assessment is required of cognitive strengths and weaknesses. Where deficits are discovered, appropriate neurorehabilitation strategies should be employed and other risk factors reduced, including assessment and support of adherence to ART. In doing so, for the majority of people living with HIV, any acquired impairment will likely remain relatively stable.

Most people living with HIV will not have access to a comprehensive neurocognitive and/or neurocognitive rehabilitation service, due to limited resources or lack of local expertise. In this chapter we have provided a framework for assessment, differential diagnosis and rehabilitation issues to be managed by the interdisciplinary care team.

We have aimed to provide clinicians with confidence to undertake tasks within their professional limits, in order to provide the most holistic and comprehensive clinical service to their clients, seeking supervision and consultation from neuropsychologist specialists when required.

Learning task

Below are different referrals you've received as a healthcare professional:

- What important information do you have already?
- What additional details would you want to collect?
- What engagement issues might there be for the client?
- What would you suggest if neurocognitive impairment was confirmed?

References

Anitinori, A., Arendt, G., Becker, J. T., Brew, B. J., Byrd, D. A., & Cherner, M. (2007). Updated research nosology for HIV associated neurocognitive disorders. *Neurology, 69,* 1789–1799.

Antiretroviral Therapy Cohort Collaboration. (2017). Survival of HIV positive patients starting antiretroviral therapy between 1996 and 2013: A collaborative analysis of cohort studies. *The Lancet HIV.*

BHIVA. (2018) British HIV Association standards of care for people living with HIV 2018, Mediscript, London.

British Psychological Society, British HIV Association and Medical Foundation for AIDS and Sexual Health. (2011). *Standards for psychological support for adults living with HIV.* London: MEDFASH.

Britton, A, & Russell, R. (2004). Multidisciplinary team intervention for delirium in patients with chronic cognitive impairment. *Cochrane Database of Systematic Reviews, 2*(2).

Chelune, G, J, Heaton, R. K., & Lehnam, R. A. (1986). Neuropsychology and personality correlates of patients' complaints of disability. In: R. E. Tarter (Ed.), *Advances in clinical neuropsychology* (3rd ed. pp. 95–126). New York: Plenum.

Cherner, M, Masliah, E., Ellis, R. J., Marcotte, T.,. D., & Moore, D. J. Grant I and HIV Neurobehavioural Research Center Group. (2002). Neurocognitive dysfunction predicts postmortem findings of HIV encephalitis. *Neurology, 50*(10), 1563–1567.

Clifford, D. B. (2017). HIV associated neurocognitive disorder. *Current Opinion in Infectious Diseases, 30*(1), 117.

Coughlan, A. K., Oddy, M., & Crawford, A. R. (2007). BIRT memory and information processing battery (BMIPB). *PSIGE Newsletter, 29,* 5.

Folstein, M., Folstein, S. E., & McHugh, P. R. (1975). "Mini-Mental State" a practical method for grading the cognitive state of patients for the clinician. *Journal of Psychiatric Research, 12*(3), 189–198.

Gray, F., Bazille, C. A., Adle-Biassette, H., Mikol, J., Moulignier, A., & Scaravilli, F. (2005). Central nervous system immune reconstitution disease in acquired immunodeficiency syndrome patients receiving highly active antiretroviral treatment. *Journal of Neurovirology, 11*, 16–22.

Heaton, R. K., Clifford, D. B., Franklin, D. R., Woods, S. P., Ake, C., Vaida, F., ... Rivera-Mindt, M. (2010). HIV-associated neurocognitive disorders persist in the era of potent antiretroviral therapy CHARTER Study. *Neurology, 75*(23), 2087–2096.

Heaton, R. K., Franklin, D. R., Ellis, R. J., McCutchan, J. A., Letendre, S. L., LeBlanc, S., ... Collier, A. C. (2011). HIV-associated neurocognitive disorders before and during the era of combination antiretroviral therapy: Differences in rates, nature, and predictors. *Journal of Neurovirology, 17*(1), 3–16.

Heaton, R. K., Marcotte, T. D., Mindt, M. R., Sadek, J., Moore, D. J., Bentley, H., ... Grant, I. (2004). The impact of HIV-associated neuropsychological impairment on everyday functioning. *Journal of the International Neuropsychological Society, 10*(03), 317–331.

Hellmuth, J., Fletcher, J. L., Valcour, V., Kroon, E., Ananworanich, J., Intasan, J., ... Krebs, S. J. (2016). Neurologic signs and symptoms frequently manifest in acute HIV I infection. *Neurology, 87*(2), 148–154.

Hsieh, S., Schubert, S., Hoon, C., Mioshi, E., & Hodges, J. R. (2013). Validation of the Addenbrooke's cognitive examination III in frontotemporal dementia and Alzheimer's disease. *Dementia and Geriatric Cognitive Disorders, 36*(3-4), 242–250.

Joska, J. A., Witten, J., Thomas, K. G., Robertson, C., Casson-Crook, M., Roosa, H., ... Sacktor, N. C. (2016). A comparison of five brief screening tools for HIV-associated neurocognitive disorders in the USA and South Africa. *AIDS and Behavior, 20*(8), 1621–1631.

Kehagia, A. A., Barker, R. A., & Robbins, T. W. (2010). Neuropsychological and clinical heterogeneity of cognitive impairment and dementia in patients with Parkinson's disease. *The Lancet Neurology, 9*(12), 1200–1213.

Laverick, R., Haddow, L., Daskalopoulou, M., Lampe, F., Gilson, R., Speakman, A., ... Rodger, A. (2017). Self-reported difficulties with everyday function, cognitive symptoms and cognitive function in people with HIV. *JAIDS Journal of Acquired Immune Deficiency Syndromes, 76*(3), 74–83.

Lawton, M. P., & Brody, E. M. (1969). Assessment of older people: Self-maintaining and instrumental activities of daily living. *Gerontologist, 9*, 179–186.

Levine, B., Robertson, I. H., Clare, L., Carter, G., Hong, J., Wilson, B. A., ... Stuss, D. T. (2000). Rehabilitation of executive functioning: An experimental – clinical validation of goal management training. *Journal of the International Neuropsychological Society, 6*(3), 299–312.

Marshall, Robert, Karow, C., Morelli, C., Iden, K., Dixon, J., & Cranfill, T. (2004). Effects of interactive strategy modelling training on problem-solving by persons with traumatic brain injury. *Aphasiology, 18*(8), 659–673.

Maruff, P., Thomas, E., Cysique, L., Brew, B., Collie, A., Snyder, P., & Pietrzak, R. H. (2009). Validity of the CogState brief battery: Relationship to standardized tests and sensitivity to cognitive impairment in mild traumatic brain injury, schizophrenia, and AIDS dementia complex. *Archives of Clinical Neuropsychology, 24*(2), 165–178.

McArthur, J. C., Hoover, D. R., Bacellar, H., Miller, E. N., Cohen, B. A., Becker, J. T., ... Visscher, B. R. (1993). Dementia in AIDS patients incidence and risk factors. *Neurology, 43*(11), 2245.

McCarthy, J., Marnoch, S., & Campbell, T. (2016). A group based approach to neurocognitive rehabilitation for people with HIV. *"Tough times for HIV services: Innovation and collaboration in the era of austerity". NHIVNA & BPS (National HIV Nurses' Association & British Psychological Society) study day, London, 19 October.*

Morgan, E. E., & Heaton, R. K. (2009). The neuropsychological approach to predicting everyday functioning. In I. Grant and K. Adams (Eds.), *Neuropsychological assessment of neuropsychiatric disorders* (3rd ed. pp. 632–651). New York: Oxford.

Nasreddine, Z. S., Phillips, N. A., Bédirian, V., Charbonneau, S., Whitehead, V., Collin, I., ... Chertkow, H. (2005). The Montreal Cognitive Assessment, MoCA: A brief screening tool for mild cognitive impairment. *Journal of the American Geriatrics Society, 53*(4), 695–699.

NHIVNA. (2017). Annual health review for people living with HIV. NHIVNA.

Nightingale, S., Winston, A., Letendre, S., Michael, B. D., McArthur, J. C., Khoo, S., & Solomon, T. (2014). Controversies in HIV-associated neurocognitive disorders. *The Lancet Neurology, 13*(11), 1139–1151.

Power, C., Selnes, O. A., Grim, J. A., & McArthur, J. C. (1995). HIV dementia scale: A rapid screening test. *JAIDS Journal of Acquired Immune Deficiency Syndromes, 8*(3), 273–278.

Rath, J. F., Hennessy, J. J., & Diller, L. (2003). Social problem solving and community integration in postacute rehabilitation outpatients with traumatic brain injury. *Rehabilitation Psychology, 48*(3), 137.

Robertson, K. R., Smurzynski, M., Parsons, T. D., Wu, K., Bosch, R. J., Wu, J., ... Ellis, R. J. (2007). The prevalence and incidence of neurocognitive impairment in the HAART era. *Aids, 21* (14), 1915–1921.

Rodkjaer, L., Gabel, C., Laursen, T., Slot, M., Leutscher, P., Christensen, N., ... Sodemann, M. (2016). Simple and practical screening approach to identify HIV-infected individuals with depression or at risk of developing depression. *HIV Medicine, 17*(10), 749–757.

Sacktor, N., Skolasky, R. L., Seaberg, E., Munro, C., Becker, J. T., Martin, E., ... Miller, E. (2016). Prevalence of HIV-associated neurocognitive disorders in the Multicenter AIDS Cohort Study. *Neurology, 86*(4), 334–340.

Sacktor, N. C., Wong, M., Nakasujja, N., Skolasky, R. L., Selnes, O. A., Musisi, S., ... Katabira, E. (2005). The international HIV dementia scale: A new rapid screening test for HIV dementia. *Aids, 19*(13), 1367–1374.

Sahakian, B. J., Elliott, R., Low, N., Mehta, M., Clark, R. T., & Pozniak, A. L. (1995). Neuropsychological deficits in tests of executive function in asymptomatic and symptomatic HIV-1 seropositive men. *Psychological Medicine, 25*(6), 1233–1246.

Simioni, S., Cavassini, M., Annoni, J. M., Abraham, A. R., Bourquin, I., Schiffer, V., ... Du Pasquier, R. A. (2010). Cognitive dysfunction in HIV patients despite long-standing suppression of viremia. *Aids, 24*(9), 1243–1250.

Skinner, S., Adewale, A. J., DeBlock, L., Gill, M. J., & Power, C. (2009). Neurocognitive screening tools in HIV/AIDS: Comparative performance among patients exposed to antiretroviral therapy. *HIV Medicine, 10*(4), 246–252.

Somerville, L. H. (2016). Searching for signatures of brain maturity: What are we searching for? *Neuron, 92*(6), 1164–1167.

Turkstra, L. S., & Flora, T. L. (2002). Compensating for executive function impairments after TBI: A single case study of functional intervention. *Journal of Communication Disorders, 35*(6), 467–482.

Turner, R. S., Chadwick, M., Horton, W. A., Simon, G. L., Jiang, X., & Esposito, G. (2016). An individual with human immunodeficiency virus, dementia, and central nervous system amyloid deposition. *Alzheimer's & Dementia: Diagnosis, Assessment & Disease Monitoring, 4*, 1–5.

Underwood, J., De Francesco, D., Post, F. A., Vera, J. H., Williams, I., Boffito, M., Mallon, P. W., Anderson, J., Sachikonye, M., Sabin, C., & Winston, A. (2017). Associations between cognitive impairments and patient-reported measures of physical/mental clinical validation HIV. *HIV Medicine, 18*, 363–369.

Vera, J. H., Cole, J. H., Boasso, A., Greathead, L., Kelleher, P., Rabiner, E. A., ... Winston, A. (2016). Neuroinflammation in treated HIV-positive individuals. *Neurology, 86*, 1–8.

Winston, A., Stöhr, W., Antinori, A., Amieva, H., Perré, P., De Wit, S., ... Grarup, J. (2017). Changes in cognitive function over 96 weeks in naive patients randomized to Darunavir – Ritonavir plus either raltegravir or tenofovir–Emtricitabine: A substudy of the NEAT001/ANRS143 Trial. *JAIDS Journal of Acquired Immune Deficiency Syndromes, 74*(2), 185–192.

Woods, S. P., Moore, D. J., Weber, E., & Grant, I. (2009). Cognitive neuropsychology of HIV-associated neurocognitive disorders. *Neuropsychology Review, 19*(2), 152–168.

Woods, S. P., Weber, E., Weisz, B. M., Twamley, E. W., & Grant, I. The HIV Neurobehavioral Research Programs Group. (2011). Prospective memory deficits are associated with unemployment in persons living with HIV infection. *Rehabilitation Psychology, 56*(1), 77–84. doi:10.1037/a0022753

Yuen, T., Brouillette, M. J., Fellows, L. K., Ellis, R. J., Letendre, S., Heaton, R., & Mayo, N. (2017). Personalized risk index for neurocognitive decline among people with well-controlled HIV infection. *JAIDS Journal of Acquired Immune Deficiency Syndromes, 76*(1), 48–54.

Zipursky, A. R., Gogolishvili, D., Rueda, S., Brunetta, J., Carvalhal, A., McCombe, J. A., ... Marcotte, T. (2013). Evaluation of brief screening tools for neurocognitive impairment in HIV/AIDS: A systematic review of the literature. *AIDS (London, England), 27*(15), 2385.

Index